Communication and Swallowing Management of Tracheostomized and Ventilator-Dependent Adults

To our greatest teachers, our parents,
from whom we will never stop learning.

Communication and Swallowing Management of Tracheostomized and Ventilator-Dependent Adults

Second Edition

KAREN J. DIKEMAN, M.A., CCC-SLP
MARTA S. KAZANDJIAN, M.A., CCC-SLP

THOMSON

DELMAR LEARNING™

Australia   Canada   Mexico   Singapore   Spain   United Kingdom   United States

THOMSON
DELMAR LEARNING

Communication and Swallowing Management of Tracheostomized and
Ventilator-Dependent Adults, Second Edition

by Karen J. Dikeman and Marta S. Kazandjian

Executive Director:
William Brottmiller

Executive Editor:
Cathy L. Esperti

Acquisitions Editor:
Candice Janco

Developmental Editor:
Deb Flis

Executive Marketing Manager:
Dawn F. Gerrain

Channel Manager:
Jennifer McAvey

Editorial Assistant:
Maria D'Angelico

Production Manager:
Barbara A. Bullock

Art/Design Coordinator:
Robert Plante

Production Coordinator:
John Mickelbank

Project Editor:
David Buddle

Library of Congress Cataloging-in-Publication Data
Dikeman, Karen J.
Communication and swallowing management of tracheostomized and ventilator-dependent adults / Karen J. Dikeman, Marta S. Kazandjian.—2nd ed.
p. ; cm.—(Dysphagia series)
Includes bibliographical references and index.
ISBN 0-7693-0245-9
1. Tracheotomy—Complications. 2. Trachea—Intubation—Complications. 3. Deglutition disorders. 4. Communicative disorders. I. Kazandjian, Marta S. II. Title. III. Series.
[DNLM: 1. Tracheostomy—rehabilitation. 2. Deglutition Disorders—rehabilitation. 3. Intermittent Positive-Pressure Ventilation. 4. Speech Disorders—rehabilitation. 5. Ventilators, Mechanical. WF 490 D575c 2003]
RF517 .D55 2003
617.5'33—dc21
2002067241

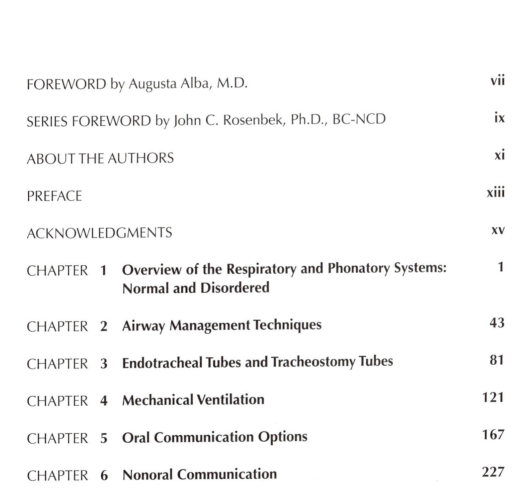

C

Contents

F

Foreword

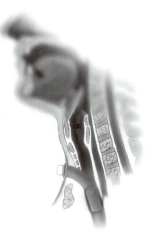

From the intensive care unit to the home, the growth of tracheostomy and tracheal intermittent positive pressure ventilation (TIPPV) as methods of prolonging life has continued. These trends began in the latter half of the 20th century; today, individuals, from neonates to the elderly, are living out a portion or all of their lives using one or both techniques. For some individuals, noninvasive ventilation is not an option because of weakness or other pathology in the upper airway; for others, invasive ventilation is a matter of choice.

Industrialized nations throughout the world have contributed to this growth by producing smaller and more reliable portable ventilators at an affordable cost and disposable accessories that meet numerous needs. Worldwide information technology and international business and travel have all played roles in refining the field of respiratory care. Public demand has led to the development of centers of excellence with emphasis on pulmonary rehabilitation, and home care services have added quality to life. The subacute ventilator unit, both in hospitals and nursing facilities, and the vent team with transdisciplinary delivery of health care are two such innovations. The importance of the management of swallowing and communication disorders in all settings has been recognized.

Among health care professionals, speech pathologists have assumed a leadership role in assessment and treatment of these disorders. We welcome the second edition of *Communication and Swallowing Management of Tracheostomized and Ventilator-Dependent Adults* as a comprehensive and lucid source of information in this field. Almost a decade has passed since the first edition of this text by two dedicated speech pathologists. They have not lost their excitement in providing the reader with explanations of the anatomy and physiology of the upper gastrointestinal and respiratory systems, along with superb photographs and illustrations. The policies and procedures necessary for the operation of a safe and effective clinical program, competencies needed by the team members, and case reports to bring it all together for the reader are included. My gratitude and congratulations go out to the authors and their publisher in giving all of us—the student, the professional, the "responaut," and the family—this valuable resource.

Augusta Alba, M.D.
Associate Professor, Clinical Rehabilitation Medicine
New York University Medical Center, N.Y.
Chief, Rehabilitation Medicine
Coler-Goldwater Specialty Hospital and Nursing Facility, N.Y.

Series Foreword

Kipling once observed that journalism was literature on the run. Some of the best is. It is equally true that the best of clinical practice is science on the run. Kazandjian and Dikeman are sprinters. The first edition of *Communication and Swallowing Management of Tracheostomized and Ventilator-Dependent Adults* became required reading for professionals responsible for managing tracheostomized patients. It did so because readers recognized that these authors seldom left the clinic, and when they did it was to go the library to find out what others were thinking about the problems they dealt with every day. The book appealed as well because readers came to trust the authors' humility, their reliance on best evidence, and their steadfast refusal to provide recipes when hypotheses were all the data and their experience could support.

Now we have the second edition. It has the first edition's virtues bolstered by the newest data and hypotheses. The same attention to detail and the same humility are obvious. The same reluctance to avoid easy answers and pat formulas appears on every page. And the authors have demonstrated that they are not sprinters. They are endurance racers. This second edition took them away from family, from friends, and from quiet, alone times. But they did it. They did it because, like scientists in love with experimentation, they are in love with clinical practice. They want patients to thrive. This second edition's content increases the likelihood that all of our patients will do just that.

John C. Rosenbek, Ph.D., BC-NCD
Clinical Professor
Department of Communicative Disorders
College of Health Professions
University of Florida

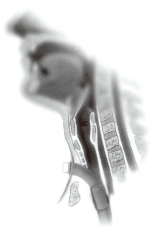

About the Authors

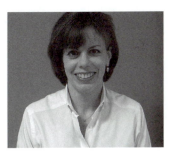

Karen Dikeman

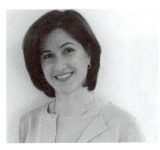

Marta Kazandjian

Karen J. Dikeman, M.A. CCC, and Marta S. Kazandjian, M.A. CCC, are speech-language pathologists who specialize in the management of adults with neurological and respiratory impairments. They have focuses their clinical skills in working with tracheostomized and ventilator-dependant adults and have shared their knowledge nationally and internationally at full-day workshops, mini-seminars, and in short courses. They are co-authors of peer-reviewed articles and book chapters and are invited contributors to medical journals.

Karen Dikeman and Marta Kazandjian received their clinical training on the pulmonary rehabilitation units of Goldwater Memorial Hospital, New York University Medical Center. They now direct programs in both acute and long-term care medical settings for Silvercrest Extended Care Facility and New York Hospital Medical Center Queens, the New York Presbyterian Healthcare System. Marta Kazandjian is also co-founder of Communication Independence for the Neurologically Impaired (CINI), a New York–based, not-for-profit organization that provides alternative communication resource information to communicatively impaired adults.

Karen Dikeman received her bachelor's degree from Valparaiso University, Valparasio Indiana, and her master's degree from Queens College, City University of New York. Marta Kazandjian received her bachelor's degree from Binghampton University, State University of New York, and her master's degree from Hunter College, City University of New York.

P

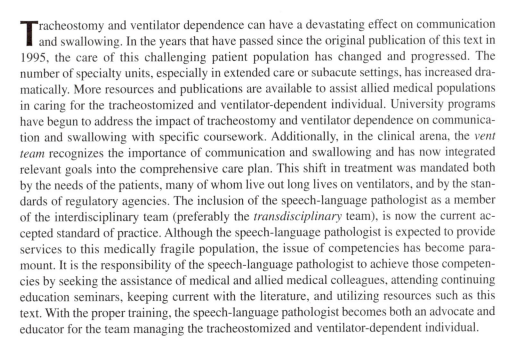

Preface

Tracheostomy and ventilator dependence can have a devastating effect on communication and swallowing. In the years that have passed since the original publication of this text in 1995, the care of this challenging patient population has changed and progressed. The number of specialty units, especially in extended care or subacute settings, has increased dramatically. More resources and publications are available to assist allied medical populations in caring for the tracheostomized and ventilator-dependent individual. University programs have begun to address the impact of tracheostomy and ventilator dependence on communication and swallowing with specific coursework. Additionally, in the clinical arena, the *vent team* recognizes the importance of communication and swallowing and has now integrated relevant goals into the comprehensive care plan. This shift in treatment was mandated both by the needs of the patients, many of whom live out long lives on ventilators, and by the standards of regulatory agencies. The inclusion of the speech-language pathologist as a member of the interdisciplinary team (preferably the *transdisciplinary* team), is now the current accepted standard of practice. Although the speech-language pathologist is expected to provide services to this medically fragile population, the issue of competencies has become paramount. It is the responsibility of the speech-language pathologist to achieve those competencies by seeking the assistance of medical and allied medical colleagues, attending continuing education seminars, keeping current with the literature, and utilizing resources such as this text. With the proper training, the speech-language pathologist becomes both an advocate and educator for the team managing the tracheostomized and ventilator-dependent individual.

The continued goal of this textbook is to integrate current theory and clinical application in the management of this challenging patient population. Therefore, although clinical in its approach, this book recognizes the need for any practitioner to understand the fundamental principles of respiratory and phonatory anatomy and physiology and the basics of airway management and mechanical ventilation as they relate to communication and swallowing. The first four chapters provide this foundation. Oral and nonoral communication and dysphagia are then addressed in a style designed to give the reader the problem-solving skills needed for assessment and intervention. The reader is also provided with sample protocols and competencies to assist in designing treatment programs and case examples to illustrate the *transdisciplinary team* approach.

Management of the tracheostomized and ventilator-dependent population can be effectively accomplished with a transdisciplinary team concept, one in which one or more team members assume the responsibility of working toward common goals set by the team. This may result in shared responsibilities; however, each discipline's scope of practice must be maintained. The terms *clinician* and *practitioner* are used in this text to refer to the speech-language pathologist and other allied medical health professionals who work with this population. This book defines the primary role of each professional working together on the transdisciplinary team. The speech-language pathologist, carrying out physician orders, has the primary responsibility for the management of communication and swallowing impairment. This includes recommendations for modifications of the tracheostomy tube and ventilator necessary to facilitate communication and swallowing. However, this is not to imply that speech-language pathologists or other allied medical health professionals perform responsibilities not within their scope of practice. As indicated by the American Speech-Language-Hearing Association (ASHA) in their 1993 position and guideline statement (ASHA, 1993), the speech-language pathologist's scope of practice does include collaboration in selecting and evaluating oral communication options and providing treatment to the tracheostomized and ventilator-dependent patient.

The loss of communication and swallowing function significantly affects the tracheostomized and ventilator-dependent patient's quality of life. Unless quality of life issues are addressed, effective treatment by all team members is compromised. It is our hope that our speech-language pathology colleagues, as well as our medical and health care practitioner colleagues, will continue to find this text helpful in their collaborative work with this challenging population.

A

Acknowledgments

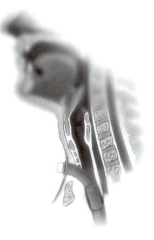

We wish to thank the manufacturers, listed in Appendix A, for their ongoing technical support and willingness to send information and product photographs.

We also wish to acknowledge our colleagues and friends who assisted by reviewing portions of this book as well as by sharing their expertise: Mel Hochman, M.D., Clifford Tracey, RRT, and John Vecchione, M.D. Our special thanks to our colleagues at Silvercrest Extended Care Facility and New York Presbyterian Healthcare System and the Vent Team, who continue to field our unending questions as we all grow and learn together. We would also like to thank our colleagues in MIS and Administration, Linda Lohrer, Damon Lee, and Lloyd Torres, who assisted us in preparing the figures for this text. We feel very lucky to have a staff of dedicated speech-language pathologists, Laura Belozerco-Tracey, Maria Schembari, Allison Harris, and Lisa Adams, who endure the crazy schedules of their department heads. We particularly appreciate the support from Patricia Leddy, R.N., Administrator, and Kenneth Carter, CEO and President, not only during the preparation of this text but during our many years at Silvercrest.

We would also like to thank Augusta Alba, M.D., our teacher, mentor, and supporter, who led us onto the respiratory/pulmonary units of Goldwater Memorial Hospital, New York University Medical Center, and shared her incredible wealth of knowledge with us. To this day we still call her and she continues to teach us!

To Jay Rosenbek, Ph.D., BC-NDC, we owe tremendous thanks, not only for his time, his clinical expertise, and his patience in reviewing this manuscript, but for his support of us not only as clinicians, but as authors.

Most especially to our families who continue to support us in all endeavors. And to Joe, Matthew, and Jack who gave us the gift of humor when it was hard to see the light at the end of the tunnel!

1

Overview of the Respiratory and Phonatory Systems: Normal and Disordered

An understanding of the normal respiratory and phonatory systems and their functions is necessary for any clinician working with the tracheostomized and ventilator-dependent patient. The complex respiratory and phonatory systems function in concert for normal breathing and voice production. Once disrupted, as with tracheostomy and ventilator-dependent patients, these systems may break down in multiple areas. For the clinician, intervention first involves identifying the disrupted areas. The identification process and the subsequent management program are not possible without a background in normal respiratory and phonatory anatomy and physiology. This chapter provides an overview of the systems the clinician encounters when intervening with the tracheostomized and ventilator-dependent patient. Normal structures and their functions will be addressed first. The disordered mechanism will then be described via examples of common diseases and conditions that affect the respiratory-phonatory systems. Although the contribution of the respiratory and phonatory systems to swallowing function will be mentioned, the reader is referred to Chapter 7 for pertinent anatomy and physiology of the swallowing mechanism.

I. RESPIRATORY AND PHONATORY SYSTEMS: NORMAL ANATOMY

The respiratory mechanism consists of the upper and lower respiratory tracts, illustrated in Figure 1-1. The **upper respiratory tract** consists of the *nasal cavity, oral pharynx,* and the *larynx.* The **lower respiratory tract,** or the *tracheobronchial tree,* incorporates the *trachea,* the *bronchi,* and the *lungs.* The following discussion will take the reader through the phonatory and respiratory systems from the nasal and oral cavities, advancing to the pharynx, larynx, and lower respiratory tract. The perspective is a direct visualization of the upper and lower respiratory system, similar to that seen during a *fiber-optic endoscopic evaluation,* where a flexible scope is inserted into the nares to view the upper respiratory tract. A *bronchoscope* is utilized to view the lower respiratory tract.

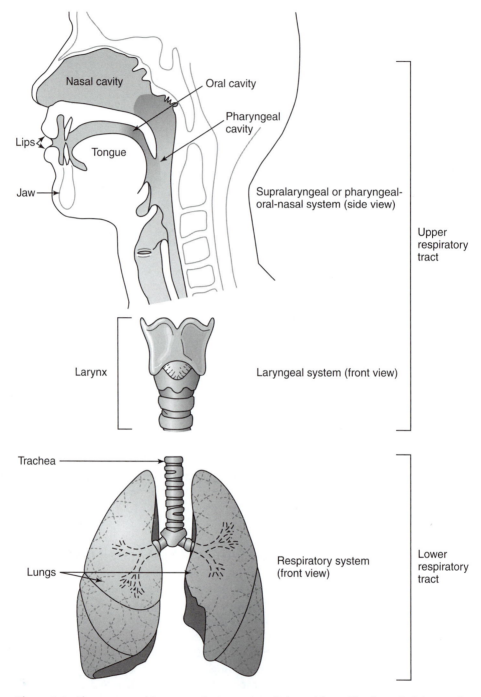

Figure 1-1. The upper and lower respiratory tracts. (Adapted from *The Speech Sciences,* by R. D. Kent, 1997, p. 57. Clifton Park, NY: Singular.)

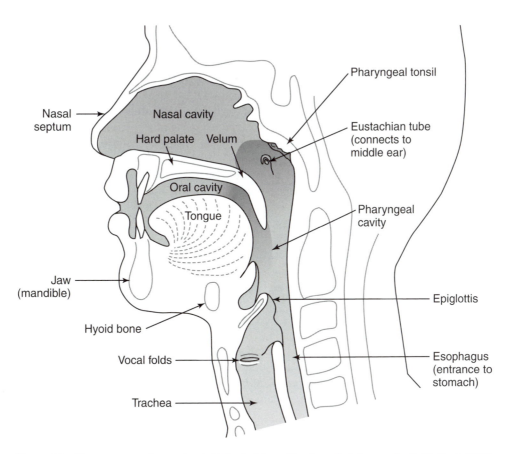

Figure 1-2. The upper respiratory tract. (Adapted from *The Speech Sciences,* by R. D. Kent, 1997, p. 142. Clifton Park, NY: Singular.)

A. Upper Respiratory Tract

The upper respiratory tract is the passageway for the breath stream to enter and leave the lungs. As air moves through the upper respiratory tract, it is warmed and humidified, and large impurities are filtered out before air reaches the lungs. The upper respiratory tract is illustrated in Figure 1-2.

1. The nose is the primary organ responsible for warming, humidifying, and filtering air for respiration. Although air filtration is the primary function of the nasal cavities, olfaction is a less vital, but nonetheless important, function.

    a. The nasal cavities at the top of the upper respiratory tract open at the two *nares* and are separated by the *nasal septum.* The *sinus cavities* are spaces that connect into the nasal cavities for drainage. Nasal breathing is normal in the adult. The structure of the nose as a filtration system does create a resistance to inspired air, created by the passage of air through the scroll-like passages of the lateral walls of the nasal cavities, the bony *nasal turbinates.* Air flows through their convoluted openings or the *nasal meatus.* This pathway is lined with a special type of epithelial cell. These sturdy cells have **cilia,** small hairs, protruding from them that assist in the movement of mucus and other material from the nose into the mouth for expectoration and swallowing. While cilia have a cleansing function, they also create additional turbulence, and therefore resistance to airflow. When there is need for greater respiratory effort, adults will switch to mouth breathing, bypassing the resistance of the nasal cavity. Mouth breathing also occurs during periods of extended speech production and when the nasal cavities are obstructed.

2. The *oral cavity* is separated from the nasal cavity by the *hard palate* and *soft palate* (i.e., the *velum*). It terminates at the **faucial arches** posteriorly and the lips anteriorly. The oral cavity, with the palate and faucial arches, is illustrated in Figure 1-3. In addition to having a *primary* respiratory role, the mouth additionally functions for both swallowing and speech. The lips, tongue, teeth, palates, cheeks, and jaw (i.e., the *mandible* and *maxilla*) form the structures of the oral cavity, and are important structures for speech production, chewing or mastication, and digestion. *Saliva,* which is secreted by the *submandibular, sublingual,* and *parotid salivary glands,* the major salivary glands, is also produced by numerous minor glands. Saliva has many important properties, in-

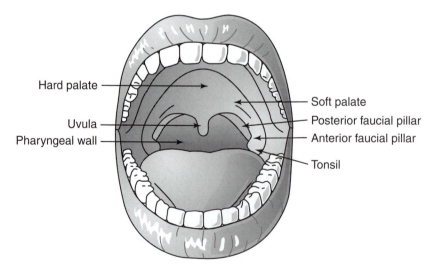

Figure 1-3. The oral cavity. (From *The Speech Sciences,* by R. D. Kent, 1997, p. 185. Clifton Park, NY: Singular.)

cluding antibacterial, antifungal, and antiviral agents. It functions to initially break down food during the oral preparatory phase of swallowing. Additionally, saliva contributes to speech production by protectively coating the articulators for ease of movement. The functional importance of saliva is clearly demonstrated when its production is depleted by medications or other influences. **Xerostomia** is a condition of extreme dry mouth that can contribute to both speech and swallowing problems. Xerostomia is often medication induced. Additionally, tracheostomized and ventilator-dependent patients often complain of dry mouth associated with the loss of the normal filtering system provided by the upper airway.

Located within the oral cavity, the tongue functions in mastication, bolus transport and control, and in articulatory speech production. The tongue is a muscular organ that does not have a skeleton of cartilage or bone. It consists of both intrinsic and extrinsic muscles, which are illustrated in Figures 1-4a and b. The functions of these muscles are described in Table 1-1. Intrinsic muscles control the fine motor muscles of the tongue necessary for articulation. Extrinsic muscles attach the tongue to other structures and control gross movements of the entire organ. The tongue can be discussed in separate regions, with its *root* or *base* particularly important to swallowing function. The tongue is also primarily responsible for the sensation of taste through its numerous sensory receptors.

3. The *pharynx* originates at the posterior portion of the nasal cavities and extends to the upper digestive tract. The pharynx is a tube-like structure consisting of three segments: the *nasopharynx* (portion of the pharynx above the velum), the *oropharynx* (portion of the pharynx from the hypopharynx to the velum), and the *hypopharynx* or *laryngopharynx* (the pharyngeal area located below the base of the tongue and the entrances into the esophagus and *larynx*).

   a. The pharynx is a dual passage for respiration and swallowing. A number of important features are present in the pharynx. Connected to each lateral side of the nasopharynx are the *eustachian tubes,* which extend into each middle ear. The eustachian tubes are normally flaccid and closed, but open to maintain equal air pressure between the ear and outside environment. They also serve to drain secretions and infectious material from the middle ear into the nasopharynx. The opening of each eustachian tube may become irritated by the presence of tubes that are medically inserted into the nasal cavity and airway for ventilation. This may cause severe, repeated middle ear infections which can contribute to conductive hearing loss.

   b. Separation of the digestive and respiratory tracts takes place in the hypopharynx. Tubes placed for feeding pass through the hypopharynx to reach the esophagus. Nasogastric tubes pass via the nasal cavity, nasopharynx,

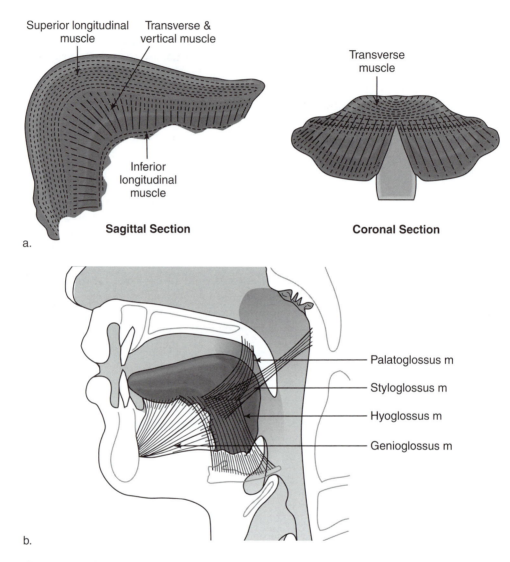

Figure 1-4a. The intrinsic muscles of the tongue. **b.** The extrinsic muscles of the tongue. (From *The Speech Sciences,* by R. D. Kent, 1997, p. 185. Clifton Park, NY: Singular.)

and oropharynx into the hypopharynx and esophagus. Protection of the pharynx from foreign objects is provided in the oropharynx, primarily by the gag reflex. When the *gag reflex* is elicited in the oropharynx, velar contraction and elevation occur, closing the entrance to the pharynx and airway. Traditionally, the gag has been used as a predictive factor in an individual's ability to swallow and manage an oral diet. However, research indicates that the gag reflex may not be present in some normal individ-

Table 1-1. Muscles of the Tongue.

NAME	PRIMARY FUNCTION
Intrinsic Muscles	
Superior longitudinal	Comprises upper layer of tongue. Elevates tip of tongue.
Inferior longitudinal	Makes up lower sides of tongue (not tongue base). Pulls tongue tip down.
Transverse	Courses from side to side. Narrows the tongue toward midline.
Vertical	Courses at right angles transverse; fibers mix with transverse. Flattens the tongue.
Extrinsic Muscles	
Palatoglossus	Connects palate and tongue. Serves to elevate tongue.
Styloglossus	Lateral tongue to temporal bone (styloid process). Pulls tongue up and back.
Hyoglossus*	Posterior tongue to hyoid bone. Lowers and retracts tongue.
Genioglossus*	Tongue surface to mandible and hyoid. Protrudes, lowers, and shapes body of tongue.

*Can also be considered laryngeal elevators.

Innervation of the intrinsic and extrinsic muscles of the tongue is by means of the hypoglossal nerve (CN XII).

uals. Leder (1996a) found that 13% (i.e., 9 of his 69 subjects) who displayed a normal swallowing pattern ("nondysphagic subjects") did not exhibit a gag reflex. While a gag is a reflex, the swallow is a mediated response. A gag does not occur during a normal swallow, and its absence is poorly predictive of dysphagia (Leder, 1997).

4. The *larynx,* a cartilaginous structure, lies inferior to the pharynx. It is located at the top of the respiratory tract, attaching to the *trachea* inferiorly and suspended superiorly from the *hyoid bone.*

   a. The supportive structure of the larynx is composed primarily of two unpaired cartilages (i.e., *cricoid, thyroid*) and one paired cartilage (i.e., arytenoids) as illustrated in Figure 1-5. The ring-shaped *cricoid cartilage* forms both the top of the trachea and the base of the larynx. The shield-shaped *thyroid cartilage* is the largest of the laryngeal cartilages. The characteristic anterior prominence of the thyroid cartilage is the anatomical landmark known as the Adam's apple or the *thyroid notch.* The thyroid cartilage articulates with the cricoid cartilage by way of the *inferior horns* of the thyroid cartilages. It is at this attachment, known as the *cricothyroid*

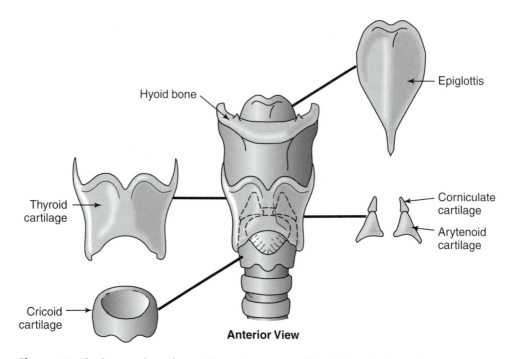

Hyoid bone

Epiglottis

Thyroid
cartilage

Corniculate
cartilage

Arytenoid
cartilage

Cricoid
cartilage

Anterior View

Figure 1-5. The laryngeal cartilages. (From *Anatomy and Physiology for Speech, Language and Hearing* [2nd ed.], by J. A. Seikel, D. W. King, & D. G. Drumright, 2000, p. 170. Clifton Park, NY: Singular.)

joint, that the cartilages rotate to lengthen and shorten the *vocal folds.* The paired pyramid-shaped *arytenoid cartilages* rest on top of the cricoid cartilage. Each arytenoid has two processes from which important muscles attach. The anterior or forward process is referred to as the *vocal process.* The lateral process is called the *muscular process.* (These structures are illustrated in Figure 1-7a). The rocking and gliding movements of the arytenoids via the *cricoarytenoid joint* (i.e., where the cricoid and arytenoid cartilages articulate) are responsible for opening (i.e., *abducting*) and closing (i.e., *adducting*) the vocal folds. The laryngeal cartilages communicate via muscles and ligaments that are covered by membranes.

b.   Smooth membranes cover the medial area of the larynx. Important in the identification of landmarks in the larynx is the *valleculae,* a mucous membrane-coated space between the tongue and the epiglottis. The *pyriform sinus* is the space between the aryepiglottic folds and the thyroid cartilages. The aryepiglottic folds comprise the upper portion of another membrane (*quadrangular membrane*) and are part of the aryepiglottic muscles. The aryepiglottic folds travel from the side of the epiglottis to the tip of the arytenoid and make up the lateral walls of the laryngeal vestibule. A vestibule is a space, and the laryngeal vestibule is the first entrance into the larynx. The vestibule ends at the *ventricular* or *false vocal folds.* Under normal phonatory conditions, the ventricular folds do not actively vibrate, but they do participate in airway closure for other functions (e.g., swallowing and heavy lifting). The next membrane-coated space in the larynx is the *laryngeal ventricle,* extending from the false vocal folds to the true vocal folds below. The true vocal folds are comprised of finer layers of tissue overlaying muscle.

The true vocal folds, ventricle, and false vocal folds, are used to functionally delineate three major regions of the larynx. The *subglottic* area runs from the lowest margin of the true vocal folds to the inside border of the cricoid cartilage. The *glottic* region is the true vocal folds. The *supraglottic* region is above the laryngeal ventricle. These areas are discussed when identifying airway obstruction or disease in tracheostomized and ventilator-dependent individuals. Landmarks of the larynx are illustrated in Figure 1-6.

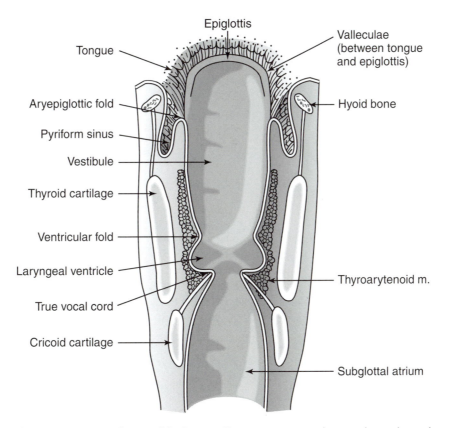

Figure 1-6. A coronal view of the larynx, illustrating pertinent laryngeal muscles and membranes. (Adapted from *Anatomy and Physiology for Speech, Language and Hearing* [2nd ed.], by J. A. Seikel, D. W. King, & D. G. Drumright, 2000, p. 171. Clifton Park, NY: Singular.)

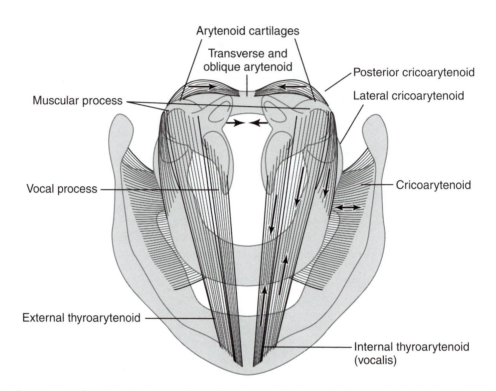

Figure 1-7a. The intrinsic laryngeal muscles. (From *The Speech Sciences,* by R. D. Kent, 1997, p. 109. Clifton Park, NY: Singular.)

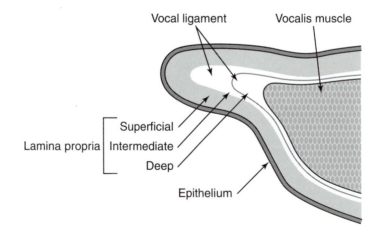

Figure 1-7b. The vocal fold, shown in coronal section and enlarged to represent its layered structure. (From *The Speech Sciences,* by R. D. Kent, 1997, p. 106. Clifton Park, NY: Singular.)

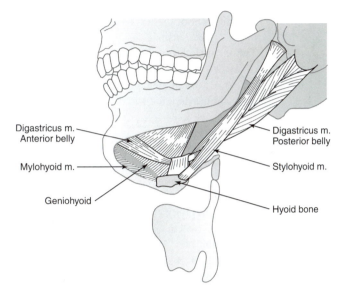

Figure 1-7c. The extrinsic muscles of the larynx (laryngeal elevators). (From *Anatomy and Physiology for Speech, Language and Hearing* [2nd ed.], by J. A. Seikel, D. W. King, & D. G. Drumright, 2000, p. 202. Clifton Park, NY: Singular.)

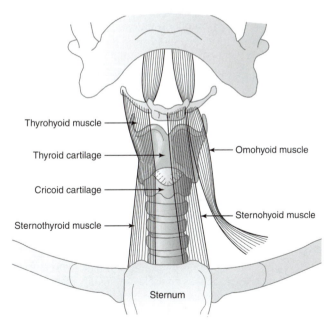

Figure 1-7d. The extrinsic muscles of the larynx (laryngeal depressors). (From *The Speech Sciences,* by R. D. Kent, 1997, p. 117. Clifton Park, NY: Singular.)

c. The muscles of the larynx are divided into two groups: *extrinsic and intrinsic*. The intrinsic laryngeal muscles are illustrated in Figure 1-7a. The intrinsic laryngeal muscles (i.e., those contained within the larynx) described above perform the finer adjustments of the larynx necessary for vocal fold movement. Specifically, these muscles function to abduct and adduct, lengthen and shorten, and alter the tension of the vocal folds.

d. The true vocal folds are part of a pair of large muscles called the *thyroarytenoids*. The *internal thyroarytenoids* (or vocalis) are covered by connective tissue layers and together compose the actual vocal folds. The *external thyroarytenoids* are the portion of the muscles that lies lateral to the internal thyroarytenoids. This portion of the external thryroarytenoids is also referred to as the thyromuscularis. The internal thyroarytenoids, or vocalis muscles, insert into the vocal process of each arytenoid muscle while the external thyroarytenoids insert into each muscular process. The outermost layer of the vocal fold is comprised of *epithelium*. The thyrovocalis muscle has a covering referred to as the *lamina propria* underlying the epithelium. The *vocal ligament* is part of the lamina propria. The true vocal folds consist of complex and multilayered muscular structures covered by connective tissue and mucous membrane. Figure 1-7b depicts the layered structure of the true vocal folds. This composition creates their unique vibratory properties as the connective and mucosal tissue move separately from the thryovocalis muscle. The vocal folds, responsible for vibrating sound for speech as well as participating in airway closure, become susceptible to damage when any medical airway intervention procedures are performed.

e. The hyoid bone is separate from the actual larynx and forms the point of attachment for many of the extrinsic laryngeal muscles (i.e., those with points of attachment outside the larynx). Consequently, many laryngeal movements will generally follow in tandem with hyoid bone movements. Selected extrinsic laryngeal muscles are shown in Figures 1-7c and d. Points of specific attachment and functions of the muscles are listed in Table 1-3. The extrinsic muscles are responsible for gross laryngeal movements of elevation and depression, as well as laryngeal stabilization. These muscles are divided into two groups, the laryngeal elevators (i.e., *suprahyoid muscle*) and the laryngeal depressors (i.e., *infrahyoid muscles*). As a group these muscles are mainly responsible for the changes in the positioning of the larynx during speech and voice production, as when altering resonance and pitch, and during swallowing.

f. Points of attachment and functions of the intrinsic and extrinsic laryngeal muscles are listed in Table 1-2 and Table 1-3. The intrinsic and extrinsic laryngeal muscles, working in concert with each other, allow the complex function of laryngeal valving for respiration, swallowing, and phonation by:

(1) opening during the inspiratory phase of respiration.

(2) providing the force needed for increased physical effort (e.g., lifting and defecation) by adducting and momentarily trapping air in the lungs and chest.

(3) closing during swallowing on several levels (i.e., ventricular and true vocal folds) to prevent foreign substances from entering the airway and lungs.

(4) sealing to trap sufficient air and increase *subglottal* air pressure so that when a protective cough is triggered by the presence of foreign substances in the larynx, those substances are then forcefully expelled.

(5) producing voice by adducting the vocal folds and then vibrating the folds by regulating the respiratory air flow and the stiffness of the vocal folds.

Normal airflow through the larynx is necessary for it to function effectively. Disruption of the airflow commonly occurs with **tracheostomy** and **ventilator dependence** and affects speech and swallowing functions in various ways.

B. Lower Respiratory Tract

The lower respiratory tract is housed in the *thoracic cavity* (i.e., *thorax*), which is formed by the 12 *thoracic vertebrae, sternum,* and *rib cage.* The thorax is divided into left and right halves by the *mediastinum,* which contains the heart, blood vessels, nerves, and esophagus. The sternum or breastbone forms the anterior attachment for the upper 10 pairs of ribs. The lower 2 pairs, although attached posteriorly to the vertebrae, remain unattached anteriorly and thus are known as the *floating ribs.* The thorax is illustrated in Figure 1-8.

1. The *lower respiratory tract* is illustrated in Figure 1-9. The *trachea* is composed of semicircular, U-shaped cartilaginous rings that extend from the larynx (i.e., cricoid cartilage) to the upper thoracic cavity. At the inferior end of the trachea, it divides into two branches called the *mainstem* or *primary bronchi.* Each tracheal ring is separated from the other by a fibroelastic membrane. The combination of firm cartilage and a flexible membrane allows the trachea to maintain its shape, to expand during inspiration, and to flex during

Table 1-2. Intrinsic Laryngeal Muscles.*

NAME	POINTS OF ATTACHMENT	FUNCTION
Thyroarytenoids	• Arytenoid cartilage to inner aspect of thyroid cartilage.	• Muscular segment of true vocal folds.
• Thyrovocalis (internal thyroarytenoid) (paired)	• Thyroid cartilage to vocal process of arytenoids.	• Vibratory portion of vocal folds; stiffens and shortens folds.
• Thyromuscularis (external thyroarytenoid) (paired)	• Thyroid cartilage to muscular process of arytenoids.	• Lateral portion of folds; decreases tension and adducts vocal folds.
Cricothyroid (paired)	• Anterior cricoid cartilage to lower edge of thyroid cartilage.	• Lengthens and stiffens vocal folds.
Lateral Cricoarytenoid (paired)	• Lateral edge of cricoid cartilage to muscular process of arytenoid cartilage.	• Primary glottal adductor.
Interarytenoids	• Posterior edge of arytenoid cartilage	• Glottal adductor
• Transverse arytenoid (unpaired)	• Horizontal across arytenoid cartilage	• Squeezes arytenoids medially.
• Oblique arytenoid (paired)	• Muscular process of one arytenoid to apex of the other; continues up to epiglottis via aryepiglottic folds.	• Pulls upper processes of arytenoids medially.
Posterior Cricoarytenoid (paired)	• Posterior portion of cricoid cartilage to muscular process of arytenoids.	• Sole glottal abductor.

*All intrinsic muscles are innervated by means of the vagus nerve (CN X).

swallowing. The inner surface of the trachea is lined with ciliated epithelial columnar cells with scattered specialized **goblet cells.** These goblet cells are mucus-secreting. These cells secrete mucus which functions as a protective and cleansing mechanism for the respiratory tract.

2. The primary *bronchi* consist of the left and right mainstem bronchi. The angles of the left and right bronchi differ considerably, with the angle to the right mainstem bronchus being less acute than to the left. The right bronchus, there-

Table 1-3. Extrinsic Laryngeal Muscles.

NAME	POINTS OF ATTACHMENT	FUNCTION
Laryngeal Elevators/Suprahyoid Muscles		
Digastric	Anterior: mandible to hyoid Posterior: temporal to hyoid	Raises hyoid bone and the entire larynx and assists in jaw depression (anterior belly).
Mylohyoid	Mandible to hyoid bone forms floor of mouth	Raises hyoid, floor of mouth and tongue and depresses jaw.
Stylohyoid	Styloid process of temporal bone to hyoid	Raises hyoid up and backwards.
Geniohyoid	Mandible to hyoid bone	Raises hyoid up and forward and depresses jaw.
Laryngeal Depressors/Infrahyoid Muscles		
Omohyoid	Inferior: scapula to sternal tendon Superior: sternal tendon to hyoid bone	Lowes the hyoid and the larynx.
Sternohyoid	Sternum to hyoid bone	Lowers and fixes the hyoid.
Thyrohyoid	Thyroid cartilage to hyoid bone	Pulls hyoid down or elevates larynx if hyoid is fixed.
Sternothyroid	Sternum to thyroid cartilage	Pulls thyroid cartilage downward.

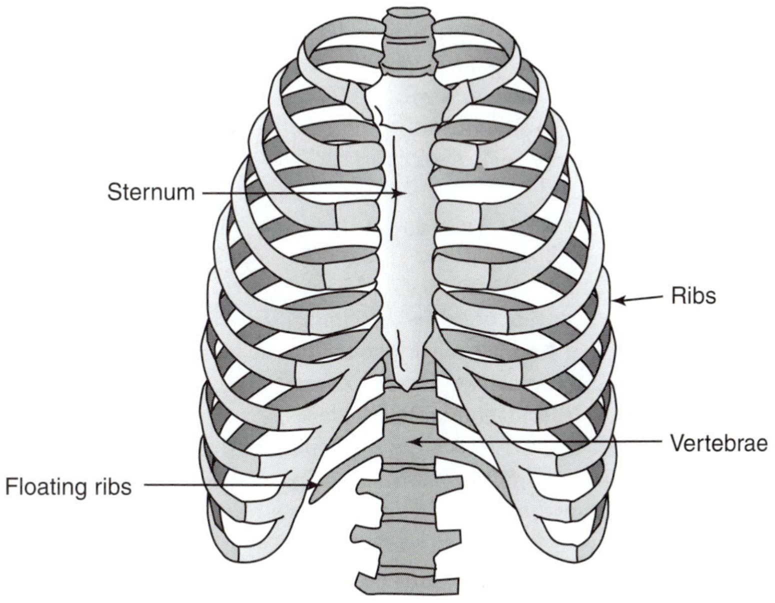

Figure 1-8. The thorax.

fore, is the more common pathway for aspirated material. The bronchi are further divided into secondary (i.e., *lobar*) and tertiary (i.e., *segmental*) groups. The bronchi separate into the *bronchioles,* with further division ending at the *terminal bronchioles* and eventually the *alveolar air sacs.* It is at the terminal bronchioles and alveoli that gas exchange with the blood stream takes place. The alveolar air sacs are illustrated in Figure 1-9.

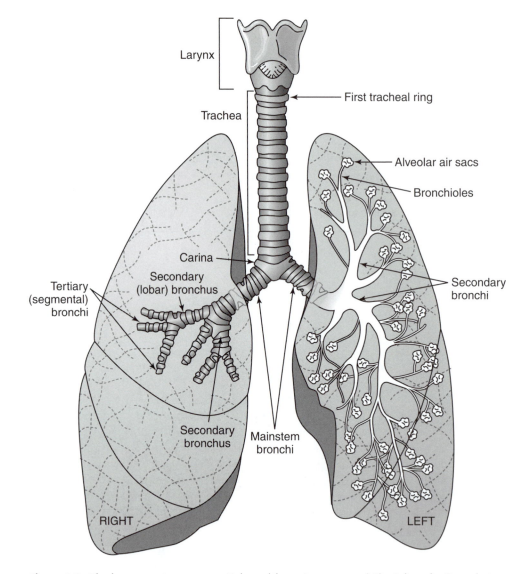

Figure 1-9. The lower respiratory tract. (Adapted from *Anatomy and Physiology for Speech, Language and Hearing* [2nd ed.], by J. A. Seikel, D. W. King, & D. G. Drumright, 2000, p. 63. Clifton Park, NY: Singular.)

3. The *lungs,* a pair of separate cone-shaped organs, fill the bulk of the thorax. They divide into smaller segments called *lobes.* Lungs consist of a spongy material with highly elastic properties. This elasticity results from a combination of the elastic fibers in the alveolar walls and the surface tension of the alveoli. Alveoli have a predisposition to collapse inward, which is prevented by a liquid called **surfactant.** Surfactant is manufactured by specialized epithelial cells of the alveoli and maintains surface tension in the alveoli throughout inspiration and expiration and provides lubrication for ease of alveolar expansion. Without surfactant, areas of alveoli would collapse and could not participate in respiration (Eubanks & Bone, 1990). Collapse of the alveolar air sacs, which can occur for a variety of reasons, is called **atelectasis.** Atelectasis usually necessitates medical intervention.

   a. Each lung is housed in an airtight sac known as the *visceral pleura.* The visceral pleura covers the lung surface while the *parietal pleura* lines the thorax or inner chest wall. The relationship of the **pleura** is illustrated in Figure 1-10. The pleurae are thin membranes which slide against one another, eased by the fluid that normally fills the **pleural cavity.** The pleural cavity is the space located between the visceral and parietal pleurae. There is negative pressure between the visceral and parietal pleura which allows the membranes to adhere to one another. This negative intrapleural pressure holds the lung tissue against the ribs, which form the chest wall. Consequently, any movement of the chest wall results in a subsequent parallel movement of the lungs. This is referred to as *pleural linkage.* The pleural fluid also protects the lungs, ensuring that abrasion is avoided during normal inspiration and expiration. Lung tissue cannot move independently of chest wall movement. The lungs would collapse inward due to their elastic nature if they were not held in place via pleural linkage. When an external fluid, or air, enters the pleural cavity, the airtight seal of the lungs is broken and their function becomes compromised. The resulting lung or lobar collapse is known as a **pneumothorax.**

4. The *respiratory musculature,* along with the design of the rib cage, is responsible for the movements of the thorax that allow for inspiration and expiration. The thorax is not a rigid structure. It expands in anterior-posterior and lateral directions, thus elevating and twisting the ribs. The cartilaginous attachment of the ribs to the sternum allows this anterior-posterior thoracic expansion created by the hinged movement of the ribs. Overall, these smooth motions result in changes in diameter to the thoracic cavity during inspiration and expiration. The respiratory musculature is illustrated in Figure 1-11. Many respiratory muscles contribute to the inspiratory/expiratory breathing cycle and thoracic expansion. They will be discussed in this section according to general anatomical location. Selected respiratory musculature are further described in Table 1-4.

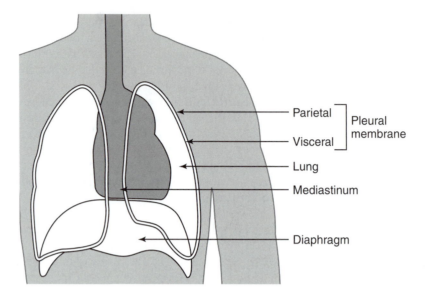

Figure 1-10. The lungs and their surrounding pleurae.

    a.   The thorax contains the *diaphragm* and the *intercostals.* The diaphragm is the major muscle of inspiration. It is an unpaired muscle which inserts into the lower portion of the rib cage and into a *central tendon* that rides over the contents of the abdomen. Although unpaired, the diaphragm is functionally divided into left and right "hemidiaphragms," each of which is supplied by the phrenic nerve on the same side. Its shape is often described as an inverted dome. The diaphragm separates the thorax and the abdomen. When the diaphragm contracts and flattens, it increases the volume of the thorax and compresses the volume of the abdomen, causing abdominal expansion. The diaphragmatic pleura, which covers the diaphragm, is important in this action as it adheres to the visceral pleurae above. As a result the lungs expand, allowing air to enter. According to Tesoriero and Dail (1990), the diaphragm is responsible for approximately 75% of the normal changes in thoracic volume during quiet inspiration. The *intercostal muscles* are located between each pair of ribs. As the name suggests, the *internal intercostal muscles* lie deep to the *external intercostals.* Contraction of the external intercostal muscles (and possibly a portion of the internal intercostals) is thought to increase thoracic volume by elevating the ribs during inspiration and to stabilize the thoracic wall. The *pectoralis major and minor* are chest muscles that function during inspiration only when the shoulder girdle and arms are fixed.

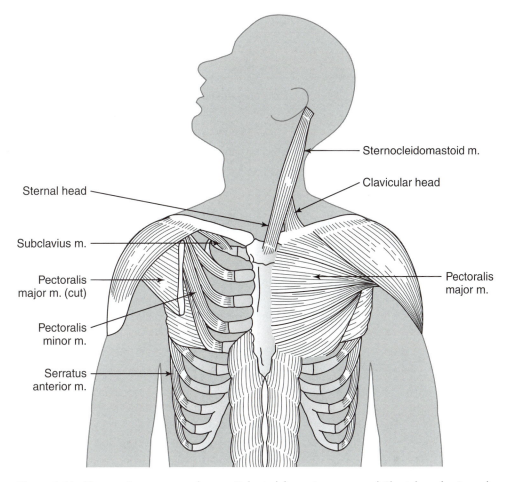

Figure 1-11. The respiratory musculature. (Adapted from *Anatomy and Physiology for Speech, Language and Hearing* [2nd ed.], by J. A. Seikel, D. W. King, & D. G. Drumright, 2000, p. 95. Clifton Park, NY: Singular.)

b. The abdominal musculature is located below the diaphragm and above the pelvis. The muscles in this group that contribute most significantly to respiration include: the *rectus abdominis, internal and external obliques,* and *transversus abdominis.* The abdominal musculature functions primarily during forced expiration to compress the abdominal contents which push against the diaphragm, assisting in a maximum exhalation. They are always active, as is the diaphragm, during respiratory function for speech. These muscles are generally relaxed during inspiration.

Table 1-4. Respiratory Musculature.

ABDOMINAL MUSCULATURE*	FUNCTION
Rectus Abdominis	Pulls sternum downward and depresses ribs during expiration, resulting in a decrease in thoracid diameter.
External Obliques	Pulls ribs downward and compresses visceral contents.
Internal Obliques	Pulls ribs downward and compresses visceral contents.
Tranversus Abdominis	Contracts abdomen, compresses visceral contents.

*All abdominal musculature aids in forced expiration

THORACIC MUSCULATURE	FUNCTION
Diaphragm	During resting inspiration, pulls central tendon forward and downward. Increases vertical diameter of the thorax.
	During resting expiration, returns to resting position as a result of recoil forces on the thorax.
External Intercostals	During inspiration, elevates ribs resulting in an increase in anterior-posterior and transverse thoracic dimension.
Internal Intercostals	Intercartilaginous portion is also a rib elevator.
	Interosseous portion functions in conjunction with abdominal musculature, depresses ribs during expiration.
Pectoralis major and pectoralis minor	Accessory muscles of inspiration, pull sternum and ribs upward when arms and shoulders are held in a fixed position; resulting in an increased anterior-posterior thoracid diameter.

NECK MUSCULATURE	FUNCTION
Sternocleidomastoid	Landmark muscle; courses from sternum and clavical uniting into mastoid process. Raises sternum and clavical during inspiration (with head fixed).
Scalene	Raises upper ribs during inspiration.

    c. The strap muscles of the neck also have a role in respiration. They include the *sternocleidomastoid* and the *scalene muscles.* Although these muscles are primarily accessory muscles of respiration, functioning to maintain head posture, they have an enhanced function in normal individuals during exercise. Along with the intercostal muscles, these accessory muscles of inspiration can compensate for a dysfunctional diaphragm. As a result, they are utilized a great deal by many patients with pulmonary disease.

C. Innervation of the Phonatory Respiratory Systems

1. The cranial nerves responsible for motor innervation of the phonatory mechanism are listed in Table 1-5. The pairs of cranial nerves that bilaterally innervate the phonatory mechanism include cranial nerves V (*trigeminal*), VII (*facial*), X (*vagus*), and XII (*hypoglossal*). The intrinsic laryngeal muscles are solely innervated by the vagus nerve (X). The vagus nerve is so named because of its wandering course through the body. The remaining three cranial nerves (V, VII, and XII) and several cervical spinal nerves innervate the extrinsic laryngeal muscles.

Table 1-5. Motor Nerve Innervation of the Phonatory Mechanism.

INTRINSIC LARYNGEAL MUSCLES	INNERVATION
Thyroarytenoid	Vagus (CN X) Recurrent laryngeal nerve branch
Lateral Cricoarytenoid	Vagus (CN X) Recurrent laryngeal nerve branch
Interarytenoids	Vagus (CN X) Recurrent laryngeal nerve branch
Posterior Cricoarytenoid	Vagus (CN X) Recurrent laryngeal nerve branch
Cricothyroid	Vagus (CN X) Recurrent laryngeal nerve branch
EXTRINIC LARYNGEAL MUSCLES	**INNERVATION**
Suprahyoid	
Digastric	Anterior: trigeminal (CN V) (mylohyoid branch) Posterior: facial (CN VII) (digastric branch)
Mylohyoid	Trigeminal (CN V) (mandibular branch)
Stylohyoid	Facial (CN VII) (mandibular branch)
Geniohyoid	Hypoglossal (geniohyoid branch)
Infrahyoid*	
Omohyoid	C1-C3 via ansa cervicalis
Sternohyoid	C2-C3 via ansa cervicalis
Thyrohyoid	C1 via hypoglossal nerve
Sternothyroid	C1-C3 via ansa cervicalis

*All innervated by cervical spinal nerves.

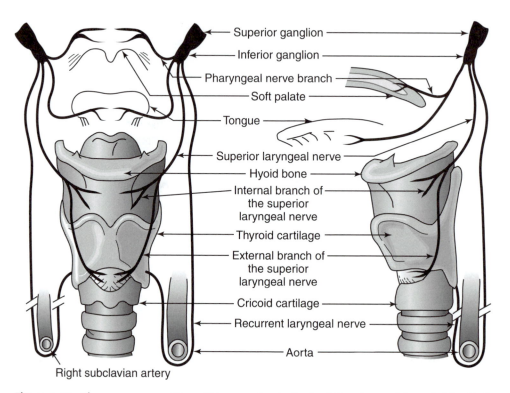

Figure 1-12. The vagus nerve. (From "Neuroanatomic Basis of Hearing and Speech," by C. R. Larson & B. E. Pfingst, 1982. In N. J. Lass, L V. McReynolds, J. L. Northern, & D. E. Yoder (Eds.), *Speech, Language and Hearing I, Normal Processes.* Philadelphia, PA: W. B. Saunders Co. Copyright 1982 C. R. Larson and N. J. Lass. Adapted with authors' permission.)

a. The vagus nerve is extremely important for vocal fold movement. Figure 1-12 illustrates the branches of the vagus nerve and their attachments to the structures they innervate. The main branch of the vagus is known as the *recurrent laryngeal nerve.* This branch innervates all of the intrinsic muscles of the larynx with the exception of the cricothyroid. It also supplies sensory innervation to the subglottic region of the larynx. The left recurrent laryngeal nerve is longer and travels below the aorta before ascending back to the larynx. Both right and left recurrent laryngeal nerves pass near the thyroid gland. Because of the structures it passes, the left recurrent laryngeal nerve is susceptible to damage during cardiac or thyroid surgery.

(1) The *superior laryngeal nerve,* which is another main branch of the vagus, also subdivides into two smaller branches. The external branch of the superior laryngeal nerve supplies motor innervation to the cricothyroid muscle. The internal branch is responsible for supraglottic laryngeal sensation.

(2) The *pharyngeal branch* of the vagus nerve is responsible for motor innervation of the pharynx and most of the soft palate, and is important in speech and swallowing function.

b. Cranial nerves V (trigeminal), VII (facial), and XII (hypoglossal) and cervical spinal nerves (C1–C3) innervate the extrinsic laryngeal musculature. These muscles are responsible for raising and lowering the larynx. The vagus innervates the intrinsic laryngeal muscles in their function to adduct and abduct the vocal folds, as well as alter vocal fold length and tension.

2. As the single most important muscle of inspiration, the diaphragm receives bilateral innervation from the *phrenic nerves.* The phrenic nerves originate from spinal nerves C3, C4, and C5 bilaterally and provide both motor and sensory information. Patients who have experienced a high spinal cord injury at this level will frequently require mechanical ventilatory support, at least temporarily. Figure 1-13 illustrates the position of the phrenic nerve relative to the heart, lungs, and diaphragm. The figure also clearly illustrates the close proximity of the heart and lungs, with the heart protected by its central placement in the body in a region known as the *mediastinum.* However, because of this proximity, cardiac and pulmonary problems often coexist. The heart, surrounded by *pericardium,* is divided into two halves, right and left. Each half

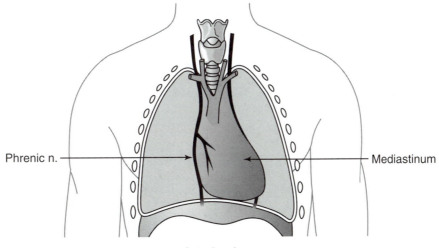

Anterior view

Figure 1-13. Relationship of the heart, lungs, and diaphragm. Note the phrenic nerve innervation of the diaphragm. (Adapted from *Anatomy and Physiology for Speech, Language and Hearing* [2nd ed.], by J. A. Seikel, D. W. King, & D. G. Drumright, 2000, p. 80. Clifton Park, NY: Singular.)

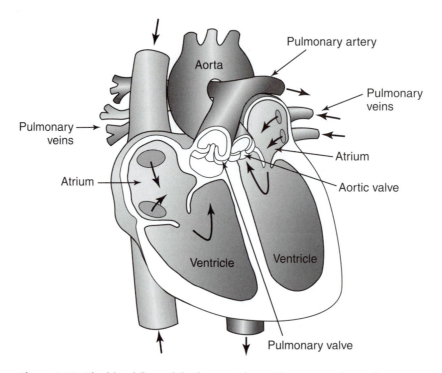

Figure 1-14. The blood flow of the heart. (Adapted from *Principles and Practices of Cardiopulmonary Physical Therapy* [3rd ed.], by D. Frownfelter & E. Dean, 1996, p. 45. St. Louis, MO: Mosby Year-Book. Copyright 1996 by Mosby Year-Book.)

has two sections. Figure 1-14 illustrates the heart with its major veins and arteries. The *atrium* receives blood from veins and the *ventricles,* which pump blood into arteries. From the right atrium blood passes to the right ventricle. The right ventricle pushes blood through the *pulmonary valve* into the *pulmonary arteries.* Blood is returned to the left atrium by *pulmonary veins,* where it passes through the left ventricle and out the *aorta,* the main artery of the body.

II. THE RESPIRATORY AND PHONATORY SYSTEMS: NORMAL FUNCTION

The mechanical event of breathing differs for quiet, forced, and speech breathing. *Quiet breathing* constitutes active inspiration and passive expiration. *Forced breathing* is active inspiration utilizing accessory inspiratory muscles (i.e., neck and chest muscles) and active expiration using abdominal muscles. *Speech breathing* is active inspiration and active expiration against the resistance of a modulated upper respiratory tract, primarily the vocal folds. Definitions of *lung volumes* and *lung capacities* are given in

Table 1-6. Lung Volumes and Capacities Defined.

Tidal Volume (TV)	Volume of air inhaled and exhaled during normal quiet breathing. Average normal value 500 ml (adult).
Inspiratory Reserve Volume (IRV)	Volume of air that can be inhaled beyond a normal tidal inspiration. Average normal value 2.5 liters (adult).
Expiratory Reserve Volume (ERV)	Volume of air that can be exhaled beyond a normal tidal expiration. Average normal value 1.5 liters (adult).
Residual Volume (RV)	Volume of air that remains in the lungs beyond a maximum forced expiration. Average normal value 1.5 liters (adult).
Functional Residual Capacity (FRC)	Volume of air that remains in the lungs beyond a normal tidal expiration. Average normal value 3 liters (adult).
Vital Capacity (VC)	Volume of air maximally exhaled after a maximum inspiration. Reflects inspiratory/expiratory muscle strength. Average value 4.5 liters (adult).
Minute Volume	Amount of air that is inspired and expired per minute. Average normal value 6–9 liters per minute (adult).

Table 1-6. These terms, used to measure and describe respiratory physiology, will be helpful in a discussion of quiet, forced, and speech breathing.

A. Quiet Breathing

Before a respiratory cycle begins, *alveolar pressure,* or the pressure within the lungs, is equal to *atmospheric pressure,* or the pressure outside the lungs. Upon inspiration, the muscles of respiration begin their action.

1. The diaphragm, previously described as the primary muscle of inspiration, contracts and flattens as it moves downward, while the intercostal muscles elevate and twist the ribs. The movement of the diaphragm serves to extend the vertical dimension of the thorax and elevate the lower ribs, decreasing intrapleural pressure, or the pressure within the lungs. Additionally, the downward movement of the diaphragm contracts the abdominal or visceral contents. This compression leads to an increase in intra-abdominal pressure. The intercostal muscles increase the thoracic diameter in both anterior-posterior and transverse directions. This increase in the thoracic dimension serves to *further* decrease intrapleural pressure and, concurrently, alveolar pressure. Alveolar

expansion is passive. As the lungs are pulled by the corresponding movements of the chest wall, the alveoli expand. As the thorax, lungs, and alveoli expand, a pressure change occurs and alveolar pressure is now less than atmospheric pressure. Air enters the airway. This inspiratory air flow continues until alveolar pressure is equal to atmospheric.

a. Unlike inspiration, expiration during quiet breathing is passive. The muscles of inspiration gradually stop contracting. Passive expiratory forces or *relaxation pressures,* gravity, *torque,* and *elastic recoil,* then come into play. Gravity acts on the raised thorax so that it moves downward. Torque is created as the ribs, twisted during inspiration, "spring" back to their normal resting posture. Additionally, the compressed abdominal viscera rebound via elastic recoil and push the diaphragm upward. The alveoli within the lungs recoil, naturally compressing the air within the air sacs. Intrapleural and alveolar pressure is now greater than the outside or atmospheric pressure; thus air leaves the lungs until alveolar and atmospheric pressures are equalized.

b. The primary goal of quiet breathing is to exchange *carbon dioxide (CO$_2$)* for *oxygen (O$_2$)* at the level of the alveolar capillaries. The air that enters the lungs during inspiration is oxygen rich. Before it reaches the lungs, it passes through the pharynx and trachea. With the exception of the alveoli, the airways are considered **dead space.** No gas exchange takes place in the airways because their walls are too thick; thus O$_2$ cannot pass into the blood supply at these upper levels. It is at the level of the alveolar air sacs, which communicate with the blood stream via thin capillary walls, that O$_2$ diffuses into the blood. In the human body, the circulatory system or blood flow provides transportation of O$_2$ to and from the cells of the body. O$_2$ is carried in red blood cells whose main component is **hemoglobin (Hb)**, a chemical compound that combines with the O$_2$ molecule. With hemoglobin, O$_2$ is carried to the heart via the small pulmonary veins, and then pumped by the left side of the heart throughout the body. Simultaneously, blood pumped by the right chambers of the heart returns to the lungs through the pulmonary artery. It now contains higher levels of CO$_2$, which has been excreted from body tissues. Again at the level of the alveolar capillaries, gas exchange takes place as CO$_2$ enters the alveoli and is exhaled from the body by the lungs. This process is illustrated in Figure 1-15. This is a constant process serving to maintain correct levels of O$_2$ and CO$_2$ in the body's blood supply. This process of gas exchange in and out of the lungs is referred to as **ventilation.**

c. The normal respiratory rate during quiet breathing is between 12–20 breaths per minute. The volume of air inhaled and exhaled during one normal quiet respiratory cycle is referred to as **tidal volume. Minute volume** is the amount of air that is inspired and expired per minute.

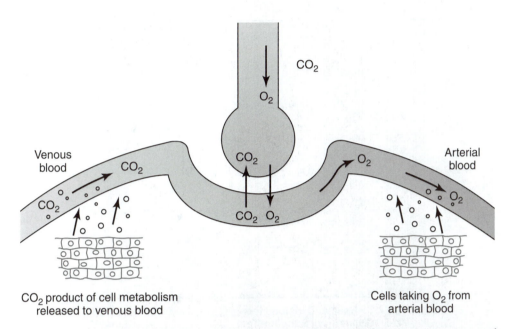

Figure 1-15. The process of gas exchange in the blood. (From "Impaired Pulmonary Function and Dysphagia," by K. J. Dikeman, M. S. Kazandjian, & R. Chua, 2000, p. 241. In R. H. Mills [Ed.], *Evaluation of Dysphagia in Adults: Expanding the Diagnostic Options* (pp. 239–282). Austin, TX: Pro-Ed. Copyright 2000 by Pro-Ed, Inc. Reprinted with permission of Pro-Ed.)

B. Forced Breathing

1. Forced breathing is necessary when the body has an increased demand for air, as during physical exertion. Forced breathing occurs with the use of primary (i.e., diaphragm, intercostals) *and* accessory (i.e., sternocleidomastoid, scalene, pectoralis) muscles of respiration. Forced expiration uses the passive forces of expiration, along with the active contraction of the muscles of expiration (i.e., the internal intercostals and abdominal musculature).

   a. During forced breathing, tidal volume increases to meet the demands of increased physical activity. *Inspiratory reserve volume* is the amount of air that can be inhaled beyond a normal tidal inspiration. *Expiratory reserve volume* is the amount of air that can be exhaled beyond a normal tidal expiration, utilizing the muscles of exhalation. *Vital capacity* is the amount of air which can be maximally expelled from the lungs after a maximum inspiration. This measure includes the tidal volume, inspiratory reserve and expiratory reserve volumes and represents the total amount of air potentially available to an individual for forced respiration. *Residual volume* is the volume of air that remains in the lungs *beyond* a maximum forced expiration. In normal healthy individuals this prevents lung collapse.

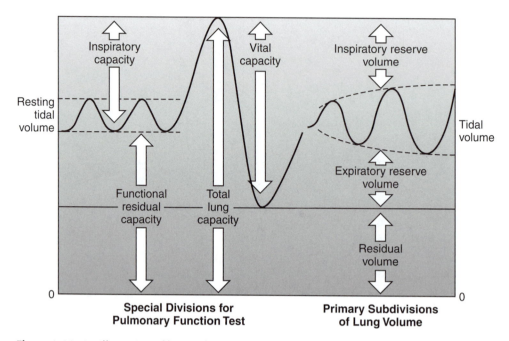

Figure 1-16. An illustration of lung volumes and lung capacities. (From *The Speech Sciences,* by R. D. Kent, 1997, p. 89. Clifton Park, NY: Singular.)

Figure 1-16 illustrates the components of each lung volume and capacity as it relates to the respiratory cycle. These measurements are obtained via **spirometry.** Spirometry is included in a battery of test called **pulmonary function tests.** These provide information about a patient's lung volumes and capacities.

C. Flow and Pressure

Normal respiration is really a system of pressure and flow working together. *Flow* can be thought of as the flow or air in and out of the lungs. Air enters the lungs when the diaphragm contracts, and leaves the lungs when the diaphragm is at rest. At the same time, changes are occurring in the lungs in terms of *pressure.* As the diaphragm contracts, alveolar pressure drops because the lungs expand. Alveolar pressure thus becomes negative. When the flow of air into the lungs has stopped, alveolar pressure is positive. Intrapleural pressure (between the parietal and visceral pleurae) is always negative but drops even more because the contracting diaphragm pulls the pleurae apart. This constantly adjusting system of flow and pressure is ventilation. Viewing ventilation as a flow-pressure system will assist the clinician in understanding the impact of mechanical ventilation as discussed in Chapter 4.

D. Speech Breathing

1. Speech breathing differs from quiet and forced breathing. During speech breathing, active inspiration and expiration take place against the resistance of a continuously modulating upper airway, primarily the vocal folds. Flow and pressure dynamics are also important in a discussion of speech breathing.

   a. When breathing for speech, the inspiratory cycle becomes shorter relative to the expiratory cycle. Phonation or production of voice occurs during the expiratory cycle. Modulation of airflow occurs at many levels along the upper and lower respiratory tracts during expiration. The articulators and the vocal folds, which create the valving system, are illustrated in Figure 1-17. They provide the greatest variability of resistance to airflow during speech. In general, speech breathing does not require a significantly

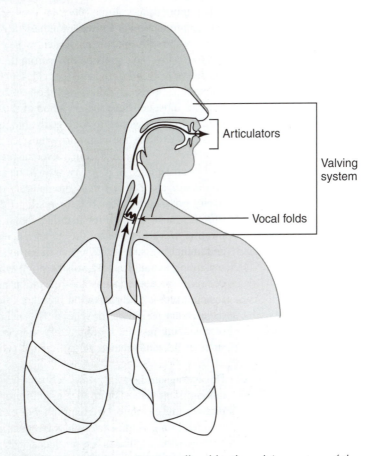

Figure 1-17. Airway resistance offered by the valving system of the articulators.

larger lung volume than quiet breathing. Adequate breath support for quiet breathing usually ensures adequate breath support for speech. However, a larger volume of inhaled air is required when speaking more loudly or saying longer phrases. Additionally, speech breathing demands a complex coordination between the airway resistance at the mouth and larynx, and between the action of inspiratory/expiratory muscles in concert with the passive expiratory forces (or relaxation pressures) of the respiratory system.

b. As noted above, volume requirements can differ in speech breathing and quiet breathing. During conversational speech breathing, air is inhaled to approximately 55–60% of vital capacity. When conversation is initiated, air is exhaled until the normal tidal volume is reached (35–40% of vital capacity). The active expiratory muscles along with the passive relaxation forces work in concert with each other during speech production. When more lung volume (alveolar pressure) is used deliberately, as for speech production at a greater loudness level (above 60% vital capacity), active inspiratory muscle movement works against the passive relaxation forces to slow the expulsion of air from the lungs. This opposing force of the active respiratory muscles provides a checking action for the passive relaxation forces. To counteract the relaxation pressures the inspiratory muscles must continue the elevation of the rib cage and expansion of the thorax. In other words, to achieve the lung volumes needed for speech or forced expiration, the inspiratory muscles must act to prevent the relaxation pressure from exceeding alveolar pressure by passively squeezing air from the lungs. In this way, air will be available for controlled speech production and not be forced prematurely from the lungs. When vital capacity goes below 35–40%, or resting tidal volume levels, expiratory muscles must function to sustain alveolar pressure. The muscles of expiration work to squeeze the abdomen, which in turn increases intra-abdominal pressure, pushing the diaphragm firmly upward to utilize the remaining available air. Until the point where lung volumes do not exceed the force exerted by the relaxation pressures and/or go below the resting volume, the relaxation pressures alone are sufficient to generate the alveolar pressures for speech. The end result of this complex process of balancing inspiratory-expiratory muscle function and relaxation pressures, is the maintenance of sufficient alveolar pressure for speech.

c. Depending on the type of speech task (e.g., conversational versus loud talking; long versus short phrases), different types of inspiratory and expiratory muscle action are required. For example, long utterances require increased lung volumes with less frequent inhalations (Kent, 1997). Conversely, shorter phrases are produced with smaller lung volumes but increased frequency of inhalation or respiratory rate. For laryngeal vibration and minimal voice production to occur, positive alveolar air pressure must

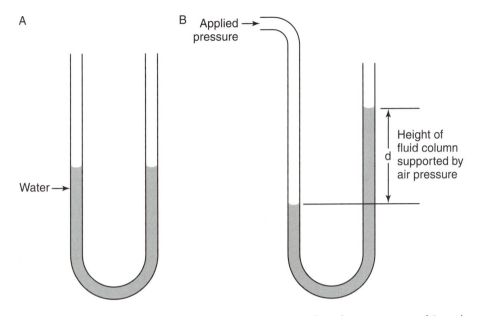

Figure 1-18. Depiction of the U-tube manometer. (From *Clinical Measurement of Speech and Voice*, by R. J. Baken & R. F. Orlikoff, 2000, p. 298. Clifton Park, NY: Singular.)

approximate 3–5 cm H_2O. Greater pressure is needed for loud speech and coughing, which is a maximum expiratory event (Netsell, 1986).

d. The air pressures for speech breathing (e.g., alveolar, subglottal, and supraglottal) also differ from quiet breathing. Subglottal pressure is the air pressure produced below the vocal folds, originating from the lungs. Indirect estimates of sustained subglottal air pressures can be measured with a simplified, oral U-tube **manometer,** a device which indicates air pressure through water displacement (Netsell & Hixon, 1978). This is illustrated in Figure 1-18. The larynx acts as valve to regulate the amount of air for phonation. The intrinsic muscles of the larynx, as previously discussed, act on the expired air to produce voice. The combination of the aerodynamics of the airway paired with the elastic properties of the connective vocal fold tissue and the intrinsic muscle action serve to achieve vocal fold adduction. As the vocal folds are closing secondary to the action of intrinsic laryngeal muscles, the glottis or space between the vocal folds becomes increasingly narrow. When this happens, air velocity increases and thus air pressure decreases between the vocal folds; the effect is to "suck" the folds together. The vocal folds quickly move medially toward the area of decreased pressure and are pulled together for phonation. When the vocal folds are together, subglottic pressure builds up until they are again blown apart or abducted.

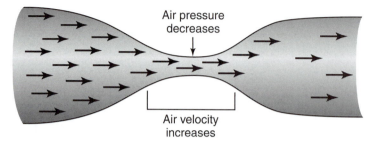

Figure 1-19. An illustration of the Bernoulli effect.

With the folds closed, functioning as a valve, subglottic pressure increases against the flow of expiratory air. Supraglottic and intraoral pressure drop, as these regions are "blocked" from the airflow below. (These pressures equalize with the vocal folds open.) When pressure reaches 3–5cm H_2O the folds open for voicing, and air again flows. Thus, the value of 3–5cm H_2O is important in measuring the adequacy of breath support for phonation. This aerodynamic principle of air pressure decreasing when air velocity increases is known as the **Bernoulli effect** and is part of the **aerodynamic-myoelastic theory** of voice production. Perkins and Kent (1986) stated, "the essence of this theory is that glottal vibration is a result of the interaction between aerodynamic forces and vocal fold muscular forces" (p. 99). The Bernoulli effect is illustrated in Figure 1-19.

E. Neurophysiology of Breathing

The mechanical events of quiet, forced, and speech breathing were previously described in the discussion of the breath cycle. The physiological control of the breath cycle can also be described during quiet breathing or during quiet breathing with additional voluntary control for such activities as speech and singing.

1. All types of breathing are controlled by the **respiratory control center** located in the *reticular formation of the brainstem* (*medulla oblongata* and *pons*). This center is responsible for maintaining stable gas exchange so that CO_2 and O_2 levels stay balanced. Eubanks and Bone (1990) stated that "the regulation of breathing is made possible by the constant analysis of the chemical state of the blood" (p. 218). The primary factor influencing this regulation and control of ventilation is CO_2 levels. Although O_2 levels are important, it is only when levels decrease to ranges significantly below normal that O_2 **chemoreceptors** respond. Oxygen chemoreceptors are a collection of specialized nerve cells in the carotid bodies which communicate information regarding the levels of O_2 in the blood to the respiratory control center. Carbon dioxide chemoreceptors in the floor of the fourth ventricle perform their func-

tion by reacting to the presence of diffused CO_2, which affects *bicarbonate* (HCO_3-) and *hydrogen* (*H+*) ion concentrations in the blood.

2. **Stretch receptors** are other types of cells which respond to the events of the respiratory cycle. They are located in the smooth muscle of the airway. Stretch receptors also contribute to cycles of ventilation by responding to the expansion and deflation of the lungs and bronchi.

3. During quiet breathing, chemoreceptors alert the respiratory control center when CO_2 levels elevate. Additionally, lung deflation triggers the stretch receptors to send feedback to the respiratory control center. The control center relays impulses to the spinal cord and ultimately to the phrenic nerve and diaphragm, as well as to additional cranial and spinal nerves which innervate the intercostal muscles. The muscles of inspiration are thus activated. As was previously described, the muscles of inspiration gradually stop their action when the alveoli are inflated and supplied with O_2. The stretch receptors also respond to lung inflation. Inspiratory muscle action is then inhibited by way of the respiratory control center. Passive expiration begins and CO_2 is exhaled.

4. During forced breathing or breathing for speech or singing, additional voluntary muscles of both inspiration and expiration are recruited. Recall that the involvement of the respiratory musculature is dependent on the particular task, nonspeech or speech breathing. The respiratory center, chemoreceptors, and stretch receptors exert the same neurological control over the inspiratory/ expiratory process. Accessory respiratory musculature participates to meet the demands of enhanced physical activity or speech. Innervation of the respiratory musculature includes cranial and spinal nerves through thoracic vertebrae XII (T12). There are 31 pair of spinal nerves. They pass between the vertebrae of the spinal cord, some by way of their anterior projections or rami. When there is damage to either the neck (i.e., cervical) or upper thoracic vertebrae, as during spinal cord injury, the function of the respiratory muscles is disrupted. The motor nerve innervation of the respiratory system is outlined in Table 1-7.

F. Physiology of Blood Gases: Acid-Base Relationships

1. One important method of determining whether adequate gas exchange or ventilation has occurred is via an analysis of the blood that measures the levels of acids and bases, or pH level, in the blood. The main base in the blood is the bicarbonate ion (HCO_3-) which, when combined with hydrogen ions (H+), forms carbonic acid (H_2CO_3). Carbonic acid is formed when a percentage of inhaled carbon dioxide mixes with water in the blood in the presence of an enzyme called carbonic anhydrase. Carbonic acid can then be broken back into its components, HCO_3- and H+. Carbonic acid is therefore another way that

Table 1-7. Motor Nerve Innervation of the Respiratory Mechanism.

MUSCLES OF RESPIRATION	INNERVATION
Thoracic Musculature	
Diaphragm	Phrenic nerves (paired C3-C5)
External Intercostals	Intercostal spinal nerves (anterior rami T2-T11)
Internal Intercostals	Internal spinal nerves (anterior rami T2-T11)
Pectoralis Major	Lateral and medial pectoral nerves (C5-C8 and T11)
Pectoralis Minor	Medial pectoral nerve (C8-T1)
Neck Musculature	
Sternocleidomastoid	Accessory nerve (CN XI; spinal root)
Scalene	Spinal nerves C2-C8 (anterior rami)
Abdominal Musculature	
Rectus Abdominis	Thoracic spinal nerves (anterior rami T6-T11)
External Obliques	Thoracic spinal nerves (anterior rami T6-T12)
Internal Obliques	Thoracic spinal nerves (anterior rami T6-T11; LI)
Transversus Abdominis	Thoracic spinal nerves (anterior rami T6-T11; LI)

CO_2 is carried in the blood. Just as the respiratory system functions to regulate carbon dioxide levels in the body by exhaling CO_2 from the lungs, the kidneys and the entire renal system must function to regulate the amount of bicarbonate in the blood. Respiratory care practitioners and physicians assess the ability of the respiratory and renal systems to perform some of their functions by analysis of oxygen, carbon dioxide, and pH levels in the blood.

2. Disorders of both respiratory and metabolic function (which affect the renal system) can affect the pH levels of the blood. If the balance of CO_2 in the body is disrupted due to respiratory or metabolic abnormalities, pH levels will rise or fall. **Hyperventilation** is a respiratory condition in which the lungs provide excessive ventilation and eliminate too much CO_2 from the body. In **hypoventilation** there is inadequate ventilation and the body retains CO_2. Both of these conditions alter pH levels. Acids and bases excreted from the body in excessive amounts cause metabolic alterations in pH (Bolton & Kline, 1994).

Blood gas analysis and pH levels will be further explained in Chapter 4, "Mechanical Ventilation." A basic understanding of blood gases will be helpful in the following discussion of diseases and conditions affecting the respiratory system.

III. DISEASES AND CONDITIONS AFFECTING THE RESPIRATORY SYSTEM

The clinician will encounter a variety of diseases and conditions of the respiratory system. These conditions can be loosely divided into those that cause intrinsic lung disease and those that affect the function of the respiratory musculature.

An overview of the most frequently encountered disorders with implications for the respiratory-phonatory system includes obstructive and restrictive diseases/conditions, neuromuscular disorders, and cardiopulmonary conditions. **Chronic obstructive pulmonary disease (COPD)** is a term that encompasses a number of irreversible lung disorders which can necessitate tracheostomy and/or ventilator support. Typical *restrictive lung disorders* include pneumonia. Many *neuromuscular conditions* impact on respiratory status by disrupting respiratory muscle function. These include spinal cord injury, amyotrophic lateral sclerosis, multiple sclerosis, Guillain-Barré syndrome, post-polio syndrome, and brainstem vascular disease. Respiratory impairment due to these disorders can cause secondary cardiac insufficiency. Disorders that primarily affect the heart and/or vascular system and cause respiratory impairment secondarily are also referred to as **cardiopulmonary disorders.**

A. Chronic Obstructive Pulmonary Disease

Chronic obstructive pulmonary disease by definition is a condition of irreversible airway obstruction caused by destruction of lung tissue. In the year 2000, the American Lung Association (ALA) estimated that more than 16 million Americans suffer from COPD. *Chronic bronchitis* and *emphysema* are included in this category.

1. **Chronic bronchitis** is defined by the presence of a productive cough for a minimum of 3 months a year for 2 consecutive years (Owens, 1992). There are excessive mucus production and narrowing of the small airways secondary to edema. Eventually, actual structural changes in the airway and lungs, with the development of tissue fibrosis, occur due to the repeated episodes of irritation and inflammation. This is usually caused by inhaled irritants such as smoke or air pollution. Cigarette smoke serves to irritate the tracheobronchial tree, stimulating the goblet cells and mucus glands to produce more mucus. The ciliary action of cleansing of the airways is also inhibited by smoke. The excessive amount of mucus that is produced, coupled with the reduced cilia movement, results in a chronic cough. The irritation of the tracheobronchial tree from smoke also results in bronchoconstriction. The bronchitic patient has been referred to as a *blue bloater* because of a characteristic presentation of **cyanosis** (lack of oxygen) due to inadequate gas exchange. The patient's low levels of oxygen in the blood trigger increased respiratory efforts. Recall that during normal gas exchange elevated CO_2 levels are the primary stimulus for ventilation. Typically, a patient with an exacerbation of chronic bronchitis presents with increased use of accessory respiratory muscles, wheezing, and

increased secretions. An arterial blood gas, if performed, would demonstrate increased carbon dioxide (CO_2), lowered oxygen, and an altered (lowered) pH. In the most extreme case, if this exacerbation is left untreated, the patient may experience respiratory failure.

2. **Emphysema** is also characterized by changes in lung tissue, specifically deterioration of the alveolar walls. Eventually, destruction of the alveolar walls leads to loss of their elastic recoil properties. As the patient inspires, high lung volumes must be used because air is trapped in the lung behind collapsed airways. The diaphragm is rendered less efficient because it is being flattened by the hyperinflated lungs. The patient works harder using the accessory muscles of respiration to lift the thorax and ventilate the alveoli. However, on expiration, the patient has difficulty exhaling air because of collapsing airways and loss of passive relaxation forces. This type of emphysematous patient has been called a *pink puffer* due to the above respiratory pattern, a thin, barrel-chested appearance, and overuse of accessory musculature. Typically, the patient with an exacerbation of emphysema complains of shortness of breath or **dyspnea.** This is why the patient utilizes accessory musculature during inspiration. These patients are often seen leaning forward, resting their forearms on a table or on their knees, to assist the accessory muscles in elevating the diaphragm. Because pockets of dead air have formed in the injured areas of the lungs, exhalation is impeded. The patient can be observed using pursed lips during expiration. When blood gases are taken, carbon dioxide is usually near normal or perhaps slightly increased, and oxygen is lowered and pH normal. However, when the patient tires from the constant overuse of the respiratory musculature, fatigue and respiratory failure can result. The "blue bloater" and "pink puffer" patterns are illustrated in Figures 1-20a and b.

3. Typically, bronchitis and emphysema co-exist to some degree in each COPD patient. Patients with COPD may require tracheostomy to facilitate elimination of airway secretions and for long-term ventilatory support. Various pharmacological agents also may ease the symptoms of COPD and improve pulmonary function.

B. Restrictive Lung Disorders

Restrictive lung disorders, unlike intrinsic disease such as COPD, involve a combination of respiratory muscle weakness or paralysis and mechanical factors involving the lungs and chest wall (Bach & Ishikawa, 2000). Patients with restrictive conditions, with an inability to take deep breaths, are described as having chronic hypoventilation of the lungs. Restrictive lung disorders typically involve reduced lung volumes and decreased lung compliance. **Compliance** refers to the amount of elasticity of the lungs and chest wall. It can be reduced by lung or neuromuscular diseases. Reduced lung compliance creates a stiff lung that is resistant to inflation. As a consequence there is decreased ventilation because sufficient volumes of air

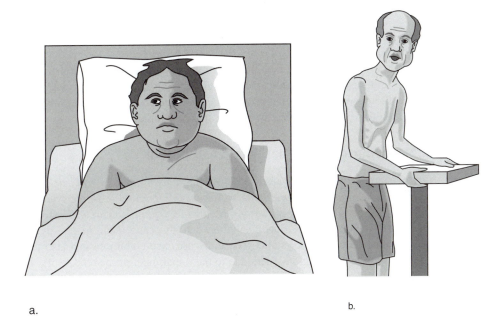

a.   b.

Figure 1-20a. "Blue bloater" breathing pattern. **b.** "Pink puffer" breathing pattern.

do not reach the alveoli. Infections and inflammation can also damage the delicate alveolar walls and impact on gas exchange. A few examples of disease processes and acute conditions that lead to restrictive pulmonary syndromes follow.

1. **Connective tissue disorders** affect lung compliance by both loss of lung tissue and fiberoptic changes in the lungs. *Scleroderma* and *systemic lupus* are included in this category. Skeletal conditions with thoracic deformities (e.g., arthritis, scoliosis) can impact lung volumes by physically reducing lung expansion. Interstitial fibrosis is an inflammatory condition of the lungs (alveolae) that can eventually cause thickening of tissue and fibrosis. The overly restrictive pattern of these conditions is that the lungs cannot fully expand (Frownfelter & Dean, 1996).

2. **Pneumonia** is an acute infection and inflammation involving the gas exchange regions of the lungs. Clinically, patients may present with fever and shortness of breath. Pneumonia is commonly caused by either viruses or bacteria. Aspiration pneumonia is common in patients with decreased swallowing function. It results from entry of foreign material such as saliva or food into

the respiratory tract. The consequences of aspiration may be a localized chemical irritation or a secondary bacterial infection in the lungs. A severe aspiration can impair respiration enough to cause a cardiopulmonary arrest. Repeated aspiration pneumonia can cause lung tissue to become increasingly fibrotic due to repeated infections and inflammations, thus decreasing lung compliance.

Individuals with worsening restrictive disorders, who are not treated with inspiratory muscle aids to assist with lung expansion, can develop significant blood gas abnormalities with altered pH, increased carbon dioxide, and lowered oxygen leading to eventual respiratory failure.

C. Neuromuscular Diseases and Conditions

Degenerative neuromuscular diseases such as *amyotrophic lateral sclerosis (ALS), multiple sclerosis (MS), muscular dystrophy (MD), Guillain-Barré syndrome,* and *poliomyelitis* affect the respiratory musculature. *Brainstem cerebral vascular accident (CVA)* and *spinal cord injury (SCI)* can also cause neurological dysfunction impacting on respiratory status. These diseases and conditions can also be classified as restrictive lung disorders due to the impairment of the respiratory muscles. Their commonality is the disturbance of the central nervous system, the regulator of breathing. Also, many of these conditions impact the pharyngeal musculature, leading to decreased cough and increased aspiration risk. Intrinsic lung disease can occur as a secondary complication of neurologic conditions.

1. *ALS* affects the motor neurons of the brain and spinal cord and consequently causes deterioration of the respiratory and laryngeal muscles. Patients can present with *hypoventilation.* This is inadequate ventilation caused in this case by weakened muscle function, often diaphragmatic paralysis. In addition to physical motor deficits, progressive respiratory and speech deterioration occur, especially when the patient presents with the *bulbar* form of the disease. This type of neurological dysfunction affects the oral, pharyngeal, and laryngeal musculature and so disrupts the function of the upper airway and swallowing as well as respiratory musculature. The majority of patients with ALS usually demonstrate intact cognitive and linguistic functioning. Typically, extraocular movements are also spared until the final stages of the disease. As oral communication and physical motor status deteriorate, patients with ALS therefore become candidates for augmentative communication systems. Most patients with ALS must make a decision regarding tracheostomy and ventilator support during the course of the disease, as diaphragm involvement and repeated aspiration-related pulmonary infections are leading causes of mortality.

2. *Multiple sclerosis* is a demyelinating disease of the white matter of the central nervous system which causes formation of plaques in the brain and spinal cord. As the disease progresses, and neuromuscular deterioration advances,

physical-motor, cognitive-linguistic, speech, and swallowing abilities are affected. Respiratory problems arise late in the disease process from plaque development in the cervical spinal cord. Respiratory musculature is thus affected and respiratory failure may result. In addition, pharyngeal stage dysphagia, poor airway protection with decreased cough, and chronic aspiration are common.

3. Respiratory impairment is a common sequelae of *muscular dystrophy* (MD), a progressive hereditary disease. Muscle deterioration begins during childhood and is progressive. Weakness affects all striated muscle groups, the heart, and diaphragm. There are a variety of types of muscular dystrophy. Each presents with a characteristic pattern of weakness. Similarly to ALS, respiratory muscle weakness is the cause of chronic hypoventilation in most patients with MD. However, a dysfunction in the respiratory center of the brain may contribute to respiratory insufficiency in myotonic muscular dystrophy (Bach, 1996). Frownfelter and Dean (1996) stated that due to chronic alveolar hypoventilation, these patients "are at risk for the development of atelectasis, impaired mucociliary transport and pneumonia" (p. 538). Pharyngeal stage dysphagia can also be seen, especially in patients with Duchenne's muscular dystrophy.

4. *Guillain-Barré syndrome* is characterized by acute onset and rapid deterioration of extremity muscle function. Two thirds of cases present with a history of preceding viral infection, surgery, immunization, or an immunologic disorder (A. Alba, personal communication, 2002). Unlike the above conditions, patients may recover completely. Although rapid physical-motor deterioration is characteristic of the disease, cognitive-linguistic abilities are spared. Speech and swallowing impairment may be evident especially in severe cases when respiratory involvement is seen. Guillain-Barré syndrome is a demyelinating disease which often leads to impaired respiratory muscle function with acute respiratory failure in at least 25% of all cases (Scanlan & Gupta, 1990). The majority of cases who receive support via a mechanical respirator or ventilator can be weaned within the first few weeks; however, a small percentage of cases with axonal involvement do not recover respiratory function and require long-term ventilatory support.

5. *Stroke* (cerebrovascular accident) can affect the central control of respiration, that is, the actual regulation of ventilation. This will occur with a brainstem stroke such as a lesion in the medulla. Cortical strokes that do not impact the brainstem have a peripheral effect on respiration. This includes changes in abdominal and thoracic muscle tone and body posture, which ultimately impact lung expansion. This directly limits lung volume and creates the restrictive respiratory pattern (Frownfelter & Dean, 1996). Depending on the site of the lesion, mechanical ventilation may be necessary on a permanent basis. Physical-motor status can be severely impaired, with resulting quadriplegia. Due to the involvement of cranial nerves IX–XII, speech and swallowing

deficits can be severe, with *anarthria* and *dysphagia* (swallowing impairment) exhibited. Anarthria is the severest form of oral-motor weakness and is characterized by absence of functional speech production. When swallow and cough are severely affected, individuals with brainstem CVAs often require a permanent tracheostomy to facilitate removal of secretions from the airway. Cognitive-linguistic functioning remains intact in cases of pure brainstem involvement; therefore, augmentative communication techniques are used frequently with this population.

6. *Poliomyelitis* is a viral disease that may cause severe muscle weakness with associated respiratory failure. Bach, Alba, Bohatiuk, Saporito, and Lee (1987) stated, "the respiratory failure associated with polio occurs either by the destruction of anterior horn cells in the spinal cord innervating respiratory muscles or by neuronal destruction of the respiratory center in the medulla or both" (p. 859). Acute poliomyelitis commonly necessitates mechanical ventilatory support. The polio epidemic in the United States during the 1940s and 1950s left survivors, many of whom were weaned from their original ventilatory support, experiencing the symptoms of postpolio syndrome. The complications associated with postpolio syndrome include respiratory insufficiency, progressive muscle weakness, and dysphagia.

7. *Spinal cord injury* (SCI) can occur at any level of the cervical or thoracic spine. Severing of the cervical spinal cord above the fourth cervical nerve renders respiratory musculature nonfunctional. The diaphragm, the primary muscle of inspiration, becomes either totally or partially paralyzed as central neural input to the phrenic nerves is severed. Cervical nerve damage below the fourth cervical vertebrae spares the diaphragm but other muscles of inspiration and expiration are impaired. Lacking the ability to use the intercostal and abdominal musculature, the quadriplegic patient is unable to utilize forced breathing. Loss of active expiration and abdominal musculature will affect the ability to forcefully push the diaphragm upward and produce an effective cough (Bach, 1996). This is characteristic of a restrictive breathing pattern. Patients with a high spinal cord injury (SCI) require mechanical ventilatory support.

D. Cardiopulmonary Conditions

Disorders of cardiovascular function impact frequently on respiratory status secondary to the close relationship between the heart and lungs. Recall that the purpose of the lungs is to accomplish gas exchange. One condition necessary for successful gas exchange is circulation of blood to the alveoli. The interdependence in the function of the heart and lungs assures that the patient maintains adequate ventilation in the presence of stable oxygen and carbon dioxide levels. Efficient circulation is often impaired in cardiovascular conditions, either because blood is not circulating or because intravascular fluids congest the lungs.

1. **Cardiopulmonary disorders** may involve either the left, the right, or both ventricles of the heart. Impairment of the left ventricle results in a pressure increase in the chambers of the heart and an increase in fluid pressure in the pulmonary vein. Fluid leaves the blood vessel and moves into lung tissue causing **pulmonary edema.** Fluid at the level at the alveoli decreases gas exchange. **Congestive heart failure** (**CHF**) occurs when the heart cannot pump out sufficient amounts of blood, and fluid begins to accumulate in the lungs. Right ventricular failure may occur secondary to left ventricular failure if the pressure changes impede passage of blood out of the right ventricle. The pressure in the pulmonary artery increases, causing *right ventricular hypertension.* This not uncommon condition in patients with COPD is referred to as **cor pulmonale** (Eubanks & Bone, 1990). In this case, cardiac failure may occur as a consequence of respiratory disease.

E. Adult Respiratory Distress Syndrome (ARDS)

Adult respiratory distress syndrome results from a variety of conditions and diseases of the lungs including stroke, trauma, infection, severe pneumonia, and inhaled toxins (Frownfelter & Dean, 1996). The hallmark of ARDS is damage to the area of oxygen transfer, the alveolar-capillary membrane, resulting in a severe impairment of the gas exchange function of the lungs. There is typically fluid leakage into alveoli, loss of surfactant, and severe *atelectasis* or collapse of the alveoli. Severe **hypoxemia** (a deficiency of oxygen in arterial blood) results with loss of pulmonary compliance, CO_2 retention, and **hypoxia.** Hypoxia refers to a lack of oxygen at the level of body tissue. Increased work of breathing, respiratory muscle fatigue, and, ultimately, respiratory failure occur from this restrictive type syndrome. Treatment is directed at stopping the damage to the alveoli and mechanically supporting ventilation (Eubanks & Bone, 1990).

The respiratory-phonatory mechanism functions primarily to ensure that the body's need for oxygen is always met and, on a secondary level, to allow phonation for communication. When airflow and gas exchange are disrupted, as they may be with a variety of diseases and conditions that affect normal structure and function, impairments in both breathing and voice production result. This may lead to the need for airway management techniques, artificial airways, and possibly mechanical ventilatory support to ensure that the primary need for oxygen is fulfilled. Clinicians who understand the basic principles of normal and disordered respiratory and phonatory physiology will be better able to utilize appropriate management techniques with their patients.

2

Airway Management Techniques

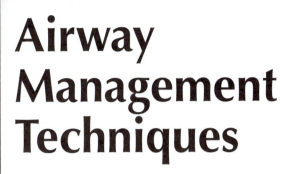

Normally, human beings pay little attention to the complex process of breathing for life and speech, a process that occurs many thousands of times a day. The clinician who manages the tracheostomized and ventilator-dependent patient, however, must have an appreciation of why and how the normal respiratory and phonatory mechanism works and how it has been disrupted. Integral to this understanding for all practitioners is an understanding of the general principles of airway management and an awareness of the medical history of the patient with respiratory insufficiency. For example, the clinician would need to know how long a patient had been intubated. For a tracheostomized patient, the clinician's history taking would include the manner in which the tracheotomy was performed, for example, emergent versus elective placement. Respiratory failure requiring intubation and/or tracheotomy may occur secondary to respiratory/pulmonary conditions, cardiac events, neurological injury or neuromuscular disease, trauma, environmental contamination, and airway obstructions. An **artificial airway** may be needed in each of these conditions. The purposes of an artificial airway are to:

- provide adequate ventilation and oxygenation
- maintain a patent airway
- eliminate airway obstruction
- reduce the potential for aspiration
- provide access to the airway/lungs for pulmonary toilet

Airway clearance and management techniques include:

- suctioning
- mask to mouth ventilation

• oral/nasal-pharyngeal and esophageal artificial airways

• endotracheal intubation

• cricothyroidotomy and tracheotomy

I. SUCTIONING

A. Indications

If a patient cannot effectively clear secretions or foreign material from the airway, they must be manually removed before an airway obstruction occurs. Patients with respiratory conditions including neuromuscular disorders, restrictive and obstructive lung diseases, and cardiopulmonary disorders may require airway **suctioning.** Secretions and, sometimes, blood and vomitus are causes of airway obstruction and must be removed from the airway with suctioning.

Clinical practitioners working with the tracheostomized patient have different roles in the suction protocol. Clinicians such as the speech-language pathologist are often called on to perform oral suctioning. During routine tracheostomy care, tracheal suctioning is usually performed by a respiratory care practitioner or nurse. In certain facilities individuals other than respiratory care practitioners and nurses do perform tracheal suctioning during their assessment and intervention. State licensure regulations vary, as do the policies and procedures of individual facilities. It is the responsibility of clinicians, such as speech-language pathologists, to be aware of these particular requirements, obtain the necessary training, and put appropriate policies and procedures into place.

B. Procedure

1. Oral/Nasal Suctioning

The equipment necessary for suctioning includes a flexible or rigid suction catheter, vacuum suction unit (either wall-mounted or portable), sterile saline solution, surgical gloves, and frequently a mask and shield for the respiratory care practitioner or nurse. The tubing is connected to the vacuum apparatus at one end. Sterile technique is maintained by avoiding air contamination and contact of the catheter tip to nonsterile surfaces. The tubing is gently introduced into the oral or nasal cavity, initially without the use of negative pressure. Lubrication may be used for nasal suctioning, by dipping the tip of the catheter in sterile water. Once the catheter tip has been placed in the mouth or nose, negative pressure is applied by occluding the proximal port of the suction catheter. Secretions are then gently removed from the mouth or nose. During oral suctioning, as the catheter is advanced into the pharynx, a gag reflex may be triggered. Negative pressure should not be maintained for extended periods

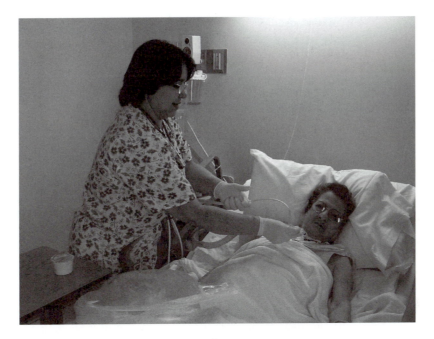

Figure 2-1. Tracheal suctioning procedure.

of time, and the suction catheter should be irrigated by sterile saline solution between introductions. This promotes easier passage of the catheter and assists in clearing any tenacious secretions from the suction tubing. Local oral and nasal suctioning is performed to remove secretions at a specific level and to enhance patient comfort. Nasal/tracheal suctioning is performed by trained medical personnel when indicated.

2. Tracheal Suctioning

The sterile technique described above is observed during tracheal suctioning. It is important to insert the flexible suction catheter gently with a slow rotational movement. Negative pressure should never be applied for more than 10–15 seconds at a time to avoid deoxygenation of a patient. The suction catheter is rotated slightly as it is slowly removed from the tracheostomy tube. The suction catheter is reinserted as needed to remove secretions, but the patient should be given an opportunity to rest between insertions. Some medical practitioners perform deep suctioning to remove secretions from the lower airways. However, the anatomical configuration of the trachea typically limits suctioning down the path of the right mainstem bronchus. Copious secretions and foreign objects must be removed from the lower airways via bronchoscopy. The tracheal suction procedure is shown in Figure 2-1. A laryngeal response

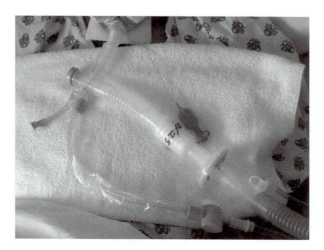

Figure 2-2. Closed suction system.

such as coughing is a normal response to insertion of the catheter but should be monitored for intensity and duration. It is possible for a patient to become hypoxemic or have reduced oxygen levels during the suctioning procedure because oxygen is being removed from the lungs. Oxygen is often given between suctioning. The same catheter should never be used for both oral/nasal and tracheal suctioning.

Specialized "closed" suction systems are available to reduce the risk of contamination of the suction catheter and the patient's airway. Figure 2-2 illustrates the closed suction system. These systems enclose the catheter within a plastic bag. The movable catheter is advanced into the tracheostomy tube without ever leaving the sterile area. Saline is introduced into the tracheostomy tube via a separate side port, to mobilize any viscous secretions. Closed suction systems are designed to decrease cross-contamination between patients and provide enhanced protection for practitioners. Some patients may find the system heavy and more cumbersome, especially if other types of tubing are in use.

C. Complications

Mucosal trauma may be a consequence of rigorous suctioning technique. The application of excessive or prolonged negative pressure can result in tearing of the mucosal lining as the catheter adheres to this delicate surface. Sometimes streaks of blood may be noted in the suctioned material. Their presence should warn the clinician that the suction pressure is too high and mucosal trauma is present. Negative pressure should not exceed -120 cm H_2O and should be monitored on the vacuum unit during the procedure. Lubrication of the catheter, use of proper negative pressure, and careful regulation of suctioning time will assist in avoiding mucosal

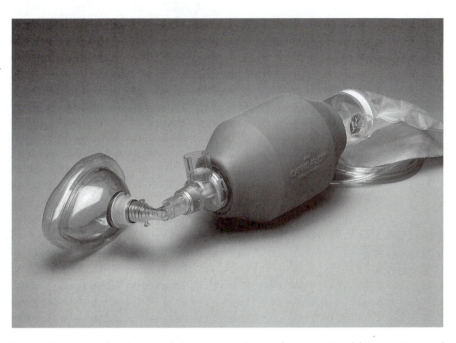

Figure 2-3. Example of manual resuscitation bag. (Photo reprinted by permission of Nellcor Puritan Bennett Inc., Pleasanton, CA)

trauma. A major limitation of tracheal suctioning is that it removes only superficial airway secretions. Secretions that accumulate below the tracheostomy tube and tracheal wall cannot be easily removed. Additionally, because the suction catheter typically is directed into the right mainstem bronchus, left lung pneumonia is common in the chronic tracheostomized and ventilator-dependent population.

It is standard practice to preoxygenate the patient prior to suctioning. After suctioning, the patient can also be told to take a deep breath. A ventilator-dependent patient can be hyperinflated or given breaths via **manual bagging.** Patients are given these extra "breaths" by using a manual resuscitation bag, a football-shaped bag with an adapter on the end depicted in Figure 2-3. Depending on the patient's status, he or she may also be given pure oxygen prior to suctioning. Proper suctioning technique will also assist in avoiding **atelectasis,** loss of oxygen from sections of the lung, as it will remove secretions and decrease the risk of mucus plugging the airway.

Cardiac arrhythmias can occur in some patients after a period of deoxygenation, especially if they have a history of cardiac involvement. **Laryngospasms,** or involuntary closure of the airway, also may occur during suctioning and are of special concern for patients with cardiac histories. Patients should be carefully monitored for this complication during the suctioning procedure.

II. NONINVASIVE AIRWAY CLEARANCE TECHNIQUES

A. Indications

Assisted cough and postural drainage are helpful in individuals with respiratory insufficiency, especially ventilator-dependent patients who are unable to produce an effective cough. Coughing consists of inspiring with a large tidal volume, contracting abdominal and intercostal muscles, increasing intrathoracic pressure by closing the glottis, and then forcefully expelling air with a rapid expiratory flow. Material, such as secretions, is removed from the airway in this manner. When pulmonary hygiene cannot be maintained through coughing, frequent suctioning is needed. Various techniques are available to assist in effective coughing. For some individuals, these techniques have lessened the need for invasive mechanical ventilation by aiding in the management of airway secretions. Postural drainage is a technique in which patients are positioned to allow their lungs to drain with the assistance of gravity. A variety of positions are utilized to facilitate drainage of the upper, middle, and lower lobes of the lungs.

B. Procedure

1. *Diaphragmatic assisted cough,* also referred to as *manual cough,* is a technique utilized for patients who present with reduced respiratory muscle strength and ineffective coughing. The clinician assists the patient during the expiratory phase of the cough by placing both hands on the lower thoracic area and supplementing the patient's own reduced abdominal compression. For individuals who have extremely low vital capacities (below 1 liter), the assisted cough may be preceded by an assisted inhalation, as with a manual resuscitation bag.

2. **Mechanical exsufflation** is a technique that uses a machine to generate a cough. A large tidal volume is supplied to the patient via positive pressure and followed by a rapid negative pressure. The positive pressure breath is delivered either by face mask or by an adapter placed over the tracheostomy tube. The patient experiences a push of air followed by a suction creating a vacuum-like effect in the airway. The change in pressure creates high expiratory flow from the lungs, mimicking a forceful cough. Secretions are expelled from the airway and can be more easily suctioned through the nose, mouth, or tracheostomy tube. Bach (1993) discusses the use of manual-assisted cough and mechanical exsufflation in facilitating airway secretion clearance for specific ventilator-dependent patients. Previously, this device was known as the cof-Flator. Currently it is marketed as the CoughAssist and is depicted in Figure 2-4.

3. **Incentive spirometry** is a technique that facilitates a deep and sustained inspiration. It is utilized for patients who have the ability to spontaneously deep

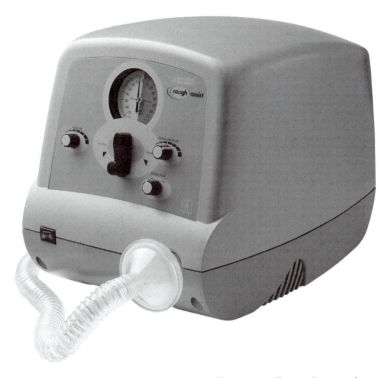

Figure 2-4. CoughAssist Mechanical Insufflation-Exsufflation device. (Photo courtesy of J. H. Emerson Company)

breathe. However, due to overall weakened physical status or reduced respiratory muscle strength, the patient does not inspire adequately to expand the lungs. As a result, the patient may be at risk of atelectasis or weakened cough. The **incentive spirometer** is a device used by the patient while the clinician encourages a maximum sustained inspiration. The patient is instructed to take a deep breath and then forcefully and maximally exhale into the mouthpiece and tube. The incentive spirometer is in essence a biofeedback tool. The patient can monitor efforts as he raises a ball on a column of air during an inspiration.

4. Before attempting *postural drainage* techniques, patients are carefully assessed regarding their tolerance for maintaining the target positions during a 3- to 10-minute session. Figures 2-5a, b, and c illustrate the typical recommended postures. While the patient is positioned, often with the aid of pillows or foam wedges, other techniques can be used to facilitate loosening and expectoration of draining secretions. These include **percussion** (vigorous clapping with a cupped hand against the patient's thorax) or **vibration** (gentle movements of the hands against the patient's chest wall). It is important to

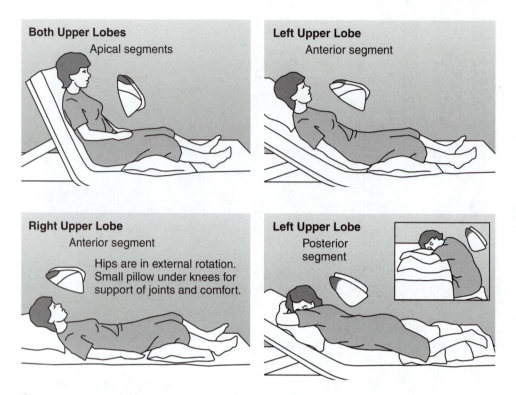

Figure 2-5a. Postural drainage positions: Upper lobes. (Adapted from *Principles and Practices of Cardiopulmonary Physical Therapy* [3rd ed.], by D. Frownfelter & E. Dean, 1996, p. 340. St. Louis, MO: Mosby Year-Book. Copyright 1996 by Mosby Year-Book.)

have suctioning equipment ready for use to remove the patient's secretions as they are mobilized. These techniques should be used *only* by trained professionals, typically respiratory care practitioners, nurses and physical therapists.

C. Complications

As with all interventions, these airways clearance techniques carry their own potential complications. Proper training is integral in both avoiding patient injury and in assuring successful outcome, in this case clearance of the patient's airway. Manual and assisted cough, for example, do apply force to the thoracic cage and if performed incorrectly could cause patient bruising, discomfort, or even rib damage. Additionally, the forceful airflow created by the assisted cough may cause uncontrollable spontaneous coughing or **bronchospasm.** The enteral feedings of patients with percutaneous endoscopic gastrostomy tubes must be timed with cough treatment so that reflux of tube feeding is not induced.

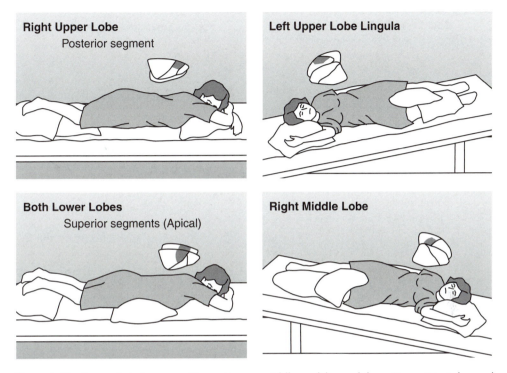

Figure 2-5b. Postural drainage positions: Upper, middle and lower lobes. (From *Principles and Practices of Cardiopulmonary Physical Therapy* [3rd ed.], by D. Frownfelter & E. Dean, 1996, p. 341. St. Louis, MO: Mosby Year-Book. Copyright 1996 by Mosby Year-Book.)

There are cautions associated with the use of mechanical exsufflation, particularly with patients with severe lung disease. Patients with a history of *bullous emphysema* (greatly enlarged air spaces in the lungs) and high risk of pneumothorax should be monitored carefully and may not be candidates for this airway clearance technique. Additionally, patients with a recent episode of barotrauma may not be considered candidates. The oxygen saturation levels of patients with cardiac instability should be closely monitored via **pulse oximetry,** which is a noninvasive technique for monitoring oxygen saturation levels.

All positions of postural drainage cannot be tolerated by all individuals. The head down position or *Trendelenburg* is contraindicated for neurosurgery patients who cannot tolerate an increase in intracranial pressures. Cardiac arrhythmia has been reported in patients following chest percussion (Hammon & Martin, 1981) and postural drainage, although as discussed by Downs (1996) it was unclear which technique may have contributed to the arrhythmia.

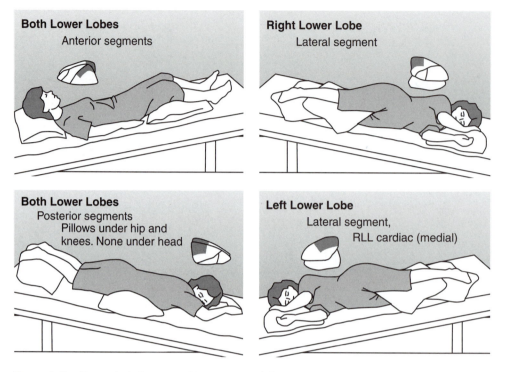

Both Lower Lobes
Anterior segments

Right Lower Lobe
Lateral segment

Both Lower Lobes
Posterior segments
Pillows under hip and
knees. None under head

Left Lower Lobe
Lateral segment,
RLL cardiac (medial)

Figure 2-5c. Postural drainage positions: Lower lobes. (From *Principles and Practices of Cardiopulmonary Physical Therapy* [3rd ed.], by D. Frownfelter & E. Dean, 1996, p. 341. St. Louis, MO: Mosby Year-Book. Copyright 1996 by Mosby Year-Book.)

III. MASK TO MOUTH VENTILATION

A. Indications

Masks are indicated to support oxygenation and ventilation, usually in spontaneously breathing patients. Oxygen is easily provided by masks which provide a tight seal to the face. Masks also can be used during resuscitation attempts and prior to tracheal intubation. The mask in this case is attached to a manual resuscitation bag.

B. Procedure

The mask is firmly sealed to the patient's face by using a forward chin tilt during placement, which ensures a patent airway by displacing the tongue. Figure 2-6 illustrates the placement of a mask over the mouth and nose. Once the mask is placed, the bag and valve device can be connected to an oxygen source or used manually with room air.

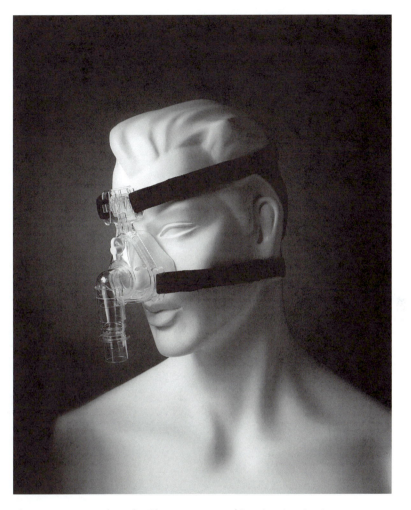

Figure 2-6. A nasal mask. (Photo courtesy of Respironics, Inc.)

IV. ORAL/NASAL PHARYNGEAL AND ESOPHAGEAL ARTIFICIAL AIRWAYS

A. Indications

Oral and nasopharyngeal airways are rubber or plastic tubes that are used for patients who have mild upper airway obstruction, perhaps secondary to the after-effects of anesthesia. They are inserted by physicians, respiratory care practitioners, and in some settings nurses. They provide a short-term means to suction secretions and blood from the pharynx and to relieve upper airway obstruction by keeping the tongue clear of the posterior pharyngeal wall. For patients whose airway protection

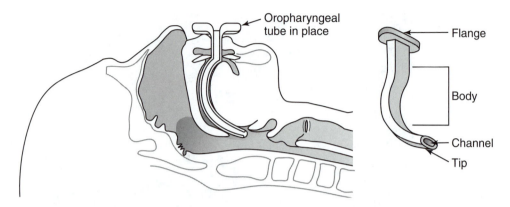

Figure 2-7. An oropharyngeal airway.

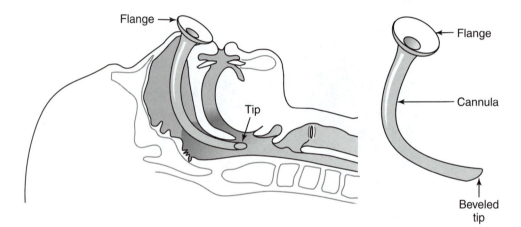

Figure 2-8. A nasopharyngeal airway.

reflexes, such as coughing, are inadequate, an artificial airway must be inserted to reduce the risk of aspiration and airway obstruction secondary to secretions (Finucane & Santora, 1988).

1. *Oropharyngeal airways* form a seal by contouring to the anatomy of the mouth. They prevent obstruction of the pharynx by the base of the tongue. Figure 2-7 illustrates the components and insertion of an oropharyngeal airway.

2. *Nasopharyngeal airways* are used with patients who are unable to relax the jaw sufficiently to accommodate an oral airway. Figure 2-8 illustrates a nasopharyngeal airway and its insertion into the airway. For patients who have an active gag reflex, nasopharyngeal airways may be easier to tolerate than oral airways. These airways also permit suctioning of the nasopharynx.

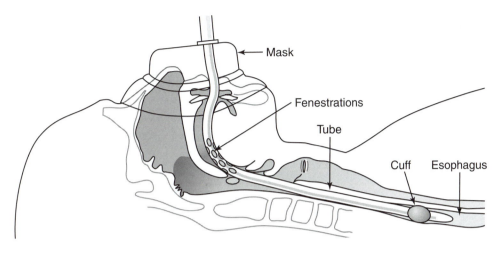

Figure 2-9. An esophageal obturator airway.

3. An *esophageal airway* consists of a tube or obturator approximately 37 centimeters long. At the proximal end of the obturator, a mask covers the mouth and nose. At the distal end, the tube is cuffed. A **cuff** is an internal balloon which surrounds the tube. It is made of a soft material which expands with air and seals to the surrounding structures, in this case, the walls of the esophagus. The cuffed portion of the tube lies in the esophagus. When the patient is ventilated through the mask, air is directed into the trachea through side ports in the obturator. Air does not enter the esophagus due to the inflated cuff. Esophageal airways are used only in unconscious patients and when an emergency airway is needed. They are used when endotracheal airways can not be inserted. This type of airway reduces the risk of aspiration of refluxed gastric contents (Donen, Tweed, Dashfsky, & Guttormson, 1983). Figure 2-9 illustrates the esophageal airway.

B. Procedure

1. Oropharyngeal airways are inserted into the mouth as the tongue is held anteriorly with a tongue depressor. They can also be inserted by tilting the jaw, positioning the tube up against the hard palate and rotating it 180° back over the tongue (Eubanks & Bone, 1990; Simmons, 1990).

2. Nasal airways are inserted transnasally after lubrication of the airway. The design of the tube, with a flange or ring at the proximal end, prevents the accidental entry of the tube into the trachea (Eubanks & Bone, 1990; Simmons, 1990).

3. Esophageal obturator airways follow the natural curve of the pharynx into the esophagus and for that reason are considered easier to insert than endotracheal

airways, which must pass through the vocal folds. The esophageal airway can be inserted into the mouth without direct visualization of the larynx. With the tube in place in the esophagus, the mask is sealed to the face and ventilation is begun. Assurance of correct placement is obtained via **auscultation** of the lungs, listening to ensure that breath sounds are heard (Eubanks & Bone, 1990; Simmons, 1990).

C. Complications

The use of any artificial airway carries with it certain risks and complications. Oral airways can trigger gagging or vomiting and are therefore inserted when the patient is unconscious and these reflexes are less likely to be activated. Nasal airways may be less likely to trigger a gag; however, complications such as abrasion of nasal tissue, epistaxis (nose bleed), or vomiting are possible. Esophageal airways, which are quite long, are inserted through the entire pharynx. They can be misplaced into the larynx or can cause esophageal trauma. Laryngospasm and vomiting are other possible side effects.

V. ENDOTRACHEAL INTUBATION

A. Indications

Endotracheal intubation is the insertion of a tube into the mouth or nose, passing through the pharynx and vocal folds into the trachea in order to provide an artificial airway and to connect the patient with mechanical ventilation. Endotracheal intubation is illustrated in Figure 2-10. The tubes are usually constructed from a semirigid polyvinyl chloride plastic so that they maintain their shape in the airway. During respiratory distress and after initial medical intervention, an endotracheal tube is normally the method of airway management. Intubation is indicated when there is need for airway protection and mechanical ventilation. Most endotracheal tubes have cuffs which are inflated in the trachea to form a seal and prevent air from escaping around the tube when the patient is connected to a ventilator. Figure 2-11 pictures a standard endotracheal tube with a cuff. Intubation, which can be done fairly quickly by experienced personnel, carries the least immediate risk to the patient while establishing a temporary airway. Situations such as tracheal stenosis and tumors may exist which prevent passage of an endotracheal tube. Other airway management techniques, such as surgical procedures, must then be used.

Endotracheal airways are considered temporary secondary to patient comfort levels and potential complications. There are multiple reports in the literature regarding the optimal length of time for intubation prior to performing a **tracheotomy,** or surgical creation of an opening in the trachea (Bishop, 1989; Brook, Sherman, Malen, & Kollef, 2000; Heffner, 1989; Marsh, Gillespie, & Baumgartner, 1989). In current practice, if an individual cannot be extubated within 14 to 21 days, if there are no

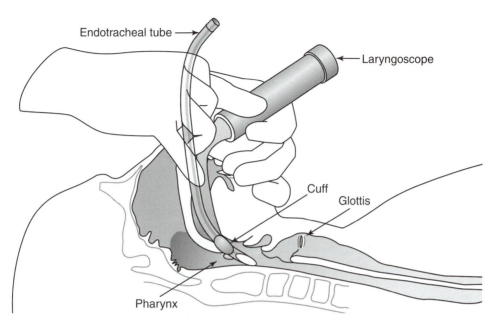

Endotracheal tube

Laryngoscope

Cuff

Glottis

Pharynx

Figure 2-10. Endotracheal intubation.

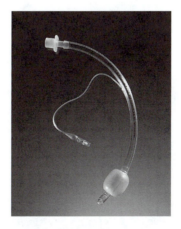

Figure 2-11. A cuffed endotracheal tube. (Photo reprinted by permission of Nellcor Puritan Bennett Inc., Pleasanton, CA)

factors contraindicating a tracheotomy, and weaning from the artificial airway is not imminent, a tracheotomy typically is performed and the endotracheal tube removed. Later in this chapter this traditional outlook regarding the change from intubation to tracheotomy will be discussed, and differing viewpoints presented.

B. Procedure

Endotracheal intubation most commonly is performed by a physician. In some settings and circumstances, the procedure may be carried out by an emergency medical technician or respiratory care practitioner. During both oral and nasal intubation the patient must first be properly positioned so that the mouth, pharynx, and larynx are aligned. This allows the glottis to be visualized and facilitates passage of the tube. Since the patient is often in respiratory distress as this procedure is being performed, 100% oxygen is normally provided via a manual resuscitation bag and face mask.

1. Equipment necessary for oral intubation includes a **laryngoscope.** This is an instrument that contains a light source allowing for direct visualization of the glottis. It is illustrated in Figure 2-12. The laryngoscope blade, which will guide the placement of the tube, is inserted over the midline portion of the tongue, advanced to displace the epiglottis and then to fully visualize the vocal folds. The endotracheal tube is then inserted. Most endotracheal tubes have cuffs. Once the cuff has passed between the vocal folds, the tube is advanced approximately another 3 centimeters. The cuff is inflated after it is placed in the trachea. Confirmation of correct placement is commonly obtained by auscultation of the chest. The endotracheal tube is then secured in place to the

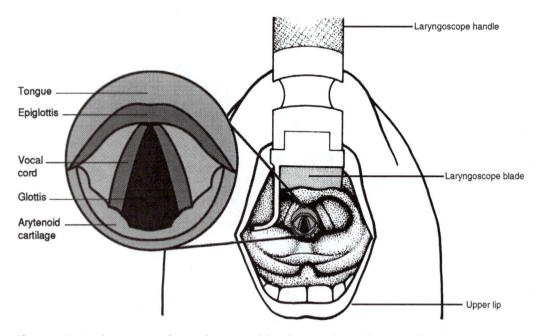

Figure 2-12. Intubation procedure with a view of the glottis. (Adapted from *Cardiopulmonary Resuscitation,* by P. D. Ellis & M. D. Billings, 1980. St. Louis, MO: Mosby.)

side of the mouth by adhesive tape (Finucane & Santora, 1988; Simmons, 1990).

2. Nasal intubation can be carried out with direct visualization via a fiberoptic or bronchoscope or laryngoscope (Simmons, 1990). Bronchoscopy is performed to directly visualize the airway, that is, the trachea and bronchi. It is performed with either a rigid or flexible bronchoscope. In a spontaneously breathing patient, it may be performed blindly, without visualizing the vocal folds. The equipment is similar to that needed for oral intubation. A local anesthetic is usually sprayed into the nasal passages for vasoconstriction or shrinkage of tiny blood vessels to prevent excessive bleeding. The end of the tube is lubricated for easier insertion. The tube is directed downward into the oropharynx and is passed through the vocal cords, usually with special forceps. The cuff is advanced and inflated, and its position is confirmed as with oral intubation. The tube tip is secured with tape at the side of the nose.

Blind nasal intubation is used when the airway cannot be visualized because the patient is unable to open the mouth or when significant trauma has occurred to the oral cavity. The patient must be able to breathe spontaneously in order for this technique to be utilized because breath sounds guide the successful passage of the tube (Finucane & Santora, 1988).

C. Complications

There are immediate and long-term complications associated with endotracheal intubation.

1. Immediate Complications

a. Oral intubation
(1) Complications related to the actual procedure of oral intubation may include trauma to the teeth and gums and abrasion of the lips, tongue, pharynx, and larynx. Tearing of the mucous membranes in the region of the posterior oropharynx can occur and result in a temporary throat pain for the patient.

(2) Damage to the vocal folds may occur secondary to trauma from the endotracheal tube. This is usually related to use of a large endotracheal tube during the procedure or to cuff overinflation immediately after intubation. Cuff overinflation is caused by introducing an excessive amount of air into the balloon so that it actually impedes on the tracheal walls as illustrated in Figure 2-13. The inflammation, edema, and resultant hoarseness are usually transient and will resolve. Rarely, damage to the recurrent laryngeal nerve will occur, again related to significant trauma to the nerve as it courses through the larynx. Large endotracheal tubes, unmonitored cuff pressures, or poor

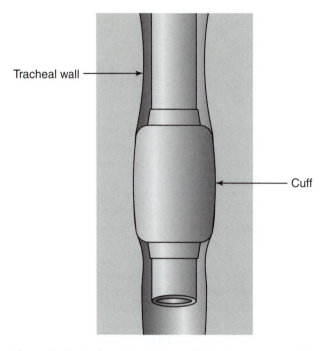

Figure 2-13. Endotracheal tube cuff impingement on the tracheal walls.

positioning of the head during the procedure may be implicated. According to Finucane and Santora (1988), laryngeal trauma can cause a more significant medical complication referred to as *subcutaneous emphysem*a, a collection of subcutaneous air caused by tearing of the tracheal wall. Air becomes trapped in the soft tissues of the face, neck, and chest walls. It usually is not a life-threatening complication but is cosmetically unsightly and uncomfortable for the patient. Conetta, Barman, Iakovou, and Masakayan (1993) reported one case of ventilatory failure caused by subcutaneous emphysema where gas collected in the soft tissues of the thorax, and the chest wall was unable to move freely.

(3) Another serious complication includes hypoxemia. Hypoxemia occurs when the quantity of oxygen that is available to the tissues is below normal. Oxygen deprivation to brain cells for more than 3 minutes significantly increases the risk of brain damage (Finucane & Santora, 1988). One cause of hypoxemia is **aspiration** of gastric contents into the trachea during the intubation process. This is usually secondary to vomiting or regurgitation. This type of aspiration is potentially serious due to the pH level of the aspirated material. A pH of less than 3.0 causes actual chemical burning of the airway and lungs (Kirsch

& Sanders, 1988). Hypoxemia can also occur on removal of the endotracheal tube. If a significant laryngospasm occurs at this time, airway obstruction and a decreased oxygen supply to body tissues can result.

(4) If the endotracheal tube is directed through the trachea and into the bronchi, left lung collapse may result. The angle of the right mainstem bronchus to the trachea predisposes the entry of the tube to the right lung, as objects in the airway are naturally directed to the right.

(5) A complication associated with the intubation procedure is esophageal intubation, or inadvertent passage of the endotracheal tube into the esophagus. This misplacement is often detected during auscultation. However, Finucane and Santora (1988) note that the presence or absence of breath sounds will not rule out esophageal intubation and that observation of the patient's respiratory status following intubation is paramount. Proper placement of the tube should be confirmed any time a patient is moved significantly. Objective devices that assist in measuring the percentages of oxygen and carbon dioxide in the blood can be helpful in establishing proper placement of the airway.

(6) Rupture of the esophagus is a rare, but potentially life-threatening, complication of intubation. It usually occurs during a difficult intubation when repeated attempts are made to pass the endotracheal tube.

(7) Cardiac complications can occur because introduction of the endotracheal tube often precipitates an increase in blood pressure and heart rate, which is usually temporary. However, this complication should be carefully monitored in hypertensive patients. Increases in intracranial pressure may also be a risk of endotracheal intubation and are of particular concern in a patient with a cerebral aneurysm (Finucane & Santora, 1988).

b. Nasal intubation

As with oral intubation, the complications just discussed are also risks of nasal intubation. There are additional complications which are specific consequences of nasotracheal intubation.

(1) Trauma to the nasal passages occurs when the tube abrades the nasal septum. Eventually, necrosis may result. Introduction of a poorly lubricated tube can precipitate nose bleed during the procedure. Removal of the endotracheal tube may be associated with epistaxis (i.e., nose bleed).

(2) Otitis media and conductive hearing loss are fairly common sequelae of the mechanical blockage of the eustachian tube by the endotracheal tube. The eustachian tube cannot open and drain properly. Additionally, movement of the endotracheal tube in even a semiconscious patient may cause irritation in this area.

2. Long-term Complications

Studies in the literature today cite difficulty in quantifying the long-term effects of intubation; however, the risk of laryngeal trauma and other complications is clear (Bishop, 1989; Colice, Stukel, & Dain, 1989; Heffner, 1993). The risk of significant tracheal injury also exists, although modifications of endotracheal tubes have lessened its incidence. A discussion of potential causes of longer-term complications of endotracheal intubation will be divided into the resultant laryngeal or tracheal trauma.

a. Laryngeal trauma
(1) Pressure necrosis

The pressure of the translaryngeal endotracheal tube against the fragile laryngeal mucosa can potentially create a tissue necrosis. The degree of irritation varies proportionately with the size of the endotracheal tube. The amount of surface contact of the tube to the laryngeal area increases the degree of damage. Therefore, although large tubes have the advantage of providing a more open airway and lower resistance to airflow, they carry an increased risk of laryngeal abrasion (Bishop, 1989). In other words, although it may be easier to ventilate the patient with the larger tubes, the risk of other complications must be weighed when they are used.

An additional source of pressure against the laryngeal mucosa has been described by Bishop, Weymuller, and Fink (1984). It is created by the interaction of the shape of the endotracheal tube relative to the shape of the larynx. The larynx is pentagon-shaped, bounded by the thyroid cartilage anteriorly and the arytenoids and cricoid cartilage posteriorly. The endotracheal tube is circular. This relationship is illustrated in Figure 2-14. When the endotracheal tube is inserted, it contacts three key areas: the two vocal processes and the cricoid cartilage. The circular shape of the tube resting in a pentagon-shaped larynx exerts significant force onto the laryngeal mucosa, concentrated at these key locations, primarily at the posterolateral site of the larynx. This relationship was described by Quartararo and Bishop (1990). According to Bishop et al. (1984), the pressure exerted by the endotracheal tube may reach up to 400 mm Hg. Once external pressures exceed the normal capillary perfusion pressures of 25–30 mm Hg, ischemic damage of the mucosa becomes evident. In other words, the capillary walls cannot maintain their integrity against the continual external force of the endotracheal tube. As a result, breakdown occurs.

The movement of the endotracheal tube against the laryngeal mucosa is an additional source of tissue irritation and potential abrasion. As

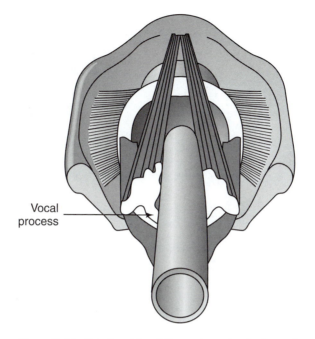

Vocal
process

Figure 2-14. Relationship of the endotracheal tube and
the shape of the glottis.

patients make even limited movements in a bed, produce a cough,
attempt to swallow, or take each breath, the endotracheal tube shifts
oppositionally to the movements of the larynx. The effect is, therefore, to have the rigid surface of the tube continuously rubbing against
the delicate mucosal tissue.

The composition of the endotracheal tube is an additional factor in
the development of complications, especially pressure necrosis. Both
polyvinyl chloride and silicone endotracheal tubes are used today.
Polyvinyl chloride tubes are inexpensive and maintain their shape
well. However, some practitioners are advocating the use of silicone
tubes, especially for prolonged intubation. Silicone plastic contains
fewer chemical additives and, by its composition, is also less likely
to permit bacteria to adhere to its surface (Weymuller, 1992).

These laryngeal complications may or may not lead to eventual long-
term clinical symptoms (Beckford, Mayo, Wilkinson, & Tierney,
1990). Hoarseness and stridor can therefore be transient effects of
intubation, but in some cases, as with intubation granuloma, they
may be clinical indicators of longer-lasting damage.

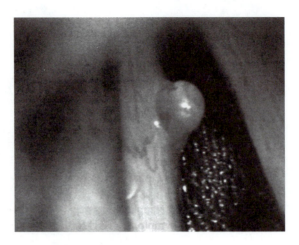

Figure 2-15. A sessile polyp on the middle third of the vocal fold.

(2) Granulomas

Postintubation **granulomas** form as injured laryngeal mucosa attempts to heal. Granulation is itself a form of tissue healing, but a slower form, occurring when the abraded or ulcerated area attempts to cover itself in the presence of damaged supporting epithelium. The cause of this abnormal healing, with its resultant scarring in some patients, may be related to the severity of the laryngeal injury. The resultant granuloma, which may develop into a **polyp,** usually occurs on the posterior third of the larynx, and often develops on the right side due to the way the tube is secured from the mouth. A polyp is an area on the vocal fold where the mucosa has loosened from the vocal ligament and has developed a large mass greater than its base attachment to the vocal fold (Aronson, 1985). It is depicted in Figure 2-15. The severest extent of granuloma may create airway obstruction. Clinical symptoms include vocal hoarseness, stridor, and pain. The persistence of these symptoms should prompt a laryngeal examination. If the granuloma does not resolve following extubation, surgical removal may be necessary. Colice (1992) noted that 4 out of 51 patients in a clinical study developed granulomas. He also noted that persistent hoarseness, beyond 4 weeks post extubation, is a clinical indicator of a potential laryngeal granuloma and that surgical intervention could be indicated in such a case. In general, healing of the damaged laryngeal mucosa occurred within 8 weeks post extubation without significant clinical complications. Balestrieri and Watson (1982) noted that, although intubation granulomas are not a common consequence of endotracheal intubation, they can be encountered with the intubated patient.

(3) **Stenosis**

Stenosis, the narrowing of the airway, is a less common consequence of the healing and tightening of epithelial tissue in the glottic and subglottic areas and trachea. Dilation, laser removal, or placement of a laryngeal stent (a small wedge placed between the vocal folds to separate them) may be necessary in cases where these problems do not resolve spontaneously. The length of intubation time does not appear to correlate with the development of either laryngeal granuloma or stenosis (Colice, 1992; Stauffer, Olson, & Petty, 1981).

(4) **Laryngeal web**

Abraded tissue may form a laryngeal web in the glottic area, potentially leading to airway obstruction. This membranous formation attaches to the margins of the vocal folds and connects them.

(5) **Glottic incompetence**

Long-term intubation can interfere with the normal protective responses of the larynx. These include laryngeal closure and the ability to clear aspirated material from the airway. Glottic incompetence may relate to actual structural damage of the vocal folds. In the absence of actual paralysis of the folds, the lack of airflow through the system appears to disrupt normal reflexes. Glottic incompetence may resolve with time with therapy but can predispose a patient to aspiration or entry of material into the airway.

b. **Tracheal trauma**

(1) **Endotracheal tube cuffs**

The major cause of tracheal trauma from endotracheal intubation is cuff overinflation. However, the incidence of injury has been drastically lessened by the use of low pressure endotracheal cuffs (Bishop, 1989). The cuff is an internal balloon which surrounds the translaryngeal tube and approximates the tracheal walls. (This was illustrated in Figure 2-13.) It is designed to provide a seal to reduce air leakage during mechanical ventilation and reduce the risk of aspiration. Excessive cuff pressures are identified as pressures that exceed 25–30 mm Hg or normal capillary wall pressure (Eubanks & Bone, 1990). When pressures are maintained below these normal levels, permanent tracheal damage should not occur. Endotracheal tube cuffs should be periodically deflated to remove the pressure against the tracheal walls and allow blood flow to, at least briefly, normalize at the cuff site. One manufacturer of tracheostomy tubes markets a standard double-cuffed tube (Portex, Inc.). With this device, each cuff can be alternately inflated and deflated, theoretically decreasing the risk of edema in one area.

(2) **Tracheal stenosis**

Cuff overinflation is a contributing factor to tracheal stenosis. Stenosis occurs any time irritated tissue attempts to heal itself, with resultant scarring and tightening. Granulation tissue formation often will occur at the site of the tracheal trauma. Cuff overinflation, paired with the movement of the endotracheal tube in relation to the trachea, creates an abrading movement and subsequently a potential for granulation formation.

VI. CRICOTHYROIDOTOMY

A. Indications

1. **Cricothyroidotomy** is an airway management procedure usually performed in an emergency situation by a physician when a patient's anatomy will not permit the creation of a tracheotomy. It involves the surgical creation of an opening into the cricothyroid membrane. This procedure is normally performed only after other nonsurgical methods of airway management have failed. In general, this is secondary to upper airway obstruction that cannot be cleared. As with any airway management procedure, additional indications for cricothyroidotomy include need for mechanical ventilation and airway suctioning. Most patients do not receive a cricothyroidotomy electively, as there appear to be more long-term complications with this procedure. Brantigan and Grow (1976, 1980) suggested that cricothyroidotomy does not carry any additional risks than tracheotomy and that this procedure may be indicated as an elective method of airway management unless there is existing laryngeal pathology. Cole and Aguilar (1988) responded to the increase in elective cricothyroidotomies with a review of the literature and a report of their own experience with the procedure. They concluded that cricothyroidotomy should *not* be recommended electively. In their conclusion, Cole and Aguilar referred to chronic vocal changes "as a common sequela of cricothyroidotomy" (p. 134).

2. Needle cricothyroidotomy or transtracheal catheterization is the most common emergency means of airway management used when intubation fails. It involves providing oxygenation through a catheter inserted into the cricothyroid membrane via a needle. This procedure is faster than traditional cricothyroidotomy in securing the airway, but is not as secure.

B. Procedure

1. Cricothyroidotomy is a surgical procedure. It is considered less complex than other surgical airway management techniques, such as tracheotomy, but still carries risks to the patient. The patient is preoxygenated usually via a face mask. The neck is extended and the skin prepared (Figure 2-16). Finucane and Santora (1988) indicate that a local anesthetic can be infiltrated into the skin if the patient is not in acute distress. With a surgical knife, an incision is made

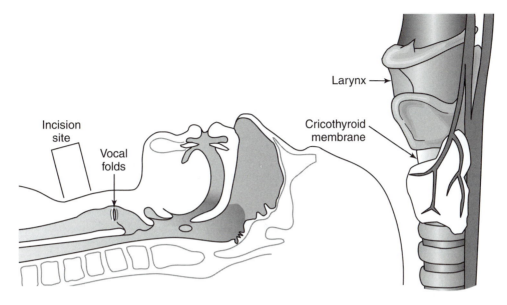

Figure 2-16. Incision site for cricothyroidotomy.

through the skin, underlying tissue, and then through the cricothyroid membrane. As the incision is held open, a tube is inserted to maintain a patent airway and allow for mechanical ventilation.

2. Needle cricothyroidotomy or transtracheal catheterization involves similar preoxygenation, positioning, and skin preparation. A needle and catheter are inserted into the midline of the cricothyroid membrane. The catheter can be connected to either manual or mechanical ventilation. This technique can allow for temporary oxygenation of the patient until airway obstruction can be cleared or until the patient is stable enough for a more permanent surgical procedure.

C. Complications

1. Immediate Complications

a. Cricothyroidotomy is a surgical procedure which carries with it the inherent risks of such an operation. These include injury to the trachea and larynx and bleeding. Damage to the trachea and larynx, specifically to the cricoid cartilage, may occur during the procedure especially if a less experienced surgeon is forced to perform the procedure quickly and inadvertently cuts beyond the specified area. Patients may develop hoarseness immediately following the procedure due to localized edema.

    b. Needle catheterization cricothyroidotomy carries complications associated with the procedure itself. Esophageal perforation is a potential complication when a needle is inserted through the larynx. Expiratory obstruction is an additional risk if the upper airway is obstructed and the oxygen which is delivered via the narrow needle cannot passively escape through the upper airway. In this instance, overinflation of the lungs becomes a significant complication as air continues to accumulate (Finucane & Santora, 1988).

    Perforation of the posterior wall of the trachea has been associated with the use of a transtracheal catheter during the delivery of oxygen therapy (Menon, Carlin, & Kaplan, 1993). This perforation may have occurred during the initial needle placement or developed as a complication of concentrated oxygen flow through the needle catheter, which impacted on the tracheal wall.

2. Long-term Complications

    a. **Subglottal stenosis** can be a long-term complication of cricothyroidotomy in patients with preexisting laryngeal pathologies. For example, laryngeal trauma secondary to endotracheal intubation has been cited as a contraindication for cricothyroidotomy because of the potential for further infection and ulceration (Heffner, Miller, & Sahn, 1986b).

    b. Vocal cord injury is a potential long-term complication because the incision site is immediately anterior to the vocal folds. Chronic hoarseness is the resulting vocal characteristic.

VII. TRACHEOTOMY

Tracheotomy involves the surgical placement of a plastic or metal tube into the trachea to create an airway, by a physician. A tracheostomy tube is depicted in situ in Figure 2-17. Tracheotomy is performed when there is an extended need for an artificial airway. This need may be secondary to upper airway obstruction, poor secretion management and inadequate airway protection, and connection to mechanical ventilation. The timing of tracheotomy following endotracheal intubation is patient specific; however, the procedure should be considered because it provides substantial benefits for long-term airway management. Tracheotomy creates an altered airway with the patient relying on air obtained via the tracheotomy stoma rather than the upper airway. This will impair phonation as air is diverted away from the vocal folds. On inspiration, air enters the tracheotomy and lower respiratory tract, bypassing the upper airway. Although the tracheostomy tube is placed to reduce the airflow resistance offered by the upper airway, and so lessen the patient's effort during breathing, the tracheostomy tube itself does provide resistance to inspired air (Yung & Snowdon, 1984).

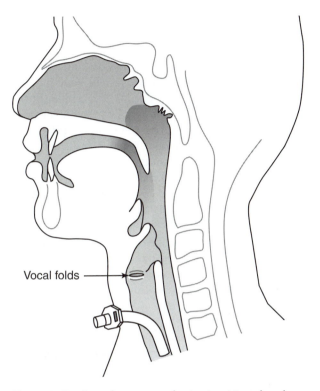

Figure 2-17. A tracheostomy tube in situ. Note the placement below the level of the vocal folds.

Vocal folds

A. Indications

The benefits of tracheotomy over other airway management techniques include:

1. Decreased risk of accidental removal of the tracheostomy tube. Inadvertent **decannulation** (i.e., removal) of a secured tracheostomy tube is less common than accidental extubation of an endotracheal tube.

2. Secretion removal is more easily accomplished via a tracheostomy tube that allows access to the lower respiratory tract. Additionally, when a nasal or oral endotracheal tube is removed, secretions can be suctioned from the nose and the mouth. Patients also can be taught to mobilize their own secretions as vocal fold adduction permits coughing and airway clearance.

3. A properly performed tracheotomy reduces the risk of the laryngeal complications associated with intubation. Tracheotomy is performed *below* the level of the vocal folds.

4. Improved **weaning,** or discontinuation from mechanical ventilation, is accomplished more effectively when a tracheostomy tube is in place. The resistance to airflow provided by a transtracheal endotracheal tube is higher than a standard tracheostomy tube (Wright, Marini, & Bernard, 1989). The endotracheal tube is longer and must be angled to fit in the curved airway. This increases turbulent airflow. The mechanics of airflow through the endotracheal tube, in addition to the presence of obstructing secretions, may impact on a patient's work of breathing and so affect their ability to be weaned. This is especially true in individuals with significant lung disease (Heffner, 1993). The design and placement of the tracheostomy tube lessens this resistance. It also decreases the amount of dead space in the airway. Dead space refers to areas of the airway that do not participate in gas exchange. Air volume is thus delivered more effectively, directly to the lungs.

5. Patient comfort will be increased with a tracheostomy tube as opposed to endotracheal intubation. Either the nasal or oral route of intubation is physically more restricting and irritating and causes increased stress to the alert patient. Observation of reduced anxiety levels is common when the patient is changed from an endotracheal tube to a tracheostomy tube.

6. Options for oral communication and oral feeding are greatly expanded with tracheostomy tube placement versus endotracheal intubation.

B. Procedure

1. A tracheotomy should be performed only by a surgeon skilled in the operation and only after the airway has been secured by other nonsurgical techniques. Most patients will already have a stabilized airway which will remain in place as long as possible during the procedure. The patient's skin is prepared and the head hyperextended. An incision is made through skin, underlying tissue, and relevant musculature to expose the thyroid isthmus. Caution must be used when working near the thyroid because it is a vascular structure and the risk of bleeding is high. The incision into the trachea is made at the level of the second or third tracheal rings as illustrated in Figure 2-18.

    a. Incision type and placement are important. The vertical skin incision is most commonly performed to permit easier insertion and removal of the tracheostomy tube, as well as to allow more normal laryngeal excursion to occur. The horizontal skin incision, although performed for many years because it was more cosmetically acceptable than the vertical type, is rarely utilized today. It is considered more physically restricting to the larynx and impedes the proper angle of the tracheostomy tube (Simmons, 1990).

    b. Placement of the tracheostomy tube above or below the second and third tracheal rings can lead to specific complications. An incision too close to

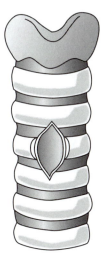

Figure 2-18. Incision site for tracheotomy.

the first tracheal ring may cause damage to the cricoid cartilage. Conversely, an incision below the fourth tracheal ring increases the risk of vascular erosion and hemorrhage due to damage of the innominate artery (Heffner et al., 1986b). This artery crosses the trachea at the level of the upper portion of the sternum. It is therefore vulnerable to damage by a tracheostomy tube situated in the lower tracheal rings.

2. The size of the tracheostomy tube is selected based on the patient's age, weight, and height. The tracheostomy tube is prepared for insertion in the newly created stoma. At this point the endotracheal tube can be removed. The tracheostomy tube is then inserted into the stoma and the patient reconnected to mechanical ventilation, if indicated. The tracheostomy tube cuff is then inflated and the tube is secured in place by the tracheostomy ties. Sutures are rarely used to hold the tube in place. The position of the tube is commonly confirmed with a chest radiograph.

C. Complications

1. Immediate Complications

a. Pneumothorax is a potential complication of tracheotomy since the pleura may be punctured during the surgery. Patients with emphysema are at a higher risk of developing pneumothorax due to their distended chest wall and the higher position of the pleura relative to the tracheotomy incision.

    b. Bleeding is another potentially serious complication that may arise particularly during the ligation near the highly vascular thyroid gland.

    c. Displacement of the tracheostomy tube may result from inadequate securing of the tracheostomy tube around the patient's neck although this is not as common as accidental extubation with endotracheal tubes.

    d. Incorrect placement of the tracheostomy tube can lead to cardiorespiratory arrest if the airway is not secured in a timely manner. Overall, tracheotomy has a mortality rate ranging from 0 to 5% (Simmons, 1990).

2. Long-term Complications

    a. Tracheal granuloma is a common complication of tracheotomy, although symptoms of airway obstruction are not always apparent (Law, Barnhart, Rowlett, de la Rocha, & Lowenberg, 1993). Granuloma is also a complication of endotracheal intubation. Tracheal granulomas are related to abrasion at the stoma site from the tracheostomy tube as illustrated in Figure 2-19. Law et al. (1993) documented tracheal granuloma in 58% of patients with long-term tracheotomies. The removal of tracheal granuloma in even apparently asymptomatic tracheotomized patients led to later successful decannulation, or removal of the tracheostomy tube, in 20 out of 25 individuals. These authors concluded that, for a large number of patients with long-term tracheostomy tubes, tracheal granulomas were a significant complication and did impact on the patient's airway. They

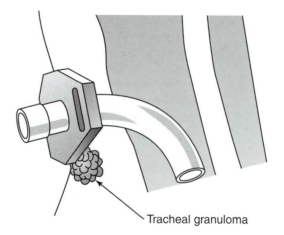

Tracheal granuloma

Figure 2-19. Tracheal granuloma at the stoma site.

noted that these patients require more than simply routine examination of the upper airway to document the presence of tracheal granuloma.

b. **Tracheomalacia,** the softening of the cartilaginous structure of the trachea, is caused by erosion of the tracheal rings. This may be secondary to any trauma to the tracheal walls that exposes cartilage and leads to tissue breakdown. Recall that the structure of the trachea is such that, although it maintains a definite shape, it is able to expand and contract according to the respiratory cycle. As the cartilaginous framework of the trachea is damaged, collapse of the structure may occur during the inspiratory phase of breathing. Tracheomalacia is often associated with tracheal stenosis.

c. **Tracheal stenosis** associated with longer-term tracheotomy may occur from various causes. Stenosis is a narrowing that occurs when the tracheal rings begin to heal following trauma. Stenosis can occur at the tracheal stoma and cuff site. Stenosis at the stoma may be related to:

- frequent infections.

- tube changes.

- continuous tugging on the tracheostomy tube from the ventilatory tubing.

- a stoma that is too large and attempts to heal and close itself.

Narrowing that develops near the cuff site results from:

- unrelieved pressure on the tracheal mucosa.

- abrasive movement of the cuff as the tube moves within the trachea (Simmons, 1990).

The incision site also may encourage development of stenosis. A tracheotomy incision made too close to the level of the cricoid cartilage may result in subglottic narrowing as the cartilage heals at that area. Tracheal stenosis may manifest subsequent clinical symptoms such as difficulty mobilizing secretions, coughing, and shortness of breath. The tracheal lumen must be reduced by 75% before these obvious clinical symptoms become evident (Heffner et al., 1986b). Management of severe tracheal stenosis is primarily surgical and may involve dilation, laser removal, stenting, or resection.

d. Tracheoesophageal and tracheoinnominate **fistulae** are serious although relatively uncommon complications of long-term tracheostomy. A tracheoesophageal fistula occurs when the tracheal and esophageal walls become necrotic and connected, forming a passageway from the gastrointestinal tract into the airway. An over-inflated tracheostomy tube cuff in

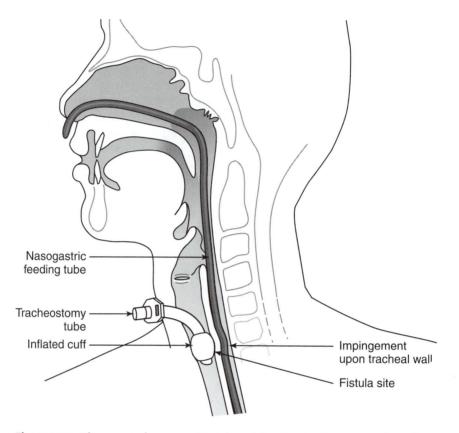

Nasogastric
feeding tube

Tracheostomy
tube

Inflated cuff

Impingement
upon tracheal wall

Fistula site

Figure 2-20. Placement of a nasogastric tube relative to a tracheostomy tube cuff.

the presence of a large nasogastric feeding tube can create this complication, especially in the presence of other predisposing factors such as poor nutrition and repeated infections. As illustrated in Figure 2-20, the pressure of the cuff on the tracheal wall meeting the unyielding nasogastric tube ulcerates and destroys the communicating wall. Clinical symptomatology of tracheoesophageal fistulae includes history of aspiration pneumonia and purulent or copious secretions related to the repeated insult to the trachea and lungs. Abdominal distention is another presenting symptom of a fistula. The distention occurs as air leaks from the trachea into the esophagus when the patient is on mechanical ventilation. The air from the ventilator, which is initially directed into the trachea, is channeled into the esophagus through the connecting fistula. A tracheoesophageal fistula must be surgically closed.

A tracheoinnominate fistula, which was previously described in the procedural section, occurs when the tracheotomy incision is made below the fourth tracheal ring. This places the distal end of the tracheostomy tube at a level to impinge on the innominate artery, causing eventual erosion, creation of a fistula, and potentially life-threatening hemorrhage. Tracheoinnominate fistula, fortunately, is not a common complication of tracheotomy.

VIII. PERCUTANEOUS TRACHEOTOMY

A. Indications

1. **Percutaneous tracheotomy** (also referred to as percutaneous dilational tracheotomy) is an airway management technique that is typically performed in the intensive care setting (ICU) with adult, intubated patients. Percutaneous tracheotomy is performed with patients who require tracheotomy but are critically ill, would be at risk of complications surrounding transfer to a surgical operating room suite, and can be managed within the ICU setting (Pothmann, Tonner, & Schulte am Esch, 1997). The bedside percutaneous technique is simpler and also less costly as compared to surgical tracheotomy. It also has a lower incidence of intraoperative and postoperative complications comparatively. Anatomical prerequisites include an ability to palpate the cricoid cartilage above the thyroid notch. Therefore, patients with neck masses or large thyroid glands are usually better suited for surgical tracheotomies. Morbid obesity is also a contraindication, as it can lead to false passage of the tube into the soft tissue of the neck. With this procedure, the patient's head must be hyperextended. However, successful percutaneous tracheotomy has also been reported in patients who could not have their necks extended, as is common in trauma patients (Mayberry, Goldman, & Rehm, 1999).

B. Procedure

1. Percutaneous tracheotomy techniques normally require from three to four skilled individuals, usually a surgeon/critical care physician, nurse and respiratory care practitioner. Individual facilities will develop their own protocols, but the procedure is usually performed under bronchoscopy. This ensures proper placement of the equipment. Percutaneous tracheotomy tube kits are commercially available. The PerFit set by Portex, Inc. is shown in Figure 2-21. The size of the tube selected is normally based on the size of the endotracheal tube, and is correct if it occupies between two thirds and three quarters of the internal diameter of the trachea.

2. Sedation and local anesthesia are required for percutaneous tracheotomy (in some settings, an anesthesiologist or anesthetist may be present). The patient's neck is extended, and 100% oxygen is delivered via mechanical ventilation. After identification of landmarks, a small 1.5 to 2.0-cm incision is made at

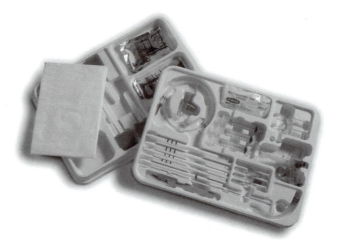

Figure 2-21. A percutaneous dilational tracheostomy kit. (Photo courtesy of Portex, Inc.)

either the cricoid cartilage and the first tracheal ring or at the first and second tracheal rings. The bronchoscope is inserted and the endotracheal tube and bronchoscope are positioned. The bronchoscope light should be seen through the incision. A catheter needle followed by a dilator with a guide wire is placed through the incision to assist placement of a guiding catheter. Progressive dilations of the trachea are then performed (Pothmann et al., 1997). Finally, a tracheostomy tube with its inner cannula replaced by a dilator is inserted. The dilator is then removed and replaced with an inner cannula; the patient is then connected to the ventilator (Kost, 1998). This process is depicted in Figures 2-22a, b, and c. Typically, less scarring is present after decannulation because this technique utilizes a small incision (1.5–2.0 cm).

C. Complications

1. Immediate

   a. Complications of percutaneous tracheotomy parallel those of surgical tracheotomy. These include intraoperative or postoperative bleeding, false passage of the tube, infection and tracheal wall injury. Most authors cite lower complication rates for percutaneous tracheotomy performed with bronchoscopic visualization, with the most common complication being accidental decannulation. Figure 2-22d depicts the complication of displacement of the tracheostomy tube out of the trachea and into the soft tissues. Mayberry et al. (1999) surveyed the literature and reported a general complication rate of 11%. However, Conlan and Kopec (2000) reported that the percutaneous tracheotomy process has several associated

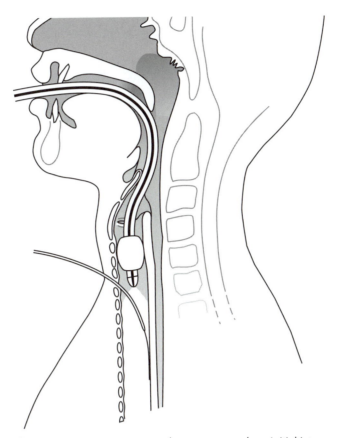

Figure 2-22a. Percutaneous tracheotomy procedure: Initial introduction of guiding catheter. (From *Tracheotomy; Airway Management, Communication and Swallowing*, by E. N. Myers, J. T. Johnson, and T. Murry, 1998, p. 82. Clifton Park, NY: Singular.)

unique risks. Accidental extubation is a potentially life-threatening hazard unless a skilled assistant secures the airway. With the proper placement of the endotracheal tube, puncturing of the tracheal wall by the catheter needle during the procedure should be minimized.

2. **Long Term**

   a. Long-term complications associated with percutaneous tracheotomy are similar to those of surgical tracheotomies. These include tracheal granuloma, stenosis, and tracheomalacia. A study performed by Law, Carney, and Manara (1997) followed 41 patients who had undergone dilation percutaneous tracheotomy at least 6 months prior to their follow-up evaluation of their airway anatomy and assessment via spirometry. All of the patients were asymptomatic. There was significant tracheal stenosis

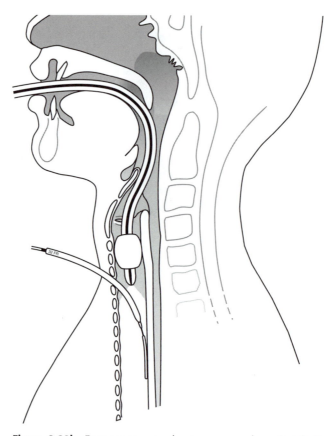

Figure 2-22b. Percutaneous tracheotomy procedure: Serial dilatations creating tracheotomy site. (From *Tracheotomy; Airway Management, Communication and Swallowing,* by E. N. Myers, J. T. Johnson, and T. Murry, 1998, p. 83. Clifton Park, NY: Singular.)

(>10%) in 4 patients, but only 2 patients demonstrated any spirometric evidence of obstruction. The authors concluded that long-term outcome is at least as good as surgical tracheotomy.

IX. CURRENT TRENDS: TIMING OF TRACHEOTOMY

The timing of tracheotomy in the intubated patient requiring long-term ventilatory support continues to be reviewed (Brook et al., 2000; Colice, 1992; Heffner, 1993). Traditionally, the medical community had operated with the premise that endotracheal intubation should not be maintained for longer than 3 weeks so as to minimize the airway complications. However, Bishop (1989) stated that the performance of a tracheotomy following such a period of intubation is "the worst possible combination for the larynx" (p. 186), predisposing it to increased scarring and decreased mobility of the vocal folds.

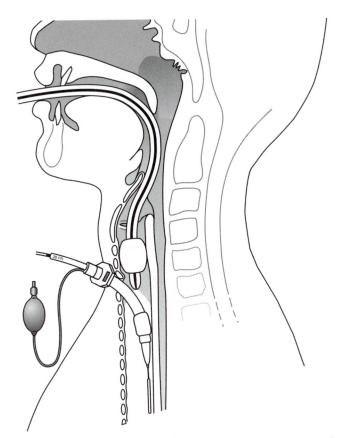

Figure 2-22c. Percutaneous tracheotomy procedure: Insertion of tracheostomy tube over guiding catheter. (From *Tracheotomy; Airway Management, Communication and Swallowing,* by E. N. Myers, J. T. Johnson, and T. Murry, 1998, p. 83. Clifton Park, NY: Singular.)

He further noted that the removal of translaryngeal intubation for early tracheotomy must be considered in light of the incidence of stomal stenosis associated with tracheotomy. Other researchers have agreed that there is no precise time limit for the change from intubation to tracheostomy. Heffner (1993) discussed the need for surgeons to consider the overall patient profile in deciding the need for the change over to tracheostomy. The anticipated time the artificial airway will be needed and the social and nutritional needs of the patient should factor into the decision. Colice (1992) reported that the laryngeal injury that can occur during extubation usually resolves within 8 weeks without persistent remaining clinical sequelae. He concluded that previous studies which assessed laryngeal injury were inadequately controlled. Brook, Sherman, Malen, and Kollef (2000) provide an extensive review of the literature regarding timing of tracheotomy. Their prospective observational study looked at the influence of the timing of tracheotomy on patient outcome as well as factors that influenced mortality in patients with acute respiratory failure. The results of their study indicated a "strong

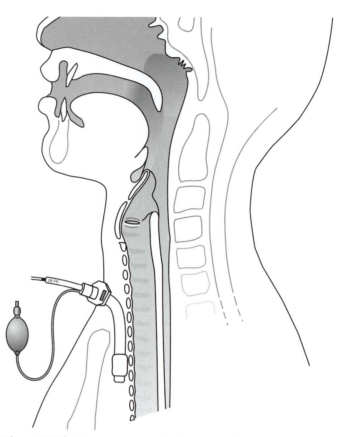

Figure 2-22d. Percutaneous tracheotomy procedure: Common complication: displacement of tracheotomy tube. (From *Tracheotomy; Airway Management, Communication and Swallowing,* by E. N. Myers, J. T. Johnson, and T. Murry, 1998, p. 82. Clifton Park, N.: Singular.)

association between early tracheotomy and improved outcome for patients in the medical ICU who require prolonged mechanical ventilation" (p. 359). Early tracheotomy was defined as the procedure performed by day 10 of mechanical ventilation. Late tracheotomy was defined as the procedure after day 10. Despite the varying definition of early tracheotomy in their review of the literature, the authors concluded that their study supported the case for early tracheotomy for better outcomes and overall reduced cost of care.

The practitioner should be aware of these various schools of thought and resulting management techniques when evaluating the tracheostomized patient. An understanding of each patient's individual clinical course and the airway management techniques utilized will assist clinicians in providing effective communication and swallowing treatment when persistent clinical complications exist.

3

Endotracheal Tubes and Tracheostomy Tubes

Effective communication management of the patient with an artificial airway demands a comprehensive understanding of endotracheal and tracheostomy tube design including materials, types, and manufacturer variations. These tracheal airways, which are associated with numerous potential complications, especially during long-term use, have a significant impact on communication and swallowing. Swallowing impairment associated with endotracheal tubes and tracheostomy will be discussed in detail in Chapters 7 and 8. This chapter provides an extensive review of endotracheal and tracheostomy tubes and introduces the impact of tracheostomy on the respiratory/phonatory mechanism. The technical information provided in this chapter is intended to assist physicians or allied health care practitioners in making informed choices and recommendations regarding tube selection for their patients with communication and swallowing disorders. This chapter aims to facilitate the problem-solving process by discussing the specific aspects of tracheostomy tube design.

I. ENDOTRACHEAL TUBES

A. Materials

As previously discussed, an endotracheal tube is a semirigid tube that is passed into the trachea via the nose or the mouth. It is usually constructed from either a *polyvinyl chloride (PVC)* or *silicone plastic*. The material is designed to be somewhat flexible yet retain its shape in the airway to avoid kinking or collapse, which would greatly increase the resistance to airflow. Due to the flexible composition of the silicone plastic, endotracheal tubes made of this material must be inserted into the airway with a rigid **stylet** and are reinforced with steel wire. There are differences between PVC and silicone plastic. PVC is a durable and inexpensive material that is widely used in the construction of endotracheal tubes (and tracheostomy tubes). It retains its shape well but will soften in heat, as with body temperature. Tubes made from PVC should be changed and disposed of approximately every 28 to 30 days. Silicone is also a durable plastic that is softer in composition than PVC. This type of plastic contains fewer chemical additives than PVC plastic, and therefore, there may be less risk of leaking of chemicals into tracheal tissues. Additionally, the composition of silicone reduces the chance of encrustation of secretions and the tendency of bacteria to adhere to the tube. Silicone can be sterilized and reused by **autoclaving** and **gas sterilization.** Plastic tubes are tested for tissue toxicity. An imprint with the abbreviations "I.T. or implant tested" and Z-79 indicates that the tube material has met the standards of the Committee of the American National Standards Institute (ANSI) for lack of toxicity.

B. Design

Specialized types of endotracheal tubes are available, which are generally used for patients who are difficult to intubate or for particular anesthesia applications. This discussion will focus on the standard endotracheal tube.

1. Figure 3-1 illustrates the components of the standard endotracheal tube. The tubes vary in internal and external diameter (mm) as well as length (cm). The proximal end of the tube is connected to a *15-mm adapter* for mechanical ventilation purposes. The 15-mm size is the standard measurement allowing for

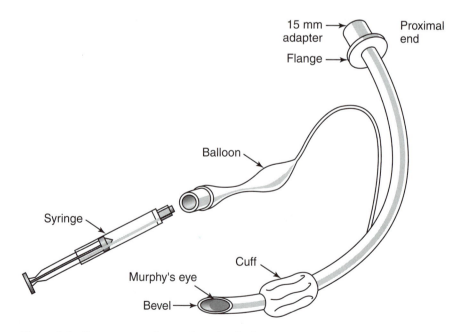

Figure 3-1. Components of an endotracheal tube.

connection from all types of endotracheal and tracheostomy tubes to various ventilatory tubings and adapters. The adapter has a **flange** or lip, which helps to prevent the proximal end of the tube from accidentally advancing into the nose or mouth. The endotracheal tube is curved to facilitate insertion. Along the body of the tube there are incremental markings that indicate length. This guides the physician during tube insertion by indicating how far the tube has been inserted into the airway.

2. At the distal end of the tube, or *tip,* there is a *beveled* or slanted opening that allows air to enter the airway. The beveled design reduces the risk of tissue damage during tube insertion. Most tubes also have a side opening commonly referred to as a *Murphy eye.* This side port allows air to continue to flow even if the main port is obstructed with mucus or blood or becomes positioned against the tracheal wall. Also located at the tube tip is a **cuff**. The cuff is connected to an external line which leads to the *external pilot balloon.* The external pilot balloon indicates how much the internal cuff is inflated. When the internal cuff is inflated, it fills the trachea like a balloon and blocks the passage of air from under the endotracheal tube into the upper airway. It will also partially stop the passage of secretions from the upper to the lower airway. A *spring-loaded valve* is located at the base of the external pilot balloon. It is here that a *syringe* is connected and air is injected to inflate the cuff and subsequently the balloon. The valve also serves to prevent inadvertent deflation of the cuff via air leakage from the balloon. During cuff deflation, the syringe is reattached, the valve opened, and air is removed. This also deflates the internal balloon, allowing the upper and lower airways to communicate.

II. TRACHEOSTOMY TUBES

Tracheostomy tubes are used to maintain the tracheal opening after the surgical procedure is performed. They will be discussed in terms of their composition or *materials, design,* and *type.*

A. Materials

Tracheostomy tubes are constructed of either polyvinyl chloride (PVC) or silicone, a mixture of these plastics, or metal. These tubes can be separated into *disposable* or *nondisposable* types.

1. *Disposable* tracheostomy tubes are plastic. The plastics used today to manufacture tracheostomy tubes are polyvinyl chloride and silicone. The two may also be mixed to achieve a particular composition. PVC alone or PVC mixed with silicone tubes are disposable. (PVC tubes are designed for single patient use; however, silicone tubes may be sterilized and reused.) The plastics used to manufacture tracheostomy tubes are designed to avoid tissue reaction and

are called medical grade plastic. However, PVC plastics contain chemicals that may cause allergic or tissue reaction in some patients. Plastics are more compliant than traditional nondisposable, metal tubes, that is, they are more adaptable and are designed to be less traumatic to the flexible airway. Silicone is intrinsically a softer material than the semirigid polyvinyl chloride plastic. Overall, due to their more compliant qualities, plastic tubes are generally favored over the more rigid metal tracheostomy tubes to enhance patient comfort. Figure 3-2a pictures a standard, disposable plastic tracheostomy tube.

2. *Nondisposable* tracheostomy tubes are metal, usually silver or stainless steel, or silicone. They are reusable and must be routinely sterilized between tracheostomy tube changes. The metal tracheostomy tubes are very rigid and heavier than the plastic. Metal tubes are more likely to cause irritation, especially at the stoma site. In addition, the metal tubes react to temperature, retaining and transmitting heat and cold. However, a metal tracheostomy tube is considered more sanitary than a PVC tube due to its composition and is often used by patients in the home care setting (S. Rothstein, personal communication, March 1994). The porous plastic PVC tubes can retain bacteria and therefore cannot be sterilized and reused, unlike metal. Many metal tracheostomy tubes do not have the 15-mm hub as a standard component; however, 15-mm adapters can be ordered. Metal tracheostomy tubes generally are not used for mechanically ventilated patients because they do not have cuffs. Although a cuff can be attached to the metal tube, the potential of dislodgment then becomes a risk factor. Figure 3-2b pictures a standard, nondisposable, metal tracheostomy tube.

    a. Silicone tracheostomy tubes can also be sterilized and reused. The nature of the silicone, different in composition from PVC, resists adherence of bacteria (Sottile et al., 1986). Silicone also retains its shape under various temperature conditions. It is therefore commonly used as a material for endotracheal and tracheostomy tubes. Figure 3-2c pictures a silicone tracheostomy tube. When silicone and PVC are mixed, the plastic is softer than PVC alone, but the tube cannot be reused.

B. Design

Standard tracheostomy tubes have similar component parts. These include the **outer cannula, inner cannula, flange, obturator, and button.** Figure 3-3 illustrates the parts of a tracheostomy tube.

1. Outer and Inner Cannulas

    a. The **outer cannula** is the outside wall of the tracheostomy tube which provides its basic structure. The **inner cannula,** which is available in a variety of sizes, fits snugly inside this outer wall. The inner cannula can

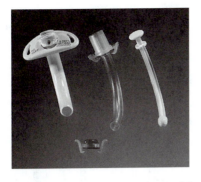

Figure 3-2a. Standard plastic disposable tracheostomy tube made from polyvinyl chloride. (Photo reprinted by permission of Nellcor Puritan Bennett Inc., Pleasanton, CA)

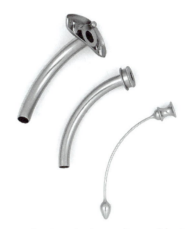

Figure 3-2b. Standard nondisposable tracheostomy tube made from metal. (Photo courtesy of Pilling Surgical)

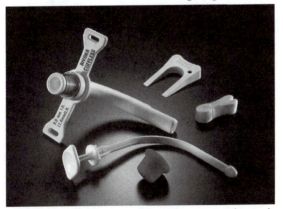

Figure 3-2c. Standard reusable tracheostomy tube made from silicone. (Photo courtesy of Portex, Inc./Bivona)

be removed for cleaning or if it becomes clogged with secretions, while the outer cannula remains in place to maintain the airway. The inner cannula is removed, soaked, and then scrubbed with a small wire brush to remove any dried or viscous material. *Disposable inner cannulas* are not cleaned and replaced in the outer cannula, but are discarded on at least a daily basis or when clogged. If the disposable inner cannula is shorter than the outer cannula and leaves a gap between the end of the tube and end of the inner cannula, there may be more potential for dried secretions to form at the distal area and block the tracheostomy tube opening; careful tracheostomy care should lessen this potential.

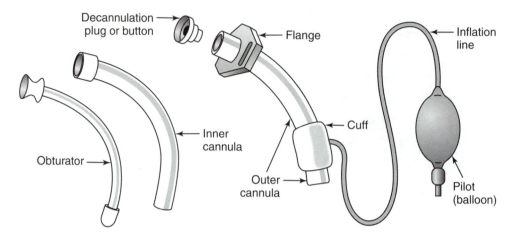

Figure 3-3. Parts of a standard tracheostomy tube.

b. Inner cannulas can be attached to the outer cannula in three ways. The disposable inner cannulas are either clipped into place by flexible prongs on each side of the 15-mm hub or are snapped securely by a coiled ring at the tip. The reusable inner cannulas are fitted into place with a rotational movement that locks the inner cannula into place on the proximal end of the outer cannula. Figures 3-4a, b, and c picture different inner cannulas with snap, clip, and lock connections. Inner cannulas are usually sized to the standard 15 mm measurement for attachment to resuscitation devices or ventilatory tubing, although there are variations among manufacturers which will be discussed later in this chapter, such as the low profile inner cannulas.

c. The inner cannula can be quickly removed in cases of obstruction, such as a mucous plug. Use of inner cannulas is therefore favored by many clinical practitioners to decrease the risk of an occluded tracheostomy tube. Silicone tracheostomy tubes are not manufactured with inner cannulas. The composition of the silicone, which was developed to decrease the potential for encrustation of secretions, decreases the need for the inner cannula. Siliconized PVC tracheostomy tubes are available with optional inner cannulas. The presence of an inner cannula will decrease the inner diameter of the tracheostomy tube and will increase airway resistance. Figure 3-5 illustrates a cross section of the inner cannula in relation to the outer cannula. Less air can pass through the tracheostomy tube because, in essence, it has been made smaller. This may increase the **work of breathing** or effort that it takes for the patient to obtain an adequate amount of air upon inspiration.

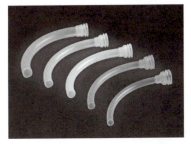

a.

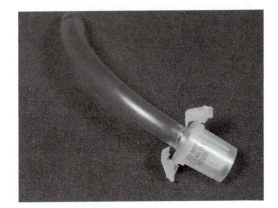

b.

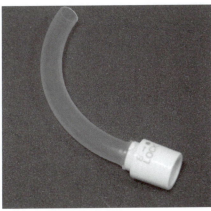

c.

Figure 3-4a. Disposable inner cannulas with snap/coiled connectors, shown with siliconized PVC tracheostomy tubes. (Photo courtesy of Portex, Inc./Bivona). **b.** A disposable inner cannula with clip connection. **c.** A nondisposable inner cannula with lock connection.

d. The relationship of the inner to the outer cannula in the tracheostomy tube is described by the *inner* and *outer diameter* measurements. The outer diameter measurement is the distance between the two outside walls of the tracheostomy tube itself. The inner diameter is the distance between the inside walls of the tracheostomy tube. The presence of an inner cannula reduces the inner diameter of the tracheostomy tube. Inner and outer diameters are expressed in millimeters. Another measurement that varies between tracheostomy tubes is the *length,* also indicated in millimeters. When selecting a tube for a particular patient, the physician is guided by these three parameters, inner and outer diameter and length.

e. Although standards for selection of tracheostomy tube size vary among practitioners, there are common guidelines for sizing. During the initial placement the physician will consider the patient's weight and general

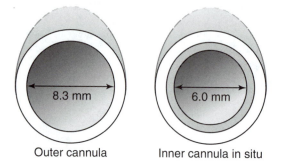

8.3 mm   6.0 mm

Outer cannula   Inner cannula in situ

Figure 3-5. A cross section of a tracheostomy tube with and without the inner cannula. Note the decrease in overall tube diameter with the inner cannula.

anatomy. Although the physician will not want to place a tube that is too large, therefore increasing the risk of complications associated with tracheal abrasion, the patient's ability to tolerate airflow resistance must be considered. In other words, the goal is to find a tracheostomy tube that provides sufficient airflow but is not too large for the patient's trachea. Generally, the tracheostomy tube should fill no more than two thirds to three quarters of the tracheal lumen (Simmons, 1990). In view of their generally larger anatomy, men usually receive larger size tracheostomy tubes than women. The decision regarding tube size is often based on clinical judgment. For ventilator-dependent patients, airflow resistance can be assessed via pressure readings of the ventilator. Tracheostomy tube size is an important consideration during communication intervention. Implications of tracheostomy tube size will be discussed in Chapter 5, "Oral Communication Options."

2. Flange

The flange is the neck plate that allows the tracheostomy tube to be held securely in place around the patient's neck. Tracheostomy tube size with the corresponding outer and inner diameter measures is indicated on the flange. The flange extends laterally and has two slits for the tie which threads through and is fastened around the patient's neck, as pictured in Figure 3-6. A flange may be either rigid or more flexible and vary in length. The flange attaches to the outer cannula and rests against the patient's stoma preventing the tube from slipping into or out of the trachea. The attachment of the outer cannula to the flange varies according to manufacturer design. Variations in flange design will be discussed further in this chapter. String ties should be securely fastened to the flange to prevent accidental **decannulation** or removal of the tracheostomy tube.

3. Obturator

The **obturator** is the portion of the tube that is used only during the insertion process and is removed immediately thereafter. It assists the physician or respiratory care practitioner in guiding the tube through the tracheal opening. The obturator is a curved piece which, when inserted into the tracheostomy tube, extends beyond the distal part of the tube to create a rounded end. It is easier to insert this rounded portion of the obturator into the trachea than to attempt to pass the blunt edge of the tube itself. Trauma to the mucosal tissue is thus lessened, especially when the obturator tip is properly lubricated. Figure 3-7 illustrates the placement of the obturator in the outer cannula.

4. Button

The tracheostomy *button* has also been referred to as a plug, cap, or cork. The button or plug comes in several forms. One example is a small, round piece of plastic that is placed into the tracheostomy tube occluding the opening and effectively closing off the tracheostomy tube. Mallinckrodt manufactures a low profile inner cannula that has a closed lumen (or opening) that is used with

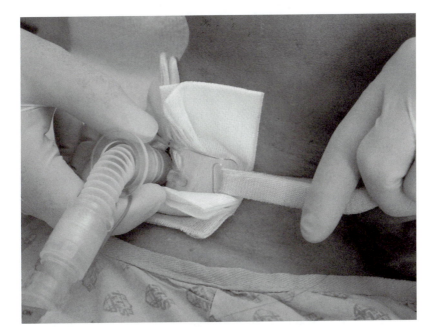

Figure 3-6. A flange securing the tracheostomy tube in place.

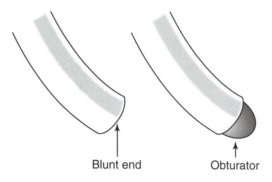

Figure 3-7. An obturator in the outer cannula.

a cuffless tracheostomy tube in order to seal off the tube. If the tracheostomy tube has an inner cannula, it must be removed before the button can be placed into the opening left by the outer cannula. Another variation, a tracheostomy cap, is placed over a fenestrated inner cannula. All of these buttons are used for patients who are learning to breathe on their own, during the weaning and decannulation process. Plugs can be quickly removed for suctioning if the patient is having trouble breathing through the upper airway and must return to using the tracheal airway. Since decannulation plugs are normally used with smaller fenestrated or cuffless tracheostomy tubes, they are often not provided in kits with cuffed, nonfenestrated tracheostomy tubes.

5. Cuff

The cuff has been previously described as an internal balloon which surrounds the outer cannula or body of the tracheostomy tube. The basic structure of the cuff and its components is the same as described above for endotracheal tubes. It is also shown in a detailed diagram in Figure 3-8. The cuff is attached internally to an *inflation line,* which provides the pathway for air to inflate and deflate the balloon. This line leads externally to a *pilot balloon,* which indicates how much air is in the cuff. This pilot balloon contains a spring-loaded valve designed to prevent inadvertent air escape from the cuff. Air is introduced or removed through this valve using a *syringe,* as pictured in Figure 3-9a. A cuff is designed to prevent air from escaping around the tube from the lower to upper airway, especially during mechanical ventilation, and to reduce the risk of aspirated secretions from the upper airway entering the trachea. Figure 3-9b depicts a tracheostomy tube cuff in both deflated and inflated states. Note that the inflated cuff prevents the passage of air to the upper airway. Typically, cuff inflation is required for more medically compromised individuals who cannot tolerate the loss of volume supplied from mechanical ventilation when air is removed from the tracheostomy tube.

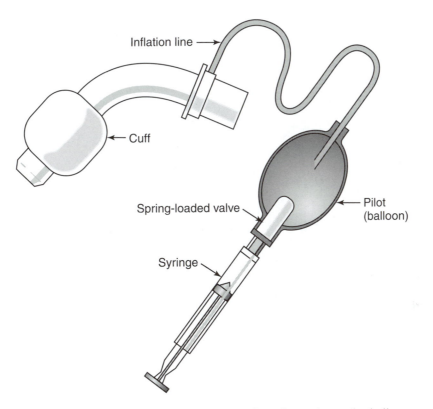

Inflation line

Cuff

Spring-loaded valve

Pilot (balloon)

Syringe

Figure 3-8. Components of a cuff, including the inflation line, pilot balloon, spring-loaded valve, and syringe.

A tracheostomy tube with a double cuff is pictured in Figure 3-10. This tube permits alternate inflation of the cuffs to lessen irritation on one area of the tracheal wall, possibly reducing the danger of tissue necrosis or tracheal malacia.

C. Types of Tracheostomy Tubes

The various features of tracheostomy tubes discussed below are provided on the manufacturer packaging and on the flange of the tube itself. For example, a package will indicate that it contains a cuffed, fenestrated #4 tracheostomy tube with a disposable inner cannula, as pictured in Figure 3-11.

1. Nonfenestrated/Fenestrated

The *nonfenestrated* tracheostomy tube is the standard tube. It may be cuffed or cuffless. A *fenestrated* tracheostomy tube has the addition of a window or

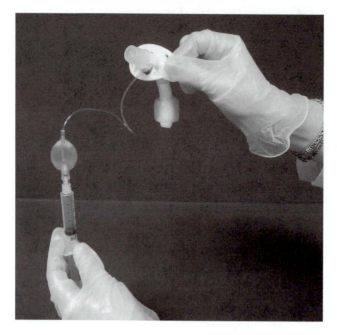

Figure 3-9a. Insertion of air into a cuff.

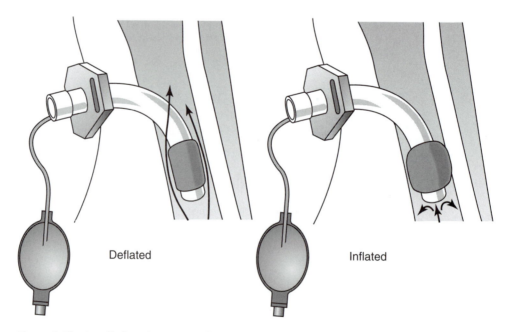

Deflated

Inflated

Figure 3-9b. A cuffed tracheostomy tube in situ, both deflated and inflated.

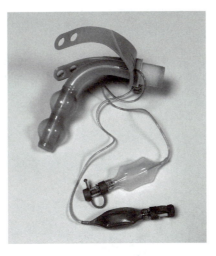

Figure 3-10. A double cuffed tracheostomy tube.

hole on the body of the outer cannula. The **fenestration** may be single or multiple. Figures 3-12a and b picture tracheostomy tubes with single and multiple fenestrations. The purpose of the fenestration is to allow air to pass from the trachea through the fenestration to the vocal folds as illustrated in Figure 3-13. Fenestrated tubes are often ordered by physicians to improve phonation because air that would otherwise pass in and out of the tracheostomy tube can travel through the fenestration to reach the vocal folds. Fenestrated tubes generally are not used in patients at high risk for aspiration due to the risk of passage of secretions or food through the fenestration and into the airway. The fenestration, while providing a path for air upward, can also channel foreign material downward into the tracheostomy and lower airway. Fenestrated tubes are also often used as part of the decannulation process. As a patient's respiratory status improves, the inner cannula can be removed, the tracheostomy tube capped, and the patient allowed to use the upper airway rather than the tracheostomy. When the patient is "capped," air travels upward both around the sides of the tube and through the fenestration.

a. Several important points must be considered when using a fenestrated tracheostomy tube. With currently available double lumen disposable tracheostomy tubes, the inner cannula must be removed if the fenestration is to be utilized. Prefabricated fenestrated inner cannulas are now marketed, but are not disposable. When a nonfenestrated inner cannula is in place, it occludes the opening(s) on the outer cannula. Figure 3-14 illustrates the fenestration open for the passage of air. The addition of the nonfenestrated inner cannula eliminates the use of the fenestration.

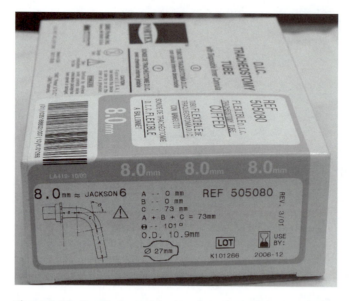

Figure 3-11. Detail of a standard tracheostomy package with size and type information.

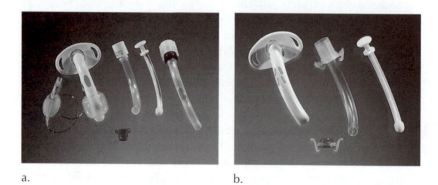

a.   b.

Figure 3-12a. A tracheostomy tube with a single fenestration. (Photo reprinted by permission of Nellcor Puritan Bennett Inc., Pleasanton, CA). **b.** A tracheostomy tube with multiple fenestrations. (Photo reprinted by permission of Nellcor Puritan Bennett Inc., Pleasanton, CA)

The development of the *fenestrated inner cannula* provides the advantage of the fenestration in the presence of a double lumen tube and 15-mm universal hub, as pictured in Figure 3-15. Metal tracheostomy tubes can be specially ordered with fenestrated outer and inner cannulas, so that the inner cannula can be left in place while utilizing the fenestration.

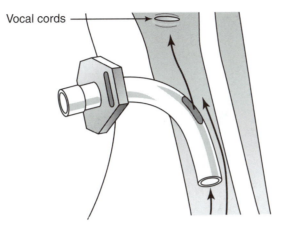

Vocal cords

Figure 3-13. A fenestrated tracheostomy tube in situ.
Airflow passes through the single fenestration.

b. Another issue with the use of fenestrations concerns the *placement of the fenestration* in relation to the tracheal wall. Standard fenestrated tracheostomy tubes are premanufactured. If individual airway variations or size is not taken into account, a potential poor fit of the fenestration can result. The fenestration may be occluded by the tracheal wall so that air will be unable to travel through the opening; this will render the fenestration ineffective. The alignment of the fenestration can be visualized by directing a light into the tracheostomy tube and then, during direct visualization, checking to see if the light can be detected from the fenestration. The difficulty of achieving proper placement of the fenestration in the airway has led some practitioners to custom fenestrate the standard tracheostomy tube. This is attempted by measuring the distance from the stoma site to the anterior inside wall of the trachea (proximal end of the fenestration) and then from the anterior to posterior wall (distal end of the fenestration) (Simmons, 1990). The fenestration is then situated in an unoccluded area. Tracheostomy tube manufacturers concerned with liability issues will often void the product warranty on the tracheostomy tube if physicians manipulate the standard product. Custom fenestrating is not an exact science. Many manufacturers will attempt to custom fenestrate for an individual patient if provided with measurements and physician prescription.

c. *Improperly aligned fenestrations* may result in the development of granulation tissue at the fenestration site. This is due to the rubbing of the edges of the fenestration against the tracheal mucosa. As a result, the tracheostomy tube may become anchored to the tracheal wall and cause significant problems due to associated bleeding during tracheostomy tube

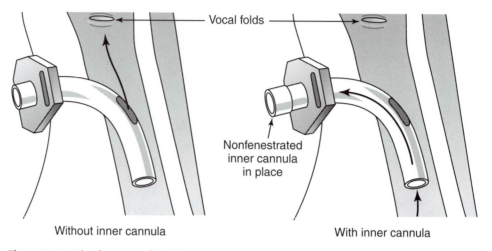

Vocal folds

Nonfenestrated
inner cannula
in place

Without inner cannula   With inner cannula

Figure 3-14. The fenestrated tracheostomy tube. Placement of a nonfenestrated inner cannula blocks the fenestration.

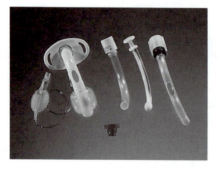

Figure 3-15. A fenestrated inner cannula. (Photo reprinted by permission of Nellcor Puritan Bennett Inc., Pleasanton, CA)

changes. Multiple, smaller fenestrations were developed in an effort to reduce the risk of concentrated tracheal abrasion and the development of granulation in a specific area. Additionally, multiple fenestrations permit the patient to be suctioned without removing the fenestrated inner cannula. Otherwise, the risk would exist that the suction catheter could be directed through the fenestration and not through the length of the tracheostomy tube.

2. Cuffless/Cuffed Tracheostomy Tubes

The **cuffless** tracheostomy tube may be fenestrated or nonfenestrated. *Cuffed* tracheostomy tubes can also be fenestrated or nonfenestrated. The most frequently used tracheostomy tube cuff is the *high volume, low pressure* cuff. This type of cuff, which has been used by the medical community since the 1970s, is designed to lessen the pressure exerted on the tracheal wall even when the cuff is inflated. Simmons (1990) stated that since the diameter of the low pressure cuff is designed to be *greater* than the tracheal diameter, a seal against the tracheal wall can be achieved without the cuff being maximally inflated. In other words, the cuff walls are designed to seal the mucosa without excess pressure and are also designed to evenly distribute pressure. Heffner, Miller, and Sahn (1986b) described this type of cuff as being "floppy" when deflated and noted that, when inflated, the cuff seals the airway without exceeding the capillary perfusion pressure (20–30 mm Hg). The risk of tracheal ischemia is therefore theoretically lessened. Prior to the development of the low pressure cuff, *low volume, high pressure* cuffs were used. These were associated with a much higher incidence of tracheal wall damage because a higher level of cuff pressure was required to achieve the same airway seal. *Pressure-controlled cuffs* are available and have safety valves which are designed to prevent cuff pressures from exceeding 20 mm Hg.

3. Single/Double Lumen Tracheostomy Tubes

Single lumen tubes refer to tracheostomy tubes that consist of only the outer cannula. These tracheostomy tubes are usually used to provide the least amount of airway resistance. The placement of the inner cannula decreases the area available for airflow, although it also provides an additional safety factor in that it can be quickly removed, leaving the airway intact. *Double lumen tubes* are those designed to be used with an outer and an inner cannula, such as a fenestrated tube. This is the standard tracheostomy tube, which has been previously described.

4. Extra Long Tracheostomy Tubes

Extra long tracheostomy tubes are tracheostomy (single lumen) tubes that are used primarily for patients who have special airway needs secondary to changes in their anatomy (e.g., stenosis, tracheal malacia). These tubes are not only longer in length, but can have a proportionately smaller outer diameter. Significant tracheal stenosis or tracheal granuloma, which has developed at the level of the standard length tracheostomy tube, may narrow the airway and cause an unacceptably high upper airway resistance. Placement of an extra long tube bypasses the stenotic area and increases the potential for healing at the irritated site. Additional indications include patients with extensive anatomical changes due to surgical procedures or trauma such as severe burns. Figure 3-16 depicts one type of extra long tube which can actually be adjusted to conform to unusual airway configurations.

D. Manufacturer Variations

Differences among manufacturers may affect the selection of a tracheostomy tube for a particular patient. Variations will be discussed in terms of size, tube angle, cuffs, flanges, and inner cannulas.

1. Size

It is important to understand that tracheostomy tube manufacturers follow different sizing guidelines. The Portex tracheostomy tubes use the inner diameter measurement to identify the size of their tracheostomy tube. For example, a size 6 Portex tracheostomy tube has an inner diameter of 6.0 mm and an outer diameter of 8.5 mm. Conversely, the Shiley tracheostomy tube utilizes the British (Jackson) sizing system for its double lumen tube. Tracheostomy tube size is identified on the tube packaging and on the flange of the tracheostomy tube itself. A clinician recommending change of the tracheostomy tube, either for downsizing during the weaning process or to take advantage of a particular manufacturer's feature, should be aware that one size 6 tracheostomy tube is not necessarily the same as another. The most accurate way to assess tube size is to compare outer and inner diameter measurements. Table 3-1 provides a sample of manufacturer variations with tracheostomy tube size.

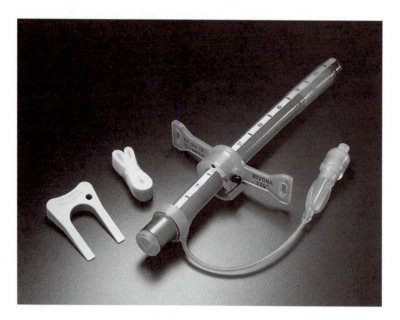

Figure 3-16. Bivona HyperFlex™ tracheostomy tube adjustable for airway angle and length. (Photo courtesy of Portex, Inc./Bivona)

2. Tracheostomy Tube Angle

The angle of the tracheostomy tube varies among manufacturers and material type. For example, the siliconized PVC Portex Blue Line® tracheostomy tube is contoured to a greater degree angle (anatomical curve) than the standard Jackson curve. The Jackson curve refers to the standard curvature tracheostomy tube. The angle of the tracheostomy tube can be one consideration in obtaining the proper fit for a fenestrated tracheostomy tube. If the fit of the fenestration is not satisfactory in one tube, a different tracheostomy tube may change the alignment of the fenestration to the tracheal wall. This positional change can facilitate improved passage of air and result in functional gain from the fenestration. Patient comfort is another consideration in selecting the angle of a tube and is often an individual preference often associated with anatomical configuration. For example, a particular patient may feel more comfortable with a sharper angled as opposed to a less angled tube. Portex, Inc./Bivona's Hyperflex™ tracheostomy tube, as depicted in Figure 3-16, can also be adjusted on a horizontal and vertical plane to accommodate a particular airway angle.

3. Cuffs

Cuffs also differ among manufacturers, although most are the high volume, low pressure type described earlier. Cuffs may differ in type of material, shape, or fit with the tracheostomy tube.

a. The high volume, low pressure cuffs are constructed of a soft plastic that is designed to mold to the walls of the trachea. Recall that the goal of cuff inflation is to obtain a seal against the trachea without exceeding capillary wall pressure. *Foam cuffs* are used when this type of tracheal wall trauma is of particular concern, usually in cases of tracheomalacia. In contrast to the plastic cuffs, foam cuffs are sponge-like. Similar to a sponge, the foam cuff is filled with air at resting position. The cuff will actually self-inflate to equalize cuff pressure and atmospheric pressure. The foam cuff is designed to conform to the contour of the patient's trachea. This particular property of the foam cuff explains its usefulness in cases of tracheal malacia when softening of the tracheal tissues, airway collapse, and further tracheal trauma are of concern. The cuff remains continuously inflated resisting the tendency of the tracheal walls to fall inward. As with any cuff, there are potential risks when using a foam cuff during occlusion of the tracheostomy tube. It is more difficult to completely deflate a sponge cuff. Due to its auto-expanding property, it will reinflate. Occlusion of the tracheostomy tube when any cuff is inflated will significantly increase airway resistance. When the patient tries to take a breath through the mouth or nose, air cannot pass between the tracheal wall and the cuff.

Table 3-1. Manufacturer Variations in Tracheostomy Tube Size. (Courtesy of Bivona Medical Technologies)

TRACHEOSTOMY TUBE CROSS-REFERENCE CHART

ADULT

Low Pressure Cuffed Tubes

BIVONA					SHILEY				PORTEX				
Product Code(s)		I.D. mm	O.D. mm	Length mm	Product Code	I.D. mm	O.D. mm	Length mm	Product Code	I.D. mm	O.D. mm	Length mm	
				Single Cannula				Inner Cannula					Inner Cannula
MR Aire-Cuf®	Fome-Cuf®												
750150	850150	5.0	7.3	60	4DCT	5.0	9.4	62	503060	5.0	8.5	67	
750160	850160	6.0	8.7	70	6DCT	6.5	10.8	74	503070	6.0	9.9	73	
750170	850170	7.0	10.0	80	8DCT	7.6	12.2	79	503080	7.0	11.3	78	
750180	850180	8.0	11.0	88	10DCT	8.9	13.8	79	503090	8.0	12.6	84	
750190	850190	9.0	12.3	98					503100	9.0	14.0	84	
750195	850195	9.5	13.3	98									

Cuffed Weaning or Fenestrated Tubes

BIVONA					SHILEY				PORTEX			
		I.D. mm	O.D. mm	Length mm	Product Code	I.D. mm	O.D. mm	Length mm	Product Code	I.D. mm	O.D. mm	Length mm
TTS™ Cuff				Single Cannula				Inner Cannula Low Pressure Cuff				Inner Cannula Low Pressure Cuff
670150		5.0	7.3	60	4DFEN	5.0	9.4	62	513060	5.0	8.5	67
670160		6.0	8.7	70	6DFEN	6.5	10.8	74	513070	6.0	9.9	73
670170		7.0	10.0	80	8DFEN	7.6	12.2	79	513080	7.0	11.3	78
670180		8.0	11.0	88					513100	9.0	14.0	84
670190		9.0	12.3	98								

Cuffed Single Cannula Tubes

MR Aire-Cuf®	Fome-Cuf®				Low Pressure Cuff					Single Cannula			
750150	850150	5.0	7.3	60	5SCT	5.0	7.0	58					
750160	850160	6.0	8.7	70	6SCT	6.0	8.3	67	530060	6.0	8.3	55
750170	850170	7.0	10.0	80	7SCT	7.0	9.6	80	530070	7.0	9.7	75
750180	850180	8.0	11.0	88	8SCT	8.0	10.9	89	530080	8.0	11.0	82
750190	850190	9.0	12.3	98	9SCT	9.0	12.1	99	530090	9.0	12.4	87
750195	850195	9.5	13.3	98	10SCT	10.0	13.3	105	530100	10.0	13.8	98

Cuffless Profile Tubes

TTS Cuff™	Cuffless				Inner Cannula					Single Cannula			
670150	60A150	5.0	7.3	60									
670160	60A160	6.0	8.7	70	4CFS	5.0	9.4	65	550060	6.0	8.3	55
670170	60A170	7.0	10.0	80	6CFS	6.4	10.8	76	550070	7.0	9.7	75
670180	60A180	8.0	11.0	88	8CFS	7.6	12.2	81	550080	8.0	11.0	82
670190	60A190	9.0	12.3	98	10CFS	8.9	13.8	81	550090	9.0	12.4	87
670195	60A195	9.5	13.3	98					530100	10.0	13.8	98

Adjustable Hyperflex

TTS™ Cuff	MR Aire-Cuf®			Maximum Usable Length (mm)
67HA60	75HA60	6.0	8.7	110
67HA70	75HA70	7.0	10.0	120
67HA80	75HA80	8.0	11.0	130
67HA90	75HA90	9.0	12.3	140

In addition, the occlusion of the tracheostomy stoma eliminates use of the tube. Therefore, both the upper and lower respiratory tracts are rendered ineffective. For that reason, foam cuffs are often used with patients who have special airway needs and with patients whose tubes will not be occluded. Portex, Inc./Bivona is the manufacturer of the Bivona Fome-Cuf® pictured in Figure 3-17a.

b. The shape of the tracheostomy tube cuff also varies among manufacturers. Shiley tubes feature the barrel-shaped (cylindrical) cuff. In theory, this cuff is designed by the manufacturer to provide more even distribution of cuff pressures throughout the trachea. On the extra-length tracheostomy tubes, the cuff is larger and longer, again theoretically to change pressure distribution. Portex distributes a barrel-shaped cuff and also markets a spherically shaped cuff on their blue line tracheostomy tubes. It appears that, when inflated, the spherically shaped cuff contacts the tracheal wall along a smaller area than the barrel-shaped cuff. Portex, Inc./Bivona Fome-Cuf® and Aire-Cuf® are oval or egg shaped. The clinical implications of these differently shaped cuffs are not known at this time.

c. The *fit of the cuff to the tracheostomy tube* also varies among manufacturers. When most cuffs are deflated they are not flush against the tube; extra bulk does remain protruding into the trachea. Ridges from the deflated cuff may also be formed around the tracheostomy tube. This may have implications for increased secretion retention and higher airway resistance, and may be of particular concern when occluding a tracheostomy tube for oral communication or during the decannulation process. Further discussion will follow in Chapter 5. Portex, Inc./Bivona offers a unique feature they refer to as their Tight to Shaft™ cuff. This is designed to offer a cuffed tracheostomy tube that not only can be partially or fully inflated, but when fully deflated leaves no additional bulk on the outer diameter of the outer cannula. This feature may offer versatility when problems with tracheostomy occlusion and oral communication arise. The Tight to Shaft™ tracheostomy tube is pictured in Figure 3-17b.

d. All of these plastic tracheostomy tubes have the cuffs permanently molded onto the outer cannula. Cuff detachment is uncommon for this reason. Recall from the earlier discussion of metal tracheostomy tubes that metal tubes are not manufactured with cuffs. A cuff can be attached if a metal tube is being used, but the risk of detachment is heightened. This option, a metal tracheostomy tube with an attached cuff, is rarely used with tracheotomized patients.

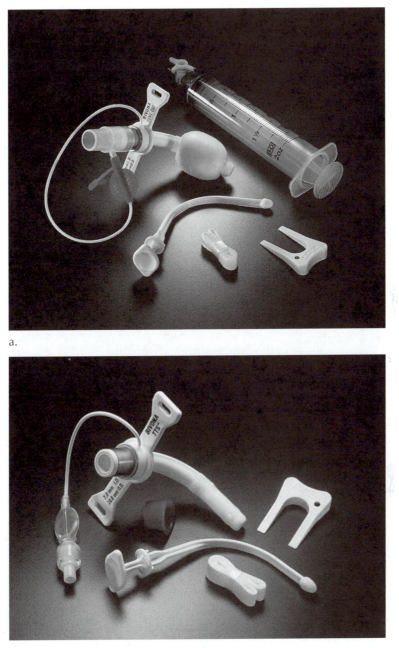

a.

b.

Figure 3-17a. A Bivona Fome-Cuf® tracheostomy tube kit. (Photo courtesy of Portex, Inc./Bivona). **b.** A Bivona TTS™ (Tight to Shaft) Aire-Cuf® tracheostomy tube. (Photo courtesy of Portex, Inc./Bivona)

4. Flange

Flanges on tracheostomy tubes differ and may affect patient comfort. They range from the more rigid types to softer and "winged" designs. Some manufacturers offer swivel attachments to allow vertical movement but minimize lateral movement of the outer cannula. The type of flange may affect the movement of the tracheostomy tube respective to the patient's movements. By nature of their composition, metal tracheostomy tubes have rigid flanges. These flanges are small and can offer a swivel attachment. For long-term tracheostomy patients the type of flange may be an issue in the patient's tolerance and comfort. A change from one type to another may help to relieve or reduce potential irritation. The patient's report of comfort with a particular tube is very important.

5. Inner Cannulas

The variations among types of inner cannulas include differences in the texture of the inner cannula, the presence or absence of the 15-mm connection, and the design of the proximal end.

a. Portex, Inc. offers a flexible, corrugated inner cannula which is designed to fit the particular angle of the Blue Line® tracheostomy tube. In contrast, smooth inner cannulas are offered by Portex and many other manufacturers of both disposable and nondisposable tubes.

b. The 15 mm connection is found on the inner rather than on the outer cannula of the Shiley and some metal tracheostomy tubes. This is important for patients who require this standard connection to mechanical ventilation. Portex and Bivona are examples of tracheostomy tubes that allow for connection to mechanical ventilation via the 15-mm hub of the outer cannula.

c. Portex offers an inner cannula with a coiled end. This end locks securely into place. Once the inner cannula is removed, however, the coil is pulled out of alignment and protrudes from the outer cannula. This design has implications for connection to oral communication devices such as speaking valves, which will be discussed in Chapter 5.

E. Variations on Standard Tracheostomy Tubes

There are numerous variations on standard tracheostomy tubes. Companies offer variations to the standard tracheostomy tube with, for example, custom fenestrations, cuff placement, or special tube length or angle. This must be ordered by physician prescription. Customizations may address specific airway management problems. For example, for the patient with an oversized tracheostoma creating excessive air leak around the sides of a tracheostomy tube, a "stoma seal" tracheostomy tube may be manufactured. A stoma seal or cuff is placed directly behind the flange of the outer cannula and can be inflated to block airflow from escaping through the stoma. Tracheostomy tube manufacturers may be contacted regarding their options for customization. Tracheostomy tubes may also be designed to assist with communication or to aid in the transitional weaning process. These variations include **talking tracheostomy tubes, tracheal buttons,** and specialty **cannulas. Laryngectomy tubes** have different indications than tracheostomy tubes and will be discussed separately.

1. Talking Tracheostomy Tubes

a. Talking tracheostomy tubes are used specifically for patients, usually ventilator dependent, who *cannot* tolerate a deflated tracheostomy tube cuff. This may occur when a patient requires maximum air from the ventilator and cannot tolerate any leak of air from the lower to the upper airway. It may also be secondary to severe, chronic aspiration of secretions. When a cuff is deflated, air can leak up through the larynx and escape through the nose and mouth. When the cuff is inflated, air does not reach the vocal folds and the patient cannot achieve voice. In this case a talking tracheostomy tube might be utilized. Talking tracheostomy tubes are generally not placed within the first 5 days following surgery because of the potential for air leakage (Heffner, Miller, & Sahn, 1986a). Figure 3-18 illustrates the components of a talking tracheostomy tube. A talking tracheostomy tube looks basically like a standard cuffed tracheostomy tube except for the addition of an external air tube that is connected to a source of compressed air. This additional tube has an opening above the level of the cuff. Air is directed through this tube into the trachea above the cuff. Air then passes up through the vocal folds. A continuous source of airflow is therefore available for phonation. With a talking tracheostomy tube, ventilation and phonation are facilitated by separate air sources. The patient is breathing with airflow supplied by the ventilator and talking on air supplied by an external source, such as a tank of oxygen. The flow is regulated by a small port on the external line. When the port is covered, air flows through the tube into the trachea and reaches the vocal folds. When the port is open, the airflow is not directed into the trachea. The talking tracheostomy tube therefore differs from the standard cuffed tracheostomy tube due to the additional air tube. A talking tracheostomy tube can allow the previously aphonic patient to voice. Further discussion of candidacy issues and techniques for use will follow in Chapter 5.

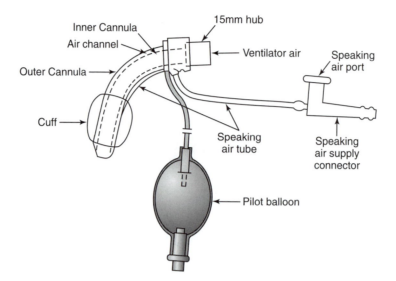

Figure 3-18. The components of the "talking" tracheostomy tube.

2. Other Specialized Tracheostomy Tubes

a. The Tucker Tube contains an inner cannula that is used with metal Jackson or Tucker tracheostomy tubes. It can facilitate phonation by way of a fenestrated silver cannula containing a hinged valve that swings open when the patient inspires, allowing air to enter the trachea. On expiration, the valve falls into a closed position and blocks off the tracheostomy tube, funneling air through the upper airway. The Tucker Tube is pictured in Figure 3-19.

b. Boston Medical Products markets Tracoe tracheostomy tubes in two types: Tracoe Comfort and Tracoe Twist tubes. The pliable Tracoe Twist tubes are designed with a swivel flange that can move both vertically and horizontally. This feature is designed to increase patient comfort. The Tracoe Comfort, a flexible clear tube, is designed to maximize patient comfort with its light weight and clear plastic design. Both tracheostomy tubes provide options for speaking valves integrated on the inner cannula. The valve allows air to enter the trachea through the inner cannula during inspiration, but closes during expiration to redirect air for phonation.

3. Tracheal Buttons

a. Tracheal buttons are prosthetic devices used to maintain an open stoma after tracheostomy tube removal. A patient who has a tracheal button in

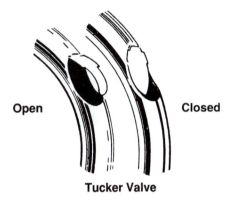

Open   **Closed**

Tucker Valve

Figure 3-19. The Tucker Tube. (Courtesy of Pilling Surgical)

place no longer breathes via the stoma. The button serves to plug the stoma. This device also maintains the opening in the anterior tracheal wall. This provides a pathway for emergency reinsertion of a tracheostomy tube. Therefore, a tracheal button is indicated for patients with neurological or pulmonary conditions that may exacerbate periodically and create a need for long-term airway suctioning or mechanical ventilation. It may also be used during the process of weaning a patient from a tracheostomy tube. Instead of requiring repeated intubations or surgical procedures, patients can use a tracheal button or closure plug over an extended period. If necessary, it can easily be replaced with a tracheostomy tube.

The Olympic Trach-Button is one example of a closure plug. Figure 3-20 pictures this type of stoma plug. The Olympic offers an adapter for suctioning or artificial ventilation. The adapter is an open cannula. When it is in place, the patient can use the now-open tracheal airway. As with an inner cannula, the adapter narrows the lumen of the closure plug. The distal end of the Trach-Button contains a petaled end which expands in the trachea, securing it in place. A properly sized tracheal button does not require a tie string to prevent it from dislodging from the stoma. Tracheal buttons must be carefully measured to ensure that the cannula extends from the stoma to the anterior tracheal wall. Because commercially available buttons come in standard sizes, the button may protrude from the stoma. Sizing rings are available to stabilize the portion of the button that extends beyond the stoma and prevent extraneous movement of the button. These sizing rings fill the gap between the tip of the button and the stoma. Due to difficulties involved with proper sizing, some physicians custom design tracheal buttons for their patients (A. Alba, personal communication, March 1989). Long and West (1981) describe the use of an

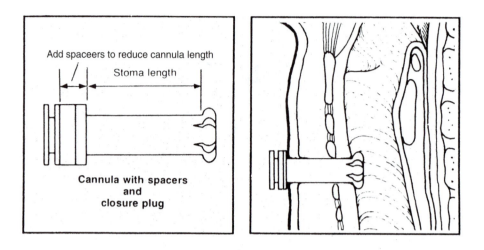

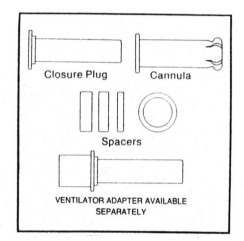

Figure 3-20. The Olympic Trach-Button™. (Courtesy of Olympic Medical Corp.)

Olympic Trach-Button following tracheostomy tube removal in patients discharged to the home care setting.

4. Specialty Cannulas

Specially designed cannula systems, which can in some cases take the place of a tracheostomy tube, also serve to maintain openings in the stoma and anterior tracheal wall. Similar to tracheal buttons, access to the tracheal airway is maintained without the presence of a tube in the trachea. The Montgomery

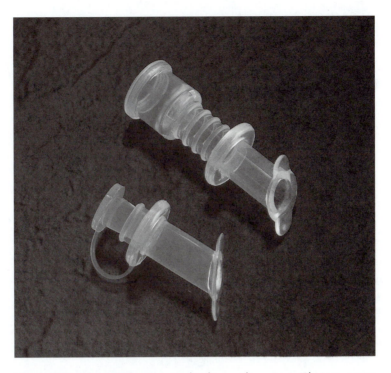

Figure 3-21. The Montgomery tracheal cannula system. (Photo courtesy of Boston Medical Products, Inc.)

cannula system, pictured in Figure 3-21, was developed as an alternative to a long-term tracheostomy tube. It is marketed with either a plug or a **speaking valve** which fits on the tracheal cannula and allows phonation. The plug closes the cannula completely, so that the patient breathes entirely through the upper airway. The speaking valve, with its flexible hinged silicone diaphragm, allows one-way airflow during inspiration and closes during expiration through the long-term cannula. The distal end of the Montgomery tracheal cannula is flanged to secure it in the trachea. Special grooves assist in maintaining secure positioning and eliminate the need for a tie string. Sizing issues are similar to those with tracheal buttons.

5. Speaking Valves

A speaking valve is a one-way valve that allows air to enter the tracheostomy tube when the patient inspires. On expiration, the valve is closed, blocking air from exiting through the cannula or tracheostomy tube. Air is directed upward through the vocal folds and is available for phonation or coughing/clearing

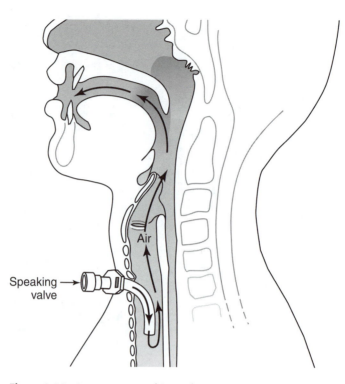

Figure 3-22. A one-way speaking valve.

of secretions. Speaking valves will be discussed in Chapter 5, including an in-depth description of one-way valves and indications for their use. Figure 3-22 illustrates the function of a one-way speaking valve.

F. Laryngectomy Tubes

Laryngectomy tubes are different from tracheostomy tubes. They are used for individuals who have had a *laryngectomy,* or removal of the larynx. This surgical procedure is usually performed on individuals who present with carcinoma in the laryngeal area. With a laryngectomy, the trachea is connected directly to the outer stoma, as pictured in Figure 3-23. Laryngectomy tubes are generally used after the initial surgical procedure and serve as a stent to maintain the newly formed stoma and maintain the airway opening. They may also be used in individuals who have difficulty keeping the stoma free of dried secretions. Laryngectomy tubes are shorter than standard tracheostomy tubes because the distance from the stoma into the trachea has been lessened by the surgical procedure. Laryngectomy tubes are also available in a variety of materials, both plastic and metal. A laryngectomy tube is pictured in Figure 3-24.

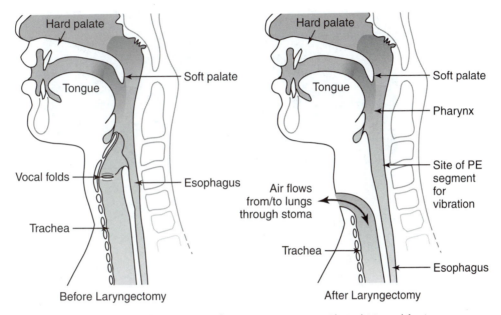

Figure 3-23. Alteration of the airway via laryngectomy. (From *Clinical Manual for Laryngectomy and Head and Neck Cancer Rehabilitation,* by J. K. Casper & R. H. Colton, 1993, p. 66. Clifton Park, NY: Singular.)

G. Impact of Tracheostomy on Phonation and Other Functions

1. Redirection of Airflow

The placement of a tracheostomy tube into the trachea impedes the normal flow of air to the larynx. Instead of air passing through the upper respiratory tract during inspiration and expiration, the majority of air enters and leaves the tracheostomy tube. This is illustrated in Figure 3-25. Because the tube is placed below the vocal folds, the air stream bypasses the larynx. However, a small air leak may permit some air to reach the vocal folds. This disturbance of airflow and interruption of normal vocal fold function has widespread implications for the entire respiratory/phonatory system.

a. Dysphonia/aphonia

The majority of airflow is redirected out of the tracheostomy tube during expiration. Residual air may pass upward toward the vocal folds but is usually insufficient to produce normal voice. Patients will therefore become *dysphonic*. If air is prevented from reaching the vocal folds at all, the patient becomes *aphonic*. Whether the patient is dys-

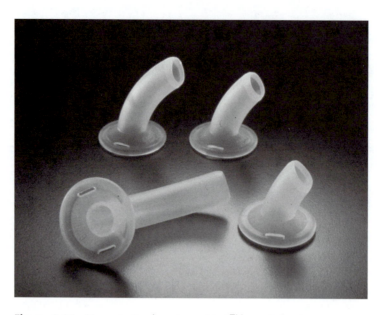

Figure 3-24. Bivona's Tracheostoma Vent™ used for laryngectomy patients. (Photo courtesy of Portex, Inc./Bivona)

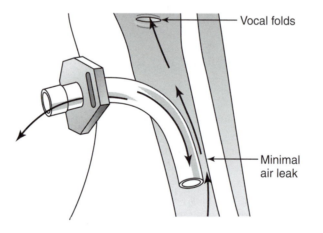

Figure 3-25. Redirection of airflow following placement of a tracheostomy tube.

phonic or aphonic at least partially depends on the size of the tracheostomy tube relative to the tracheal lumen. In other words, as the size of the tracheostomy tube increases, the space between the tube and the tracheal walls decreases. The amount of air that can potentially pass around the tracheostomy tube and reach the vocal folds will decrease proportionately.

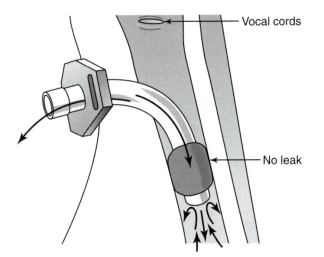

Figure 3-26. Function of the inflated cuff in stopping air-flow to the upper airway.

In addition to tracheostomy tube size, the cuff on the tracheostomy tube also has a major impact on the patient's ability to produce voice. If the cuff is deflated, at least a small amount of air may be able to pass around the tracheostomy tube and reach the vocal folds. However, the residual air is usually not sufficient to produce normal phonation. The presence of an inflated tracheostomy tube cuff usually creates aphonia as air cannot pass between the cuff and the tracheal wall. Figure 3-26 illustrates the passage of airflow through the cuffed tracheostomy tube. Airflow does not reach the upper airway.

b. Difficulty with secretion control

Oral secretion control is disrupted in several ways by the presence of a tracheostomy tube. Tracheotomized patients will often notice an increase in their secretions. This is due to the disruption of normal airflow.

(1) Since airflow through the nose and mouth is reduced with a tracheostomy tube in place, the usual process of evaporation of oral secretions cannot take place. Oral secretions therefore accumulate.

(2) The normal mucociliary process of filtration and hydration is also disrupted. Mucus is produced by the goblet cells that line the upper airway as a natural lubricant. This natural lubricant maintains a moist environment and traps small debris that enters the airway. The cilia of the *epithelial columnar cells* then act to expel this mucus and any foreign material. When the tracheostomy tube is placed, this lubrication and filtration system is bypassed. Air entering and

leaving the tracheostomy tube is not warmed or filtered, and the lower respiratory tract is more vulnerable to irritants. In addition, more secretions are produced, and there is greater chance for them to accumulate.

(3) Clearance of this increased amount of secretions is further reduced secondary to the tracheotomized patient's inability to produce an effective cough. Because air cannot reach the vocal folds, the air pressure available to forcefully exhale and clear any accumulated mucus is lessened. Oral and tracheal suctioning becomes necessary under these conditions.

c. Disruption of vocal fold function

When air is diverted away from the larynx for extended periods of time, the sensitivity of the larynx is altered. The **glottic closure response** occurs when foreign material enters the laryngeal area. Normally, the vocal folds will quickly adduct to seal off the airway below. The placement of the tracheostomy tube, with its subsequent long-term diversion of airflow away from the larynx, leads to decreased sensitivity and altered coordination of this response. Material may penetrate the larynx without eliciting this reflexive glottal closure response (Nash, 1988; Shaker, 2000). This predisposes the patient to chronic entry of secretions and/or food into the trachea, potentially leading to pulmonary infections.

d. Decreased subglottic pressure

The ability to generate pressure below the level of the vocal folds is affected in patients with tracheotomies. This reduction in subglottic pressure is due to the expulsion of air from the tracheostomy tube whenever the patient attempts to create pressure in the airway. When airflow is redirected, other activities are also affected. The ability to produce intrathoracic air pressure during maximal vocal fold closure is referred to as a **Valsalva maneuver**. The Valsalva is useful during defecation or any type of forceful lifting. Patients with unoccluded tracheostomies cannot produce an effective Valsalva maneuver.

e. Sensory impairments

The redirection of airflow affects the ability to smell and to taste. In order for a patient to maintain these senses air must travel through the nasal and oral cavities. With air, sensory molecules stimulate the chemoreceptor cells which include the olfactory receptors in the nasal mucosa and taste buds of the tongue and mouth. Tracheostomized patients often report decreased smell and taste with subsequent reduction in appetite.

H. Potential Hazards of Long-term Cuff Inflation

1. Complications

Chapter 2 described the long-term complications associated with tracheostomy and the risks associated with tracheostomy tube cuff inflation. With the advent of high volume, low pressure tracheostomy tube cuffs the incidence of tracheal stenosis has lessened. However, the risk of damage to the tracheal mucosa still exists when excessive cuff pressure is utilized. Heffner et al. (1986b) note that the soft "floppy" characteristic of the low pressure cuff is lost when air even slightly exceeds 20 mm Hg. The low pressure cuff then acts like a high pressure cuff. The description of the pressure-volume curve by Heffner et al. (1986b) explains how the high volume, low pressure cuff changes to display low volume, high pressure characteristics. This response appears to occur due to the presence of the cuff in the small confined area of the trachea. In other words, the cuff remains floppy and distensible under test conditions, but when in an enclosed area such as the trachea, even small increases in cuff volume produce subsequent high pressures. A high pressure cuff is associated with a much greater incidence of erosion of tracheal cartilage and mucosa, with the subsequent development of tracheal stenosis, tracheal malacia, and, more rarely, tracheoesophageal and tracheoinnominate fistulas. Practitioners who are not aware of the dangers of adding additional air to low pressure cuffs may place patients at risk for these significant complications. Clinically, a chronic pattern emerges where the tracheal walls around the overinflated cuff begin to soften and break down. As a result, the cuff to tracheal wall seal is destroyed. As the space around the cuff is eroded, an air leak is evidenced. The practitioner attempts to obtain a seal by injecting more air into the cuff. The pattern continues with the resultant effect on the tracheal tissue. Heffner et al. (1986b) stated, "because of the above problems, careful management of cuff inflation is imperative" (p. 432). Figure 3-27 illustrates the selected complications associated with cuff inflation.

2. Effect on Function

a. Desensitization of the larynx

The redirection of airflow by the tracheostomy tube is compounded by the long-term use of an inflated tracheostomy tube cuff. A cuff provides a seal that prevents airflow from reaching the larynx and exacerbates the complications of the tracheostomy tube. Although the maintenance of the air-tight cuff seal may be desirable for pulmonary demands, especially for the ventilator-dependent patient, the cessation of airflow through the larynx greatly impairs normal functioning. Sasaki, Suzuki, Horiuchi, and

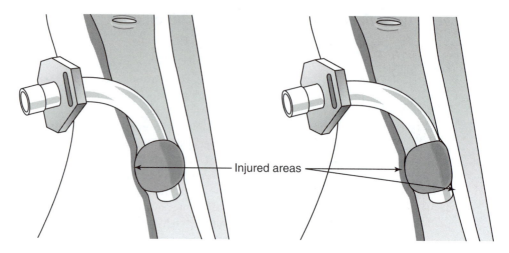

Figure 3-27. Complications of inflated cuffs.

Kirshner (1977) described the negative impact of tracheostomy on the normal laryngeal closure reflex.

(1) Unproductive cough

Individuals with tracheostomy and cuff inflation have both decreased sensitivity to the entry of foreign material into the larynx and an inability to generate the airflow needed for a productive cough. When secretions and foreign materials enter the unprotected larynx, they pool above the level of the cuff. They must be removed by tracheal suctioning because the patient's protective cough reflex has been eliminated. For patients with long-term cuff inflation, this protective function does not immediately return once the cuff is deflated. Individuals with cuffed tracheostomy tubes will also evidence a significant amount of oral secretions because airflow is not available to evaporate the patient's saliva. Oral suctioning is frequently needed to clear secretions from the oral cavity.

3. Management of Cuff Pressures

a. Measuring cuff pressures

Manipulation of the external balloon of the cuff is one method often used to determine inflation of the cuff. However, finger estimation of cuff pressure is not reliable. Fernandez, Blanch, Mancebo, Bonsoms, and Artigas (1990) demonstrated that the reliability of cuff pressure estimation by finger manipulation is very low and concluded that intracuff pressures must be objectively measured. This is done by the use of *cuff manometry*. The manometer is connected to the cuff pilot line. The amount of pressure

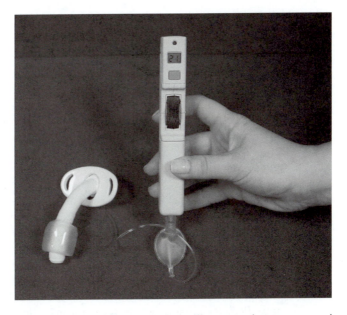

Figure 3-28. Tracheostomy tube cuff pressure being measured via manometry.

exerted on the tracheal wall is displayed on the manometer as pictured in Figure 3-28. Pressure controlled cuffs are useful in minimizing the risk of tracheal injury due to cuff overinflation.

(1) Although measuring cuff pressure is vital, the clinician must also assess cuff volume. The dynamics of each patient's airway, especially patients who are on ventilators, is different. A set cuff pressure (below 20 mm Hg) may not be ideal for each patient in all the positions, activities and so on throughout the day. The clinician must use a stethoscope to assess cuff volume to adequately ensure that cuff pressures do not place the patient at risk for tracheal injury. There are devices, such as the Posey Cufflator, that automatically control cuff pressures. The device attaches to the cuff inflation line. Intracuff pressure is displayed on a color-coded dial, and air can be added to or released from the cuff as necessary.

b. Minimal leak/minimal occluding volume techniques

The minimal leak technique and the minimal occluding volume technique are two alternatives used to safely inflate the tracheostomy tube cuff.

(1) Minimal leak technique involves the insertion of air into the cuff until an air seal is obtained. The patient exhales through the mouth and nose as the cuff is slowly inflated. A stethoscope can also be used to monitor the upper airway. When air can no longer be detected, either through the mouth or via the stethoscope, a seal is assumed. A small amount of air is then removed from the pilot balloon, creating the minimal leak.

(2) Minimal occluding volume involves inflating the cuff to the point where air can no longer be heard, via *auscultation* (with a stethoscope), escaping around the cuff into the upper airway. Once the seal is obtained, air is no longer inserted.

c. Suctioning protocol

Suctioning technique in the presence of an inflated tracheostomy tube cuff requires an understanding of the mechanism of the cuff and the potential for foreign material to collect in the airway above the level of the cuff. Suctioning a patient through the tracheostomy tube with an inflated cuff will not remove the pooled secretions and aspirated material present above the cuff itself. This is pictured in Figure 3-29. The suction catheter merely enters and clears the secretions inside and below the tracheostomy tube. Pooled secretions held by the cuff can be cleared only by suctioning via the mouth and through the vocal folds or after cuff deflation. The much preferred route is to begin with the tracheostomy tube cuff inflated, insert the suction catheter through the tracheostomy tube and into the trachea, and then deflate the cuff. This procedure should remove the majority of material that has collected above the inflated cuff. Because foreign

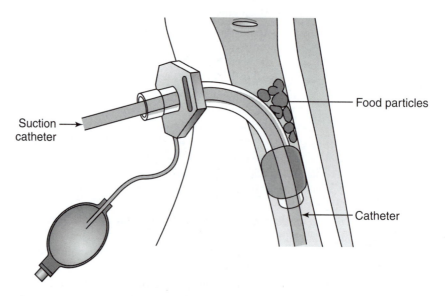

Figure 3-29. Suctioning with an inflated cuff, leaving food particles trapped on top of the cuff.

material can easily colonize undesirable bacteria if allowed to pool above the cuff, it is important to periodically deflate the cuff and suction with this technique. A small amount of material can still escape into the trachea when the catheter is placed and the cuff is deflated. Therefore, routine deflation is even more imperative to prevent the accumulation of material that collects above the cuff.

Once familiar with the various types of tracheostomy tubes available for airway management and intervention with the tracheostomized patient, the clinician will be able to make recommendations that will optimize communication and swallowing management.

4

Mechanical Ventilation

Clinicians who work with individuals who are tracheostomized and/or ventilator dependent must have an understanding of the basic principles of mechanical ventilation. The pulmonologist and respiratory care practitioner are primarily responsible for making decisions regarding the need for mechanical support and the mode of ventilation. Respiratory therapy is usually responsible for the daily operation of the ventilator, while nursing assists in assessing the patient's clinical response to particular settings. When feasible, all three disciplines work toward the ultimate goal of weaning. Other allied health professionals, such as the speech-language pathologist, recommend modifications of ventilatory settings that will facilitate speech and swallowing. Therefore, the clinician not only must be familiar with the terminology and general operating principles of the ventilator but appreciate the physiologic impact of mechanical ventilation on the airway.

This chapter will review the indications for mechanical ventilation including the causes of respiratory failure, ventilator operations, modes of ventilation, ventilator settings, equipment, and monitoring tools.

I. INDICATIONS FOR MECHANICAL VENTILATION

A patient is placed on mechanical ventilation when there is a disruption in the normal process of exchange of air in and out of the lungs. At the level of the alveoli, gas exchange is the transfer of oxygen and carbon dioxide between the pulmonary capillaries and alveoli. The terms **PAO_2** and **$PACO_2$** define alveolar gas pressure. **PaO_2** and **$PaCO_2$** are used to describe the partial pressure of oxygen and carbon dioxide dissolved in the arterial blood. **Partial pressure** refers to the force that is necessary to move the oxygen from air to blood (PAO_2) and then from blood to body tissues (PaO_2).

Table 4-1. Normal Arterial Blood Gases Values (at Sea Level on Room Air).

TERMS	NORMAL RANGE
Acid-Base Balance (pH)	7.35–7.45
Arterial Carbon Dioxide (PaCO$_2$)	35–45 mm Hg
Arterial Oxygen (PaO$_2$)	80–100 mm Hg
Bicarbonate Ion (HCO$_3$–)	22–26 mEq
Arterial Oxygen Saturation (SaO$_2$)	95%>
Hemoglobin (Hgb)	12–18 g/100 ml

Note: ABG also represents oxygen content (PaO$_2$; SaO$_2$; and Hgb)

This process is reversed for CO$_2$. The adequacy of ventilation is determined by obtaining and analyzing a patient's **arterial blood gases (ABGs).** ABGs also indicate the acid-base or pH status of the blood. Normal arterial blood gas levels are illustrated in Table 4-1. ABG results are one of the factors used in determining the need for a patient to be placed on **mechanical ventilation.**

A. Impairment of the Respiratory Mechanism

When there is failure of the respiratory system and respiratory muscles, as in diseases described in Chapter 1, the physical mechanism that moves air in and out of the lungs is impaired. Failure of the respiratory drive mechanism, at the level of the brainstem, will also impair the movement of air in and out of the lung. In both cases, carbon dioxide in the blood (PaCO$_2$) increases, and oxygen in the blood (PaO$_2$) decreases. Respiratory muscle failure per se causes accumulation of carbon dioxide resulting in underventilation or *alveolar hypoventilation.* Failure of the respiratory drive results in *central alveolar hypoventilation* despite adequate respiratory muscle strength. Hypoventilation is inadequate ventilation which will ultimately affect gas exchange at the level of the alveoli. A patient with either or both of these conditions will require some type of mechanical ventilatory support to assist in the gas exchange process, resuming the movement of air in and out of the lungs.

B. Intrinsic Lung Disease

Patients with disease at the level of the lungs may have an adequate respiratory mechanism, especially at the beginning stages of the disease. However, the change in the diseased lung tissue affects oxygen exchange at the level of the alveoli. PaO$_2$ decreases and the patient may benefit from supplemental oxygen. As the disease progresses, the PaCO$_2$ may increase. If other body systems cannot compensate, and respiratory failure occurs, the $PaCO_2$ increases to the point that the patient requires mechanical ventilatory support.

C. Understanding Arterial Blood Gases

1. Arterial blood gas values indicate the amount of oxygen in blood plasma (PaO_2), the amount of carbon dioxide in blood plasma ($PaCO_2$), and the *acid-base balance (pH)*. The normal value for PaO_2 on room air is between 80–100 mm Hg; the normal $PaCO_2$ is between 35–45 mm Hg. (The measurement mm Hg is a pressure measurement, with 1 millimeter of mercury equivalent to 1.36 centimeters of water, or cm H_2O. This represents a tension or resistance that can be measured in specific increments.) Levels of hemoglobin are also reflected in the arterial blood gas. Recall that hemoglobin is the protein by which oxygen is transported. **SaO_2** reflects "the extent to which hemoglobin is saturated with oxygen" (Hough, 1991, p. 8). The pH measures the acid-base balance of the blood and normally falls between 7.35 and 7.45. The pH is contingent upon the levels of the hydrogen ion (H+). Abnormalities in this value may be indicative of some type of respiratory status change, but may also reflect a metabolic disturbance. Disturbances in blood gas levels known as acid-base disorders are called **acidosis** and **alkalosis.** *Respiratory acidosis* or *respiratory alkalosis* is caused by dysfunction in the "ventilatory control mechanism or in the breathing apparatus itself" (Levitzky, Cairo, & Hall, 1990, p. 141). *Metabolic acidosis* or *metabolic alkalosis* can be caused by a dysfunction in normal renal function which disrupts the acid-base balance (pH) (Eubanks & Bone, 1990). Additionally, there are other metabolic causes of acidosis and alkalosis, including diabetes and sepsis, usually involving a failure of multiple body organs. Definitions of acidosis and alkalosis are provided in Table 4-2.

   a. Acidosis is a condition that can be categorized as either *respiratory* or *metabolic.* Acidosis occurs when there is a decrease in pH value to less than 7.35 indicating that there is too much acidity in the blood. Respiratory acidosis is associated with elevated $PaCO_2$ levels due to alveolar hypoventilation. Elevated $PaCO_2$ causes the pH to decrease. A blood gas reading that indicates elevated $PaCO_2$ with decreased pH (inverse relationship) indicates that the patient has an *uncompensated (acute) respiratory acidosis.* The renal system will attempt to compensate for this condition by excreting hydrogen ions (H+), as ammonia, in urine *or* by conserving bicarbonate (HCO_3). It normally takes about 24 hours for the kidneys to respond to this change in the status of the blood. If the renal system is not functioning, this compensation will not take place.

   Uncompensated (acute) metabolic acidosis as with respiratory acidosis is also associated with decreased pH. The blood gas analysis will also show increased hydrogen ion (H+) or decreased bicarbonate (HCO_3-).

Table 4-2. Definitions of Acidosis and Alkalosis.

Acidosis: a decrease in pH value, less than 7.35			
Respiratory: retention of CO_2 (hypoventilation)	pH	α	$\dfrac{[HCO_3-]}{PaCO_2}$
Metabolic: loss of HCO_3 or excess H+ ions	pH	α	$\dfrac{[HCO_3-]}{PaCO_2}$
Alkalosis: an increase in pH value, greater than 7.45			
Respiratory: elimination of CO_2 (hyperventilation)	pH	α	$\dfrac{[HCO_3-]}{PaCO_2}$
Metabolic: **accumulation of HCO_3—or loss of H+ ions**	pH	α	$\dfrac{[HCO_3-]}{PaCO_2}$

Note: α represents "proportional to"

Metabolic or nonrespiratory acidosis occurs because there is either production of too much acid in the body or excretion of too much bicarbonate. This is common in renal disease and diabetes. The respiratory system, if capable, will increase respiratory rate to compensate for this metabolic disturbance by increasing ventilation (eliminating the CO_2) and decreasing $PaCO_2$. In a healthy respiratory system, this response normally is almost immediate and may serve to correct the metabolic disturbance. However, a diseased respiratory system stressed by these demands may be inadequate to compensate for the imbalance in the pH.

b. Alkalosis is also a condition that can be either respiratory or metabolic. Alkalosis occurs when there is a drop in hydrogen ions (H+) or excessive bicarbonate (HCO_3-) in the blood leading to an *alkaline* pH, above 7.45. Respiratory alkalosis is caused by a decrease in $PaCO_2$ secondary to alveolar hyperventilation, that is, excessive ventilation with the lungs exhaling too much CO_2. Blood gas analysis indicates an *uncompensated respiratory alkalosis* if $PaCO_2$ is decreased while pH is increased (inverse relationship). A functioning renal system may be able to compensate for respiratory alkalosis, this time by excreting bicarbonate ions (HCO_3-) in the urine or retaining acid (H+).

Uncompensated (acute) metabolic alkalosis, like respiratory alkalosis, is associated with increased pH. The blood gas analysis also shows decreased H+ ions or increased bicarbonate (HCO_3-). This occurs because there is either production of excessive base or bicarbonate in the body or excretion of too much acid. The compensatory respiratory mechanism in alkalosis is the decrease in respiratory rate to conserve CO_2.

c. *Compensated (chronic) metabolic* and *respiratory acidosis* and *alkalosis* refer to a condition where the body, via the respiratory or renal systems, must continuously work toward balancing the pH at a normal level. For example, an individual in acute respiratory alkalosis may maintain a normal pH but only if the renal system can continuously excrete bicarbonate (HCO_3-). This compensates for the disordered respiratory system that is hyperventilating and exhaling too much CO_2. This individual is now in compensated respiratory alkalosis despite the ongoing respiratory condition.

2. **Hypoxemia and Hypoxia**

Other parameters will be important in the treatment of the patient with impaired ventilation and oxygenation. Hypoxemia refers to a deficiency of oxygen in arterial blood; it is indicated by a PaO_2 that is lower than the normal value (Hough, 1991). A lack of oxygen at the level of body tissue is called hypoxia. If the lack of oxygen becomes critical, it can lead to irreversible damage to cells such as brain tissue. The treatment for hypoxia is to provide oxygen (FIO_2). If the deficit in oxygenation cannot be overcome, as can happen in lungs that are damaged and have lost surfactant, assisted ventilation will then be required. The use of positive pressure breaths to maintain pressure in the lungs even at the end of expiration is necessary. This keeps the lungs and alveoli inflated to ensure oxygen delivery. This concept is referred to as **positive end expiratory pressure (PEEP)** and is described later in this chapter. There are prerequisites for successful oxygen delivery, including:

a. Adequate PAO_2 at the level of the lungs.

b. Adequate quantities/normal quality of hemoglobin.

c. Adequate cardiac output, to circulate the oxygenated hemoglobin.

d. Adequate channels (arteries/capillaries) for blood to deliver O_2 to tissues.

3. **Hypercapnia,** or alveolar hypoventilation, is indicated by a $PaCO_2$ that is higher than normal. Hypercapnia is caused by inadequate ventilation or failure to eliminate carbon dioxide from the blood. The buildup of carbon dioxide decreases the oxygen concentration in the alveoli.

The physician and respiratory care practitioner will use clinical information and blood gas analysis to determine whether the cause of the respiratory disorder is respiratory or metabolic. This will assist decision making and therapeutic intervention, and influence the choice of respiratory care provided. Mechanical ventilatory support is just one option for the pulmonologist and respiratory care practitioner in their treatment of the patient with a respiratory disorder.

D. Body Systems Related to Respiratory Failure

Patients who are ventilator dependent often have multisystem organ involvement such as renal and cardiac abnormalities as well as respiratory failure. The clinician must be aware of the ways in which these systems interrelate and may potentially impact on a patient's response to rehabilitation. When assessing a patient, the physician must complete a medical history that takes note of a renal or cardiac involvement.

1. Renal System

The renal system is responsible for regulating the arterial blood pH or acid-base content. The kidneys are the organs responsible for either excreting or retaining acids or bicarbonates. The kidneys work in conjunction with the respiratory system to balance the amount of acids or hydrogen ions (H+) and bicarbonate ions (HCO_3-) in the blood to achieve *homeostasis* or equilibrium of the internal mechanisms of the body. In other words, and as discussed above, normal kidneys will respond to certain respiratory conditions by working to maintain a balanced blood pH. A disorder of the renal system, conversely, can stress the respiratory system by disturbing both normal pH levels and the overall balance of fluids in the body.

2. Cardiac/Pulmonary System

Cardiac function is also closely interwoven with the respiratory system. The cardiovascular system is responsible for insuring that adequate levels of blood are circulated to and from the heart and through the circulatory system to deliver oxygen to body tissues. If interference with the blood flow occurs, there may be a failure of gas exchange. This can occur in **congestive heart failure (CHF)**. CHF is fluid accumulation in the lungs and other tissues due to heart failure. As described in Chapter 1, pulmonary edema is frequently a result of impaired pumping action of the heart. Severe CHF can lead to cardiac-respiratory failure due to decreased lung compliance as a result of the increased fluid retention of the lung. This results in increasing the work of breathing. In essence then, cardiac failure can result in inadequate ability to deliver oxygen to the body. Conversely, a respiratory system that is experiencing increased work of breathing may place strain on a limited cardiovascular system. Mechanical ventilation is one way to support cardiac function in a patient who is experiencing respiratory compromise.

II. VENTILATOR OPERATIONS: BASIC PRINCIPLES AND RELEVANCE TO THE CLINICIAN

The respiratory care practitioner takes the primary responsibility for the technical operation of the ventilator, and works with the physician, usually the pulmonologist, who makes the decisions regarding the mode of ventilation and settings. All allied health professionals working with the ventilator-dependent patient should have a basic understanding of the principles of ventilator operation. *However, modifications of the ventilator are performed by either the physician or the respiratory care practitioner and nurse who follow physician orders.*

A. Positive Pressure Ventilation

Positive pressure ventilation is performed with the use of a mechanical device called a *ventilator* or *respirator.* This chapter will use the term ventilator. When the ventilator provides positive pressure and inflates the lungs, it is referred to as **intermittent positive pressure ventilation (IPPV).** Positive pressure means that gas, at above atmospheric pressure, is applied to the respiratory tract with the result of pushing gas into the patient's lungs and raising intra-alveolar pressure during inspiration. This is accomplished by delivering a preset volume or pressure of gas to the lungs in order to inflate them. When the gas is no longer being delivered, the lungs begin to passively deflate and empty via the elastic recoil of the lungs and chest. As exhalation passively occurs, air leaves the lungs. The ventilator, which is programmed to cycle again, redelivers the desired amount of air. This differs from spontaneous breathing in which air enters the lungs from an area of greater pressure (atmospheric pressure) to an area of less pressure (alveolar pressure). Normal inspiration occurs as the chest wall expands due to the active function of the inspiratory muscles which creates negative intrathoracic pressure. Expiration, as in mechanically assisted breathing, is also passive. Because positive pressure ventilation is so different from the normal breathing process with pressure in the airway always higher than that in the lungs, there are numerous complications associated with the delivery of air under pressure to the lungs. These complications will be discussed later in this chapter. Two terms important in describing mechanical ventilation are *volume* and *pressure.* Volume is the amount of air delivered to the lungs (as in tidal volume). Pressure is the force of air used when delivering this volume.

1. Positive pressure ventilators are classified by the parameters which determine when the ventilator stops the delivery of inspiratory airflow. Most commonly ventilators are either volume or pressure cycled; less frequently they may be set to cycle by time. The sophisticated acute care ventilators, often found in the ICU, can be adjusted to provide a variety of these different parameters.

    a. *Volume cycled ventilators* will provide airflow for inspiration until a preset volume is delivered by the ventilator. In order to achieve this volume delivery, any pressure required will be delivered until a preset volume is reached. This is the most common type of positive pressure ventilator.

    b. *Pressure cycled ventilators* will provide inspiratory airflow until a preset pressure is met. Volume can vary from breath to breath. One form of pressure cycled mechanical ventilation, now frequently used in the ICU, is **pressure support ventilation (PSV).**

c. *Time cycled ventilators* deliver airflow for a certain amount of time during the inspiratory phase, then stop after that preset interval. This type of cycling mechanism for a positive pressure ventilator is called the *controlled mode.*

Positive pressure ventilation is delivered in a variety of different modes, depending on a patient's specific needs. These will be discussed later in this chapter.

B. High Frequency Ventilation

High frequency ventilation differs from positive pressure ventilation in delivery of air. There are different modes of high frequency ventilation, including *high frequency positive pressure ventilation* and *high frequency jet ventilation.*

1. *High frequency positive pressure ventilation* delivers conventional ventilatory support at a higher than the normal rate of 50–150 cycles/minute (Hough, 1991; Peruzzi, 1993). Hough (1991) states that tidal volume is delivered so that it just exceeds the dead space created by the normal anatomy of the airway. Dead space refers to the amount of air that does not participate in ventilation. The aim of high frequency positive pressure ventilation is adequate gas exchange at a low tidal volume. During high frequency positive pressure ventilation, air is quickly delivered in and out of the lungs at a low air volume, providing adequate gas exchange while minimizing the degree that the lungs are actually inflated.

2. *High frequency jet ventilation* provides rapid pulses of air from a high pressure source. As the air bursts are delivered into the airway, some volume is created, but remains low. Gas exchange is instead achieved by air mixing in the airways, fueled by the rapid pulses of air and resulting turbulent flow.

    a. Theoretically, both forms of high frequency ventilation depress spontaneous ventilation and decrease chest wall movement, tidal volumes, and airway pressures. Fluctuations in blood pressure, common with conventional ventilation, may be minimized. Therefore, patients with conditions such as unstable cardiac status may benefit from high frequency ventilation.

    b. Disadvantages of high frequency ventilation include a tendency toward atelectasis or collapse of portions of the lung because tidal volumes are maintained at minimal levels. The entire airway may be affected by these decreased volumes, resulting in problems in airway patency. Inadequate humidification is another disadvantage of high frequency ventilation. This is secondary to the fact that oxygen, by nature a dry gas, is also being provided at a very high rate. This limits the opportunity of the gas to receive humidification.

C. Negative Pressure Ventilation

Negative pressure ventilation is performed with the use of a *body ventilator* which surrounds a patient with adjustable negative pressure and creates a vacuum around the chest wall. This negative pressure is applied at predetermined intervals. During the periods of negative pressure, the chest wall is sucked outward and the diaphragm pulled downward. Pleural pressure falls and the lungs and alveoli expand. A pressure differential is created between air outside and inside the lungs. In essence, the application of negative pressure ventilation mimics the action of the inspiratory muscles. As with normal ventilation, expiration is passive, occurring as the displaced chest wall and diaphragm return to their normal resting position. Negative pressure is applied again, at the same predetermined setting.

D. Invasive/Noninvasive Ventilatory Techniques

Artificial positive pressure ventilation can be delivered via invasive or noninvasive means. Negative pressure ventilation is always noninvasive. Invasive techniques are those that utilize artificial airways, such as those discussed in Chapter 3. The airway is secured by either an endotracheal tube or tracheostomy tube, and positive pressure ventilation is applied. Noninvasive techniques are external, via either masks or mouthpieces, or utilizing negative pressure body ventilators (Alba & Pilkington, 1984). The trend in the medical community over the last 10 years has been to both evaluate the efficacy of noninvasive acute and long-term mechanical ventilation and to provide patients with options in the decision-making process with regard to accepting assisted ventilation (Bach 1993; Bach & Alba 1990b; Bach, Alba, Mosher, & Delaubier, 1987; Ellis, Bye, Bruderer, & Sullivan, 1987; Meyer & Hill 1994; Oppenheimer, 1993). Meyer and Hill (1994) reported that:

> Use of noninvasive positive pressure ventilation, the delivery of positive pressure mechanical ventilation to the lungs without endotracheal intubation, is increasing among patients with acute and chronic respiratory failure, mainly because of its convenience, lower cost, and morbidity-sparing potential compared with standard invasive positive pressure ventilation. (p. 760)

Noninvasive positive pressure ventilation supports or substitutes for a patient's spontaneous breathing. To utilize noninvasive ventilation, patients must present with functional upper airways and adequate airway protection/secretion management. Noninvasive mechanical support is used both for acute and chronic respiratory failure.

1. **Invasive Techniques**

    a. **Positive pressure ventilation**
        (1) **Endotracheal/tracheostomy tubes**
            Positive pressure ventilation can be accomplished via artificial air-
            ways, either endotracheal tubes or tracheostomy tubes. Often the
            primary indication for a tracheotomy is the need for prolonged me-
            chanical ventilation. Artificial airways are an effective method of
            delivering positive pressure ventilation, especially because of the
            presence of cuffs which provide a tracheal seal and prevent loss of air
            from the ventilator. Compared with masks or mouthpieces, artificial
            airways are less likely to dislodge and are therefore safer for certain
            patients. One main disadvantage of endotracheal tubes and trache-
            ostomy tubes is the disruption of communication and swallowing. In
            addition, as was discussed in Chapters 2 and 3, there are numerous
            complications which may accompany the use of artificial airways.
        (2) The use of endotracheal tubes and tracheostomy tubes is indicated
            for individuals with:

        *   altered mental status (especially coma).

        *   **hemodynamic** instability.

        *   excessive secretions/risk of aspiration (especially bulbar dys-
            function).

        *   decreased ability to cooperate with noninvasive mechanical
            ventilation.

        *   trauma to face and chest wall.

2. **Noninvasive Techniques**

    a. **Positive pressure ventilation**
        (1) **Mask or mouthpiece**
            The types of positive pressure ventilation that can be provided by
            mask or nose or mouthpiece are CPAP (continuous positive airway
            pressure), **BiPAP**™ (bilevel positive airway pressure) or mouth/nasal
            intermittent positive pressure (M/NIPPV). CPAP delivers air above
            atmospheric pressure to a spontaneously breathing patient and serves
            to maintain an open airway throughout the breath cycle. CPAP can be
            used for a variety of pulmonary problems and is usually delivered via
            nasal mask. Bilevel ventilation or BiPAP™ is a variation of CPAP.
            Both modes provide pressure support when a patient spontaneously
            breathes. Bilevel ventilation is usually considered a method to aug-
            ment ventilation. It provides an inspiratory pressure (IPAP) as well

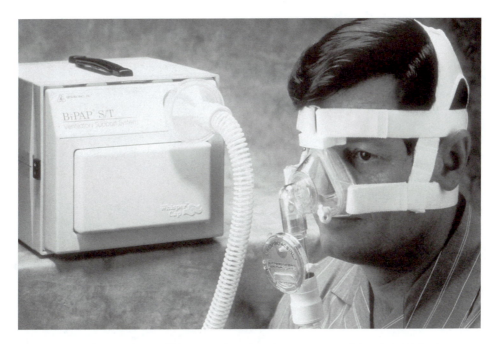

Figure 4-1. Delivery of BiPAP™ via nasal mask. (Photo courtesy of Respironics, Inc.)

as a lower expiratory pressure (EPAP). Figure 4-1 depicts a patient receiving BiPAP™ noninvasive mechanical ventilation.

b. Negative pressure ventilation (NPV)

Noninvasive negative pressure ventilation is utilized primarily with patients who have neuromuscular diseases or spinal cord injury. It is less commonly used with patients who have diseased lungs such as COPD. Negative pressure ventilation is delivered by the following techniques:

(1) Iron lung

The iron lung is an airtight tank in which the patient is completely encased except for the head. Either at the foot end, or beneath the tank, there is a large flexible bellows which expands. A photo of the iron lung is shown in Figure 4-2. An internal negative pressure is created each time the bellows expands. The negative pressure causes expansion of the chest wall and creates a pressure drop within the airway. Inspiration occurs when air then flows from the area of greater to lesser pressure. As the bellows moves inward, a valve on the top of the tank opens and allows pressure to return to atmospheric. Expiration begins as the chest returns to its normal resting position. The movement of the bellows is electrically powered but

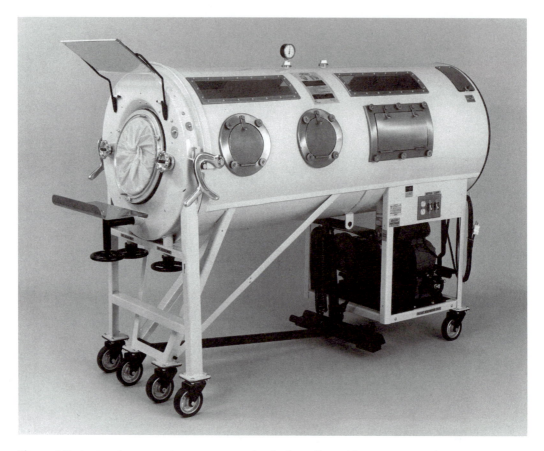

Figure 4-2. An iron lung negative pressure mechanical ventilator. (Photo courtesy of Respironics, Inc.)

can also be operated manually. Because the patient's body is completely within the tank, daily care is delivered via port holes in the sides of the ventilator.

(2) Cuirass

A cuirass is a chest piece shell which covers the patient's chest and abdomen as depicted in Figure 4-3. It was created as an alternative to the iron lung as patients are less restricted with this noninvasive method of ventilation. The cuirass has a tubing which leads to a negative pressure electric pump. The pump is the source for the negative pressure that is applied to the chest. Ventilation is controlled by adjusting the rate and amount of negative pressure. At times there may be difficulty maintaining a tight seal between the chest piece and patient's body, particularly when there are *scoliosis* and *kyphosis,* ab-

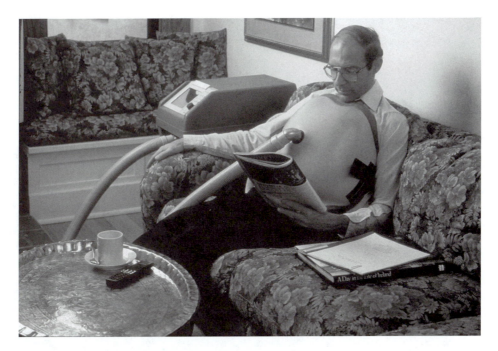

Figure 4-3. A cuirass. (Photo courtesy of Respironics, Inc.)

normalities of spine curvature. The cuirass can be used both during the day when a patient is sitting up or more commonly during the night when the patient is in bed.

(3) **Rocking bed**

The rocking bed utilizes the effects of gravity on the abdominal contents and diaphragm. The head of the bed literally rocks up and down via a motor. The supine patient is moved through a predetermined range and at a predetermined speed. When the head of the bed is raised, gravity pulls on the abdomen and displaces the diaphragm downward. When the head of the bed is lowered, the abdominal contents shift with the diaphragm, which returns to its upright resting position. The net effect is that when the head of the bed is raised the patient inhales and when it is lowered, the patient exhales. The rocking bed is considered less restrictive than the iron lung or cuirass. A photo is provided in Figure 4-4.

(4) **Pneumobelt**

The pneumobelt is similar to a corset that surrounds the abdomen. It contains a bladder section that inflates and puts pressure on the abdominal contents, pushing the diaphragm upward. The pneumobelt thus functions to assist in expiration, leaving inspiration to occur

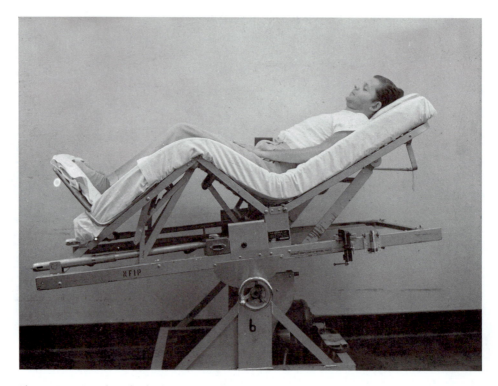

Figure 4-4. A rocking bed.

either by the action of any remaining inspiratory function or passively. The patient must be either sitting or standing upright to use this device. It leaves the face and mouth free and can be worn under clothing to maintain a more normal appearance. Figure 4-5 pictures a pneumobelt.

III. MODES OF VENTILATION

In describing mechanical ventilation, the term *mode* is used to identify the type of support being delivered by the ventilator. Chang (2001) described a ventilator mode as a set of operating characteristics that control how a ventilator functions. A ventilator operating mode is characterized by the way a ventilator is triggered into the inspiratory phase and then cycled into exhalation. It also describes other characteristics, mandatory versus spontaneous breaths and so on. Essentially, a mode describes the way the patient and the machine interact to perform the ventilatory cycle. Modes of ventilation vary according to the patient's ability to initiate and maintain independent respiration, and may be combined for patient needs.

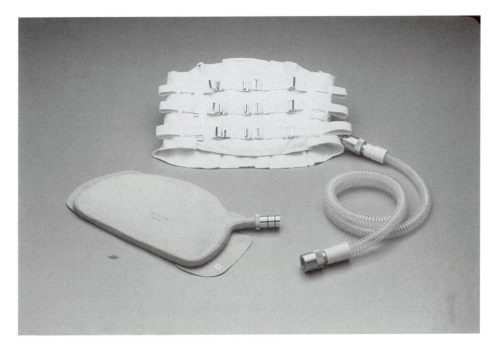

Figure 4-5. A pneumobelt. (Photo courtesy of Respironics, Inc.)

A. Controlled Mode Ventilation (CMV)

As the name suggests, **controlled mode ventilation (CMV)** provides complete control over the rate and volume of each breath provided, regardless of any inspiratory efforts on the part of the patient. CVM is a time-cycled ventilatory mode. It can be either volume controlled or delivered in a pressure support mode. More commonly it is volume controlled. It is the most precise mode of ventilation as it is totally predetermined by the ventilatory settings. Inspiration, or delivery of a specific tidal volume or pressure, is given at a preset time. The patient is not able to breathe between ventilator breaths. In order for patients to benefit from this mode of ventilation, they must often be anesthetized. Patients who are awake and alert, with the ability to breathe partially on their own, will find CMV uncomfortable and distressing because spontaneous breaths are actually "locked out." Scanlan (1990b) states that controlled ventilation is poorly tolerated because it results in "asynchronous breathing efforts against the mechanically controlled breaths, or strenuous, but futile attempts to breathe spontaneously" (p. 760). This response often necessitates sedation of the patient and is the reason why CMV is not used in individuals with any degree of spontaneous breathing. This mode of ventilation is used primarily in the operating room or with patients without respiratory drive, depressed respiratory centers, or inability to trigger the ventilator with their own inspiratory efforts (i.e., patients with spinal cord injury or advanced ALS patients).

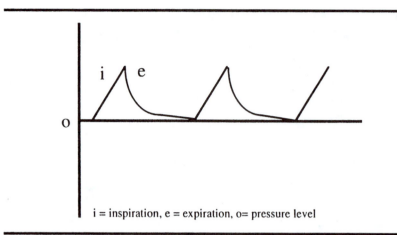

i = inspiration, e = expiration, o= pressure level

Figure 4-6. Breathing pattern for control mode of ventilation. (From "Respiratory Care," by M. F. Mason, J. I. Frey, and B. Fornoff, 1993, p. 208. In M. F. Mason [Ed.], *Speech Pathology for Tracheostomized and Ventilator Dependent Patients*, pp. 184–255. Newport Beach, CA: Voicing! Inc. Copyright 1993 by Voicing! Reprinted with permission.)

If a patient receives CMV for an extended time, respiratory muscle weakness and atrophy may result. The breathing pattern for CMV is illustrated in Figure 4-6.

B. Assist Control (A/C) Ventilation

Assist control (A/C) is variation of controlled mode ventilation. It allows the patient to participate in the breathing process. There is a sensitivity control on the ventilator that sets the amount of effort needed to initiate the machine-cycled breath. This setting must be carefully assessed so that a patient will not overly fatigue trying to reach this preset level. A/C is considered a form of *full* ventilatory support and is used for patients who are unable to maintain adequate *minute ventilation*, or *minute volume*, yet can regulate their own rate of breathing. Minute ventilation/volume refers to the total amount of air exchanged during the breathing cycle each minute. Assist control provides that preset volume or preset pressure support every time the patient initiates a spontaneous breath. In addition, the ventilator is preset to provide a minimum number of breaths, called the back-up rate, should the patient fail to trigger inspiration. For example, a patient on A/C setting of 10 with a tidal volume of 800 ml will receive air each time the ventilator senses the negative pressure caused by an inspiratory effort, regardless of how many times this inspiration has occurred. If the patient does not trigger a breath within the predetermined rate setting, the ventilator will provide the positive pressure breath of 800 ml at 10 breaths per minute. This delineates the A/C mode from the pure *assist* mode, in which there are no preset back-up breaths delivered. The breathing pattern for assist mode ventilation is illustrated in Figure 4-7.

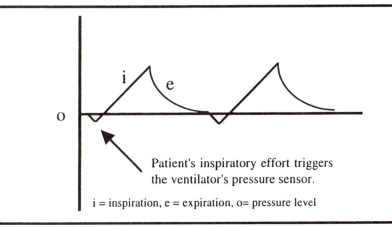

Patient's inspiratory effort triggers
the ventilator's pressure sensor.

i = inspiration, e = expiration, o= pressure level

Figure 4-7. Breathing pattern for assist control ventilation. (From "Respiratory Care," by M. F. Mason, J. I. Frey, and B. Fornoff, 1993, p. 207. In M. F. Mason [Ed.], *Speech Pathology for Tracheostomized and Ventilator Dependent Patients,* pp. 184–255. Newport Beach, CA: Voicing! Inc. Copyright 1993 by Voicing! Reprinted with permission.)

C. Assist Mode (A)

The assist mode is a patient-cycled form of ventilation where inspiration is initiated only by patient effort. There is no back-up ventilator rate set, so candidates must have intact respiratory drives. The sensitivity control must be carefully adjusted in the assist mode because this will determine how much work of breathing or patient effort is required to trigger the ventilatory breath. This mode of ventilation is usually not continuously applied but is used for shorter time periods.

D. Intermittent Mandatory Ventilation (IMV)

Intermittent mandatory ventilation (IMV) is a timed mode that permits a patient to breathe spontaneously between preset positive pressure breaths. It differs from assist control in that a patient may breathe spontaneously both at his own rate *and* volume independent of the breaths that are provided by the ventilator. In other words, the patient can breathe spontaneously between mandatory breaths. If the patient does not breathe these additional breaths, he will receive only what is preset on the ventilator. During this period of spontaneous breathing the patient is still receiving volume from the ventilator, but the patient determines how much volume by the amount of effort he initiates. IMV allows the patient to take on some of the work of breathing, contributing to rate and minute volume. Oxygen (FIO_2) levels are predetermined. The ability to spontaneously breathe and contribute to the tidal volume obtained from the ventilator allows for the maintenance of muscle tone and ventilatory drive. The breathing pattern for IMV is illustrated in Figure 4-8.

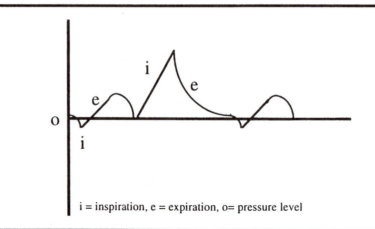

i = inspiration, e = expiration, o= pressure level

Figure 4-8. Breathing pattern for intermittent mandatory mode of ventilation. (From "Respiratory Care," by M. F. Mason, J. I. Frey, and B. Fornoff, 1993, p. 209. In M. F. Mason [Ed.], *Speech Pathology for Tracheostomized and Ventilator Dependent Patients,* pp. 184–255. Newport Beach, CA: Voicing! Inc. Copyright 1993 by Voicing! Reprinted with permission.)

Some practitioners use IMV and **synchronized intermittent mandatory ventilation (SIMV)** during weaning. IMV may begin the steps in the weaning process in these instances. IMV allows a patient learning to breathe spontaneously to take spontaneous breaths between machine breaths. However, although the "mandatory" ventilation ensures that the preset number of breaths are given regardless of patient effort, it also provides those breaths without regard for what the patient is doing. This is a possible disadvantage of IMV as a patient may have just initiated an inspiration when another is delivered by the ventilator. This is referred to as *breath stacking.* This was the rationale for the development of synchronized intermittent mandatory ventilation (SIMV).

E. Synchronized Intermittent Mandatory Ventilation (SIMV)

SIMV is a modification of IMV that coincides the mandatory machine breaths to occur with the patient's inspiratory efforts, if they are present. This mode of ventilation waits for the patient to breathe (within a certain preset time frame) and then delivers a preset volume in conjunction with the patient's effort. Again, if the patient fails to inspire, the ventilator will deliver a breath. However, the ventilator will not provide this breath on top of the patient's breath; rather the ventilator synchronizes with the patient's efforts. SIMV, as compared to IMV, will theoretically reduce the potential for breaths to stack one on top of the other, and should be more comfortable for a patient. SIMV is usually used as a weaning mode because it requires a patient to take on some of the work of breathing. Inadequate settings of IMV and

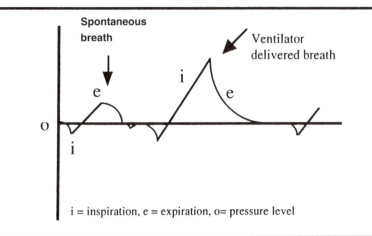

Figure 4-9. Breathing pattern for synchronized intermittent mandatory ventilation. (From "Respiratory Care," by M. F. Mason, J. I. Frey, and B. Fornoff, 1993, p. 210. In M. F. Mason [Ed.], *Speech Pathology for Tracheostomized and Ventilator Dependent Patients,* pp. 184–255. Newport Beach, CA: Voicing! Inc. Copyright 1993 by Voicing! Reprinted with permission.)

SIMV may contribute to respiratory muscle fatigue. The breathing pattern for SIMV is illustrated in Figure 4-9.

F. Continuous Positive Airway Pressure (CPAP)

Continuous positive airway pressure provides a constant flow of air (continuous positive pressure) during both the inspiratory and expiratory phases without providing cycled or intermittent mechanical ventilatory assistance. The patient must have the ability to maintain sufficient tidal volume and breathing rate. However, if the patient is unable to sustain adequate oxygenation, CPAP can provide this via the connection to a continuous supply of oxygen. CPAP's function is to keep the alveoli inflated at an enhanced volume which provides a safeguard against alveolar collapse and a source of improved oxygenation. CPAP is also used as a weaning modality and can be combined with other methods of ventilatory support such as **pressure support ventilation (PSV).**

G. Pressure Support Ventilation (PSV)

Pressure support is a mode of ventilation that supplements the patient's spontaneous inspiration with a preset amount of positive airway pressure. The pressure is delivered throughout the entire inspiration. Because pressure support assists during spontaneous breaths, the patient determines the rate, duration of the breath, and the volume of air received. This mode must be used for spontaneously breathing patients and is useful for patients with respiratory muscle weakness because it reduces the work of breathing, especially at higher levels of pressure support. As pressure support levels increase, delivering greater amounts of positive pressure to the airway, the patient will work less during breathing. In part, this is due to the higher amounts of tidal volume that will usually result from higher pressure support levels. However, the tidal volume received and subsequently the work of breathing will vary, depending on patient's lung compliance and respiratory effort. Pressure support can also be useful in compensating for high airway resistance, as with small artificial airways, and for the mechanical dead space provided by the ventilatory tubing. The pressure provided by pressure support ventilation will be set above any levels of **positive end expiratory pressure (PEEP)** if this mode is also being used.

H. Positive End Expiratory Pressure (PEEP)

Positive end expiratory pressure (PEEP) refers to the maintenance of positive pressure at the end of **expiration.** It ensures that the airway pressure never falls below a set value. PEEP serves to keep the lungs and subsequently the alveoli inflated at the end of expiration. Airway pressures are maintained and do not fall to atmospheric pressure when expiration is completed. The effect of this pressure maintenance is to reduce the potential for alveolar collapse and improve oxygenation levels. Oxygen levels generally rise because the patient never exhales to a zero airway pressure but instead preserves a constant and enhanced amount of gas in the lungs. PEEP is, therefore, useful for patients who have difficulty maintaining adequate oxygenation and may eliminate the need for high and potentially toxic levels of applied oxygen (Hough, 1991). Common complications associated with the increased intrathoracic pressure generated by PEEP are reduced venous return and decreased cardiac output.

I. T-Piece or Trach Collar

T-pieces and *trach collars* are used for patients who still require oxygen or humidified gas, but do not require the continuous positive airway pressure that is provided by CPAP. Although the oxygenation needs of these patients are less, they are not yet ready to obtain the necessary amounts of O_2 from room air. T-piece or trach collar is usually the final stage in weaning from mechanical ventilation.

1. T-piece refers to a crossed or T-shaped connection that allows air to flow from an air source to the patient. Air then blows out the sides of the connector. This design provides the patient with a continuous source of fresh air which can be humidified as needed. The majority of the expired air is able to escape into the atmosphere. This eliminates the rebreathing of air with a high CO_2 concentration.

2. A trach collar is a clear plastic mask that is placed over the tracheostomy. It also provides an oxygen rich humidified environment for the patient to breathe.

Holes in the side of the mask lessen the accumulation of expired air that potentially could be rebreathed by the patient.

IV. VENTILATOR SETTINGS/PARAMETERS OF VENTILATION

Although ventilators vary according to manufacturer design, all devices have standard settings and parameters that can be altered according to patient need. The following settings are the most relevant to the clinician who may recommend modifications to facilitate communication and swallowing. Figure 4-10 depicts a standard portable ventilator display.

A. Tidal Volume

1. **Tidal volume** refers to the amount of air per breath that is delivered by the ventilator. It is expressed in milliliters (ml) or liters (L). Normal tidal volume settings are commonly based on ideal body weight that takes into account the dead space created by a patient's conducting airways (i.e., the upper airway, the trachea, and the larger bronchi).

2. **Exhaled tidal volume** refers to the amount of volume or air that returns through the ventilator expiratory tubing on expiration. This is measured by the ventilator to ensure that the patient did receive the proper amount of preset volume.

B. Respiratory Rate

The **respiratory rate** setting indicates the number of breath cycles the ventilator is set to deliver. In normal individuals breaths average 12 per minute (Zemlin, 1981). Respiratory rate influences the $PaCO_2$ levels because rate times tidal volume determines how quickly air is exchanged in the lungs. On a ventilator, settings vary depending on the mode of ventilation and the presence of any spontaneous breathing. For example, if a patient does not demonstrate any spontaneous breathing, is on full support or CMV, and the ventilator is set at 12, the patient will breathe at 12 breaths per minute. The set respiratory rate can be decreased as the patient moves from one mode to another, perhaps during the weaning process. For example, the respiratory rate setting of 6 for a patient on SIMV mode reflects the 6 breaths per minute that the ventilator will deliver. If the patient can take additional spontaneous breaths he may be able to breathe more frequently than the mandatory breaths provided by ventilator. As the patient takes on the majority of the work of breathing, he may require fewer mandatory breaths. Respiratory rate must be carefully monitored. If the respiratory rate is too high (rapid), a phenomenon called **auto PEEP** can occur. Because expiration is passive and positive pressure air is pushed into the lungs faster than it can be expired, air becomes trapped. This trapped gas creates auto (physiologic) PEEP.

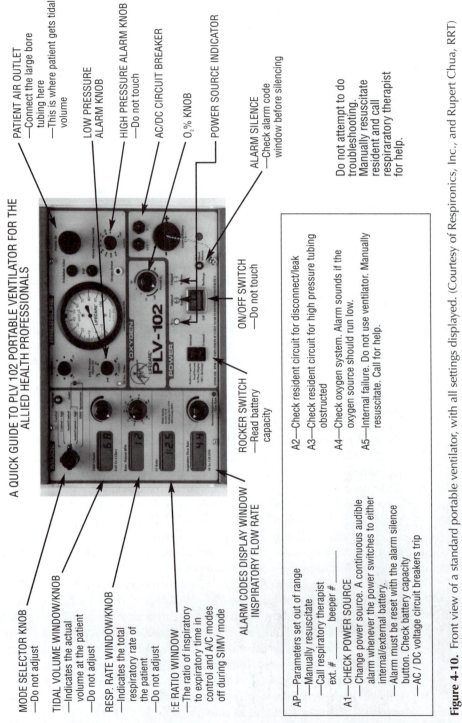

A QUICK GUIDE TO PLV 102 PORTABLE VENTILATOR FOR THE ALLIED HEALTH PROFESSIONALS

MODE SELECTOR KNOB
—Do not adjust

TIDAL VOLUME WINDOW/KNOB
—Indicates the actual volume at the patient
—Do not adjust

RESP. RATE WINDOW/KNOB
—Indicates the total respiratory rate of the patient
—Do not adjust

I:E RATIO WINDOW
—The ratio of inspiratory to expiratory time in control and A/C modes off during SIMV mode

ALARM CODES DISPLAY WINDOW
INSPIRATORY FLOW RATE

PATIENT AIR OUTLET
—Connect the large bore tubing here
—This is where patient gets tidal volume

LOW PRESSURE ALARM KNOB

HIGH PRESSURE ALARM KNOB
—Do not touch

AC/DC CIRCUIT BREAKER

O₂% KNOB

POWER SOURCE INDICATOR

ALARM SILENCE
—Check alarm code window before silencing

Do not attempt to do troubleshooting.
Manually resuscitate resident and call respiratory therapist for help.

ROCKER SWITCH
—Read battery capacity

ON/OFF SWITCH
—Do not touch

AP—Parameters set out of range
—Manually resuscitate
—Call respiratory therapist
ext. # _____ beeper # _____

A1—CHECK POWER SOURCE
—Change power source. A continuous audible alarm whenever the power switches to either internal/external battery.
—Alarm must be reset with the alarm silence button. Check battery capacity
—AC / DC voltage circuit breakers trip

A2—Check resident circuit for disconnect/leak

A3—Check resident circuit for high pressure tubing obstructed

A4—Check oxygen system. Alarm sounds if the oxygen source should run low.

A5—Internal failure. Do not use ventilator. Manually resuscitate. Call for help.

Figure 4-10. Front view of a standard portable ventilator, with all settings displayed. (Courtesy of Respironics, Inc., and Rupert Chua, RRT)

1. Minute Ventilation

Minute ventilation (minute volume) is the product of tidal volume and respiratory rate and indicates the total volume of air that is breathed in 1 minute. It is expressed in liters (L). It is adjusted based on the $PaCO_2$ levels that the patient exhibits. In CMV, A/C, and IMV/SIMV modes, the respiratory care practitioner fully determines the minimum minute ventilation received by the patient. In contrast, during the CPAP mode of ventilation, the spontaneously breathing patient regulates minute ventilation. All modes of mechanical ventilation aim to establish adequate O_2 levels and facilitate CO_2 removal by maintaining adequate minute ventilation (Williams-Colon & Thalken, 1990).

a. Alveolar ventilation

Alveolar ventilation is a product of tidal volume minus dead space times respiratory rate or frequency. It is the amount of gas that is exchanged in and out of the alveoli. Mechanical ventilatory support functions to control alveolar minute ventilation. This is accomplished by manipulating the tidal volume or respiratory rate settings of the ventilator while anatomic dead space remains relatively constant. A patient who is approaching respiratory failure will demonstrate increased respiratory rate (shallow breathing) and decreased tidal volume that will lessen alveolar ventilation. For example, if the anatomic dead space equals 150 ml and 600 ml of tidal volume is provided, total tidal volume will equal 450 ml. With a respiratory rate of 10, this would produce alveolar ventilation of 4500 ml (450 ml × 10). If, however, the respiratory rate is increased to 20 while tidal volume is lowered to 300 ml to provide the same minute ventilation, the resulting alveolar ventilation is 3000 ml (300 ml – 150 ml × 20 = 3000 ml). Alveolar ventilation is significantly lessened for this patient.

C. Inspiratory/Expiratory Ratio (I:E ratio)

The **inspiratory/expiratory ratio** indicates the time relationship between the inspiratory phase of ventilation and expiratory phase of ventilation. The *I* refers to the time spent on inspiration and the *E* refers to the time spent on expiration. This ratio is set dependent on the presenting pulmonary disease and the patient's needs for additional time in each phase. Generally, the expiratory time should be 1.5 times the length of the inspiration (Eubanks & Bone, 1990). This will allow an adequate inspiration, to deliver tidal volume, followed by a full exhalation to avoid air trapping. For example, to meet a patient's special needs an I:E ratio may be set at 1:4. A patient on this setting may present with diseased lungs and require a longer exhalation phase to prevent air from becoming trapped in the poorly elastic lung tissue. There is an interrelationship between the I:E ratio and the *inspiratory flow rate*. These parameters can be set independently, however; for example, the inspiratory flow rate must be high enough to maintain a particular I:E ratio.

D. Inspiratory Flow Rate

The inspiratory flow rate delineates the amount of gas flow in liters provided to the patient during the inspiratory cycle. It determines how long it takes to deliver the tidal volume. Normal inspiratory flow rates on the ventilator generally range between 40 and 80 L/minute to maintain an I:E ratio of at least 1:2 (Chang, 2001).

E. Fractional Inspired Oxygen Concentration (FIO$_2$)

FIO$_2$ refers to the amount of oxygen provided to the patient, usually expressed in percent. Patients who can tolerate breathing room air, where the oxygen concentration is approximately 21%, will not need supplemental oxygen delivered through the ventilator. An increase in FIO$_2$ may be needed if the patient's work of breathing is increased and/or if there is intrinsic lung disease and O$_2$ exchange does not easily occur.

F. Sensitivity

Sensitivity is a setting that regulates how much effort is needed by the patient to cycle the ventilator "on" for inspiration. The inspiration is triggered by the negative pressure created by the inspiratory effort of the patient. Therefore, this setting is relevant in the A/C and IMV/SIMV modes but not in CMV. With higher sensitivity settings (i.e., the higher numbers), the ventilator will be less sensitive to the patient's inspiratory efforts. It will be more difficult to trigger breaths from the machine, and more of the work of breathing will be imposed upon the patient. This may be desirable during the weaning process but can fatigue some individuals.

G. Sigh Breath

A *sigh* can be added to the ventilatory mode (usually CMV or A/C) to give the patient an increased amount of volume at periodic intervals. A sigh is usually one and a half to two times the tidal volume. This setting is designed to mimic the sighs that occur as part of a normal breathing pattern and functions to help prevent atelectasis or lung collapse. A sigh breath is normally not necessary when high tidal volumes or PEEP is being provided because the lungs are inherently maintained at higher levels of inflation with these modes.

H. Peak Inspiratory Pressure (Pressure limit)

The **peak inspiratory pressure** is the parameter that is preset on the ventilator to limit the amount of pressure, expressed in cm H$_2$O, that can be created in the airway during inspiration. Peak inspiratory pressure combined with inspiratory time and flow rate determines the tidal volume given to the patient. Peak inspiratory pressure greater than 30–40 cm H$_2$O increases the risk of barotrauma.

Mean airway pressure refers to the average or mean amount of pressure that is present in the patient's lungs. It is created by all of the time and pressure variables previously discussed. High mean airway pressures also increase the risk of barotrauma.

V. VENTILATOR EQUIPMENT

A. Standard Nonportable Ventilator

The standard nonportable ventilators are larger in size and therefore are not used for patients who require mobility. Some contain a visual display to represent both the settings of the ventilator and the patient's response to each breath cycle. The more sophisticated ventilators have a built-in microprocessor which computerizes the functions of the ventilator and provides preset parameters in an effort to limit human error. An example of a standard nonportable ventilator is shown in Figure 4-11.

B. Portable Ventilator

As the name implies, the portable ventilators are smaller in size and allow for increased mobility for the patient. They are often mounted to wheelchairs to provide accessibility to various environments. Certain features cannot be provided on the portable ventilator. This may limit their applicability with particular patient populations such as the patient in the early stages of weaning. Figure 4-12 shows a standard portable ventilator.

C. Ventilator Tubing/Circuit

The ventilator tubing or circuitry provides the connections between the patient and the ventilator. Additional pieces of equipment such as valves are placed in line with the tubing to serve their special functions and complete the ventilatory circuit.

1. Disposable/Nondisposable

Ventilator tubing can be either disposable or nondisposable. Sometimes adapters must be used to ensure proper completion of the circuitry if different types of tubing are used.

2. Inspiratory/Expiratory Tubing Lines

The ventilatory circuitry on most mechanical ventilators consists of two lines of tubing, one to allow inspiratory flow to the patient and the other to collect expiratory gas flow. The dual lines allow the ventilator to measure gas flows and assist in monitoring patient status. Single line circuits are also utilized, usually for patients who are on portable ventilators.

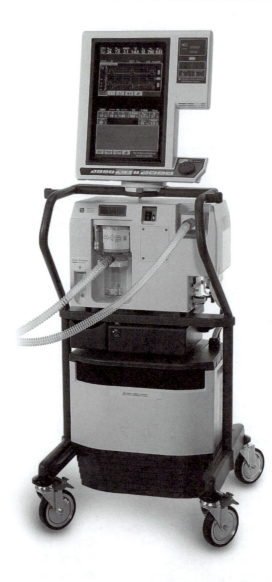

Figure 4-11. A standard nonportable ventilator. (Photo reprinted by permission of Nellcor Puritan Bennett Inc., Pleasanton, CA)

3. Exhalation Valve

The *exhalation valve* may be located in the ventilator itself or in the ventilatory tubing. The purpose of an exhalation valve is to keep the circuitry pressurized during the inspiratory phase, so that air will go to the lungs and not

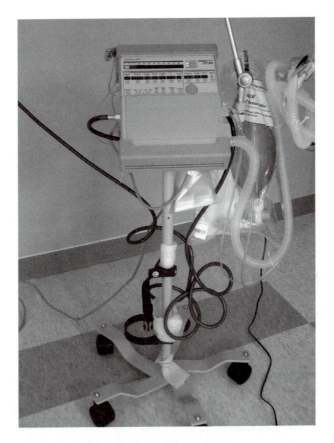

Figure 4-12. A standard portable ventilator.

escape into the tubing. During expiration, the valve opens so that air can be released from the lungs and escape into the atmosphere. Air is not trapped in the ventilatory tubing, where it could be rebreathed by the patient.

D. Humidification Systems

Humidification is necessary in the normal respiratory system and is provided by the upper airway which filters and moisturizes air. When the normal system is bypassed by an endotracheal or tracheostomy tube, drying of the respiratory mucosa and thickening of airway secretions can result. Therefore, additional sources of humidification are needed. For patients receiving mechanical ventilation, humidification is usually delivered through the ventilator circuitry.

1. *Heated humidifiers,* such as *wick type* and *cascade* humidifiers, pass gas over liquid and then deliver it to the patient through the ventilator tubing. They are

examples of evaporating devices that essentially humidify air with water vapor. Heat is used to increase the water content of gas which is delivered at near body temperature. With these systems, the nurse or respiratory care practitioner must periodically remove accumulated condensation from the ventilatory circuitry.

2. **Heat-moisture exchange filters (HME)** serve to trap moisture from air expired from the patient. When the next breath is received, the air passes through the filter and is humidified. The full exhaled tidal volume of air must pass through the HME in order for the humidification to be effective. Therefore, the presence of a leak in the system (e.g, cuff deflation) which allows air to travel through the upper airway, may decrease the usefulness of the HME. HMEs alone may not provide enough humidification for patients with thick, copious secretions.

VI. MONITORING VENTILATORY STATUS

A. Internal Devices

Ventilator alarms provide ongoing monitoring of the patient's response to the ventilator. Alarms are set to ensure that the patient is safe and receiving the desired ventilatory support. If the ventilator does not sense adequate inspiratory/expiratory flows, an alarm will sound. Each alarm provides specific information about a parameter of the ventilator's function. This provides the clinician with specific information regarding trouble shooting of the ventilator and patient condition. Most alarms are designed to be both visual and auditory to attract maximum attention. For each type of ventilator, the alarms provided and their particular parameters will be delineated on the manufacturer's specification sheets.

1. Alarms

a. Low Pressure/Disconnect

The low pressure/disconnect alarm is an internal monitoring device that indicates when the ventilator does not sense adequate pressure between the patient and the ventilator. It is a very important alarm because it senses when the patient is no longer connected to the ventilator. The ventilator is programmed to anticipate the rise and fall of pressure in conjunction with the breath cycle. The pressure will normally fall to zero or to the PEEP level if the patient is receiving PEEP. If for a given amount of time a preset pressure is not reached, the low pressure alarm will sound. Failure to reach the preset pressure may indicate disconnect from the ventilator or a leak in the ventilatory circuitry. The settings of the low pressure/disconnect alarm depend on the needs of the patient and the corresponding ventilatory settings. Low pressure alarms are usually adjusted at about 5–10 cm H_2O below the peak airway pressure.

b. High pressure

The high pressure alarm, which indicates increased airway resistance, is another important internal monitoring device. High resistance will create high airway pressure. Although a certain amount of pressure should be maintained in the ventilatory circuitry, this pressure should not significantly exceed the average peak airway pressure. The high pressure alarm sounds when there is an obstruction to airflow that causes a preset high pressure limit to be reached. Airflow can be obstructed by the presence of secretions or water in the ventilatory circuitry, bronchospasm, or kinking in the ventilatory tubing. Abnormally stiff or noncompliant lungs can also create increased airway pressure. Lung compliance impacts on airway pressure when air is not emptied from the lungs before the ventilator attempts to deliver another breath. Atelectasis can also prevent the patient from receiving air from the ventilator, so that pressure quickly builds as the ventilator cycles. High intrapulmonary pressure can be extremely dangerous to the patient as it can cause barotrauma, or actual rupture of delicate lung tissue with resulting pneumothorax. High pressure alarms can be set at different levels depending on patient status (e.g., to reflect degree of lung compliance). The high pressure alarm is usually adjusted at 10–15 cm H_2O above the peak airway pressure, and usually not higher than 50 cm H_2O.

c. Battery/ventilator inoperative/power failure

Ventilators have power indicators which indicate if the ventilator is functioning on wall current or the *internal* or *external* battery. If the ventilator is operating solely on the internal battery, battery failure will render the ventilator inoperative. A power failure that disrupts the flow of electricity from the wall socket to the ventilator should cause the internal battery to activate, as well as sounding an alarm to alert staff. Portable ventilators have the option of operating on external batteries. An alarm will indicate if that source of power becomes low. The sounding of the external battery alarm should alert someone to plug the ventilator into the wall current immediately. The internal battery should not be used for long periods of time, but should function for emergencies and when traveling short distances. When responding to a power alarm the clinician may need to manually ventilate the patient if both the internal battery and external power sources fail.

d. Exhaled tidal volume (return) alarm

The exhaled tidal volume return alarm is designed to activate when the ventilator does not sense an adequate amount of air returning through the ventilator circuitry. Tidal volume may fall below what has been designated for the patient if a portion of air is diverted from the ventilator tubing. This may occur if there is a partial leak, but not a full disconnect, in the ventilator tubing or if air is diverted as when a patient's cuff is deflated.

e. Apnea alarm

The apnea alarm is an additional safety measure that indicates if the patient has stopped spontaneously breathing. The alarm is most helpful when the patient is breathing on his own, for example, during the weaning process. If breathing ceases for any reason, the apnea alarm will sound, and the patient will be reconnected automatically to mechanical ventilation. Apnea alarms are also used when a patient is on an assist mode of ventilation and must trigger at least intermittent spontaneous breaths.

B. External Monitoring

1. Chest Movement and Auscultation

During mechanical ventilation, the importance of the clinician's observations of patient status cannot be downplayed. Chest wall movement is one parameter that provides information regarding the patient's work of breathing. For example, a patient who is experiencing an increased respiratory rate or **tachypnea** may exhibit shallow, rapid inspiratory efforts characteristic of a respiratory dysfunction.

Auscultation is also used during clinical assessment. The use of a stethoscope can detect breath sounds characteristic of specific conditions. Table 4-3 lists abnormal breath sounds and their related conditions. Speech-language pathologists can be trained to identify typical patterns that assist in identifying the conditions in their patients. This enables the speech-language pathologist to be aware of potential problems and to then alert appropriate medical practitioners.

2. Alarms

External alarms are used as additional safety measures in the event that internal alarms are rendered nonfunctional. An external alarm can also be utilized to replace internal alarming sensors such as the exhaled tidal volume alarm.

3. Arterial Blood Gases (ABG)

Arterial blood gases are obtained via an invasive procedure in which a needle is inserted into an artery. The results obtained reflect the patient's status only at the time that the sample was taken. Therefore, this is not a measure that

Table 4-3. Abnormal Breath Sounds and Related Conditions. (From *Clinical Application of Mechanical Ventilation,* 2nd ed., by D. W. Chang, 2001. Clifton Park, NY: Delmar Learning, p. 209.)

BREATH SOUND	CONDITIONS
Diminished or absent	Airway obstruction
	Atelectasis
	Main-stem intubation
	Pleural effusion
	Pneumothorax
Wheezes	Airway narrowing
Inspiratory crackles	Lung consolidation
	Pulmonary edema
Coarse crackles	Excessive secretions

records fluctuations in a patient's status over a period of time unless it is repeated periodically. However, blood gases are the most reliable and comprehensive indicator of respiratory status.

4. **Pulse Oximetry**

    Oximetry is a technique by which oxygen saturation of hemoglobin in the arterial circulation is obtained via analysis of the degree of absorbed light in the blood. Blood that has absorbed a higher amount of oxygen is bright red. Darker blood indicates less oxygenation. Although the simple observation of blood color can be a helpful clinical tool, oximetry is used to provide an objective method of determining oxygen saturation based upon light absorption in the blood (Levitsky et al., 1990).

    a. Pulse oximetry is a noninvasive tool that is commonly used for ongoing monitoring of oxygen saturation. It involves placing a probe onto a well-oxygenated area of the body, usually the nail bed of a finger or an ear lobe as pictured in Figure 4-13. The probe has two parts, one that releases wavelengths of light and one that reads those light waves. The probe is placed, and pulses of light are sent through the skin and capillaries to be read by the sensor on the other side (Figure 4-13). Some of the light waves will be absorbed, dependent upon the degree of oxygen saturation and subsequent color of the blood. The difference between the number of wavelengths of light emitted and the number of wavelengths read by the sensor is calculated by the pulse oximeter. An arterial saturation level is

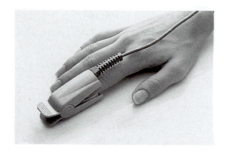

Figure 4-13. Typical placement of a pulse oximeter sensor on a finger. (Photo reprinted by permission of Nellcor Puritan Bennett Inc., Pleasanton, CA)

obtained. A digital display provides the clinician with continuous oxygen saturation levels as well as heart rate or pulse.

b. Oximetry is a very helpful monitoring tool for some parameters, but its measurements should not be regarded as absolute values. Rather, reports in the literature suggest that pulse oximetry can assess *changes* or trends in blood oxygen saturation (Escourrou, Delaperche, & Visseaux, 1990; Orenstein, Curtis, Nixon, & Hartigan, 1993). Additionally oximetry does not provide information regarding carbon dioxide levels or pH. Limitations also include inaccurate readings due to a patient's movements, the presence of extraneous light in the environment, differences between oximetry units, concentration of different types of hemoglobin in the blood, skin pigmentation, and even dark nail polish. Oximetry is most effectively utilized with other monitoring tools.

5. Capnography

Capnography is a noninvasive tool which measures the carbon dioxide levels in exhaled/end tidal CO_2 (PetCO$_2$). PetCO$_2$ will generally reflect alveolar CO_2 (i.e., PACO$_2$). In theory, the capnogram or waveform that is obtained from this analysis should correlate with the arterial carbon dioxide (i.e., PaCO$_2$). The capnogram is obtained through either infrared analysis, reading light absorption in molecules of carbon dioxide, or mass spectrometry, which counts ionized gas molecules. Capnography is performed in-line with the ventilatory tubing and can provide ongoing assessment of ventilatory status. Recent concerns regarding the correlation of PetCO$_2$ levels, obtained via capnography, with PaCO$_2$ have suggested that multiple factors may affect PetCO$_2$ and that the exhaled air may not always accurately differentiate changes in PaCO$_2$ levels (Hess, Schlottag, Levin, Mathai, & Rexrode, 1991). As with oximetry, capnography appears most effective in providing information regarding *changes* or trends in exhaled CO_2. Figure 4-14 shows a monitoring tool with combined oximetry and capnography.

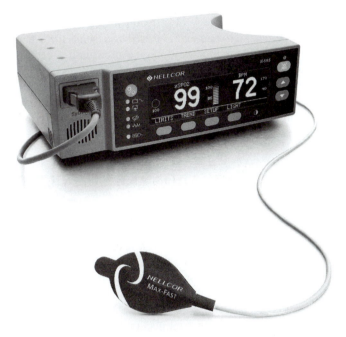

Figure 4-14. Example of a dual oximetry/capnography monitoring tool. (Photo reprinted by permission of Nellcor Puritan Bennett Inc., Pleasanton, CA)

6. Transcutaneous Oxygen/Carbon Dioxide Monitoring

Transcutaneous oxygen/carbon dioxide monitoring is another noninvasive technique which can measure PaO_2 and $PaCO_2$ via heated electrodes placed onto the skin. For O_2 monitoring, the technique is utilized more in neonates versus adults due to the differences in skin structure (Jubran & Tobin, 1994). Transcutaneous PCO_2 monitoring will usually correlate well with $PaCO_2$ levels. There are circumstances when the relationship becomes less accurate (i.e., during certain medical conditions).

7. Spirometry

Spirometry is a noninvasive technique utilized to measure the volume of air that is inhaled and exhaled. In other words, it is a measurement of vital capacity taken at the airway opening when the patient performs a vital capacity maneuver. Spirometry is often included in a battery of **pulmonary function tests (PFTs).** Pulmonary function tests provide objective information regarding pulmonary mechanics and physiology. These tests may be utilized to diagnose a pulmonary disease process, monitor the course of the disease, and establish the efficacy of a treatment regimen. In addition to its diagnostic properties, spirometry may be used to establish the patency of the upper airway. For example, spirometry may be used with a ventilator-dependent patient who is being assessed for tolerance of cuff deflation. The patient's ability to exhale through the upper airway and around the sides of the tracheostomy tube can be measured at the patient's mouth during the exhalation. The spirometer will indicate the volume of air that is exhaled through the upper airway after cuff deflation.

VII. MECHANICAL VENTILATION AND CUFF DEFLATION

A. Purpose of Cuff Inflation with Mechanical Ventilation

1. Inflated endotracheal and/or tracheostomy tube cuffs are used to prevent air which has been supplied by the ventilator from escaping through the upper airway, as illustrated in Figure 4-15. The cuff can compensate for the area in the tracheal lumen that is not filled by the tracheostomy tube itself. When a cuff is deflated, it may be difficult to maintain the tidal volume settings of the ventilator. Air escapes on inspiration and travels through the upper airway, instead of remaining in a closed loop between the ventilator and patient. Air

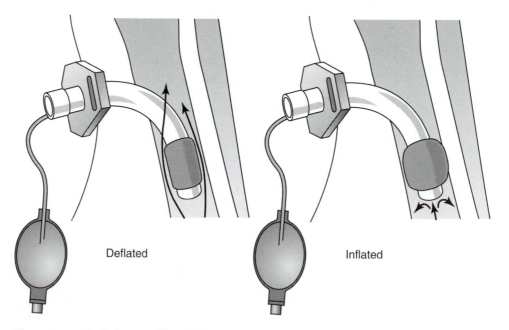

Deflated   Inflated

Figure 4-15. The leak created by a deflated tracheostomy tube cuff contrasted with the seal of an inflated cuff.

leakage will occur during all periods of ventilator connection, whether the patient is awake or asleep. When this happens, the tidal volume or exhaled return volume alarm will usually sound, indicating that the set volume that has been delivered to the patient is not returning to the ventilator. The cuff seal will vary according to the phases of respiration as the pressure under the cuff increases during the delivery of a mechanical breath. Both intracuff pressure and cuff-to-tracheal pressure increase during this time. Therefore, the pressure exerted by an overinflated cuff will become even greater.

2. Ventilator-dependent patients present with multiple factors predisposing them to aspiration. Bach and Alba (1990a) state that "the cuff is often left inflated because it is thought to prevent aspiration of food, gastric contents and upper airway secretions" (p. 680). An inflated cuff will *reduce* the amount of aspirated material that passes around the sides of the tracheostomy tube into the trachea by providing a mechanical block. It *does not* provide an air tight seal and should not be thought of as a solution to the problem of aspiration.

B. Benefits of Cuff Deflation

The potential contraindications of cuff overinflation and long-term cuff inflation have previously been discussed in Chapters 2 and 3. Cuff *deflation* provides:

1. More complete access to the upper airway during suctioning.

2. Normalized airflow through the upper airway for the preservation of airway protection reflexes.

3. Reduced risk of trauma to the mucosal tissue during tracheostomy and ventilator dependence.

4. Decreased interference with laryngeal elevation during swallowing.

5. Potential for oral communication options.

C. Effective Ventilation in the Presence of a Deflated Cuff

1. Cuff deflation may reduce the tidal volume delivered to the lungs by the ventilator. To compensate for the leakage of air, changes can be made to ventilatory settings that will not compromise adequate ventilation. The following modifications of ventilator settings have proved effective (Bach & Alba, 1990a; Dikeman, Kazandjian, and Chua, 2000):

   a. Increase tidal volume so that the patient receives the prescribed amount of air. This increase can be estimated via spirometry or by exhaled tidal volume.

b. Decrease or increase respiratory rate to more easily coordinate phonation with the cycles of the ventilator.

c. Provide increased pressure support or oxygen levels to reduce the work of breathing.

d. Increase tracheostomy tube size to reduce airway resistance and provide more air from the ventilator on each breath. This reduces the work of breathing. This option is usually used for patients who are not candidates for weaning.

2. The patient is carefully monitored during the process of cuff deflation. Noninvasive and invasive monitoring tools such as pulse oximetry, capnography, spirometry, and blood gas analysis are used. The clinical observations made by the clinicians are as valuable as these objective measurements determine whether a patient can tolerate cuff deflation.

The benefits of cuff deflation for both speech and swallowing will be covered in depth in Chapters 5, 7, and 8.

VIII. SELECTED COMPLICATIONS ASSOCIATED WITH POSITIVE PRESSURE VENTILATION

Numerous complications are associated with mechanical ventilation, specifically with positive pressure ventilation. Positive pressure ventilation is an artificial method of breathing in which pressure is applied to the airway. Types of complications include pulmonary, cardiac, and infectious etiologies.

A. Pulmonary

1. Barotrauma

Barotrauma results from overinflation and subsequent rupture of the alveoli. It is a risk of IPPV, particularly in the diseased lung. When a lung is poorly compliant, it is more sensitive to the continuous pressure exerted by mechanical ventilation. It is for this reason that peak airway pressure should be carefully monitored.

2. Atelectasis

Atelectasis or collapse of a lung or lobe may result from inadequate ventilation to portions of the lung. It is sometimes caused by an imbalance of ventilation-perfusion where air is supplied but is not well distributed to each area of the lung (Levitsky, 1982). This may be secondary to trauma, or to a mechanical obstruction (i.e., secretions or a tumor). It also may result from small ventilatory volumes without use of a periodic sigh breath. In theory, the use of a sigh or at least periodic larger volumes of air will help prevent lung collapse.

B. Cardiac

Cardiac complications commonly result from a decreased return of blood from the venous system into the right side of the heart. This is secondary to the positive pressure that is created in the chest by IPPV. The increased pressure compresses the veins that normally channel blood to the heart. This decreased blood supply can reduce cardiac output (Hough, 1991). As the amount of blood moving through the pulmonary/respiratory system is reduced, the patient may present with **hypotension** or blood pressure that is below normal values.

C. Infection

1. Infection that is acquired in the hospital setting is possible when proper disinfection and hand washing techniques are not employed. The hands of health care workers are only one site for the colonization of bacteria. The moist environment of the respiratory circuitry also provides a breeding ground for bacteria which can be easily introduced into the patient's respiratory system, commonly during suctioning. Routine use of gloves and hand washing are essential in reducing this risk.

2. Ventilator-dependent individuals in institutional settings will have a higher risk of colonizing bacteria at the tracheobronchial site. Neiderman, Ferranti, Zeigler, Merrill, and Reynolds (1984) noted that hospitalized patients with long-term tracheostomies and mechanical ventilation demonstrated persistent bacterial colonization of the lower respiratory tract. These patients tended to develop more infectious complications. Additionally, oropharyngeal colonization of bacteria increases in patients with less stable medical status (Kirsch & Sanders, 1988). These bacteria found in the oropharynx can be aspirated along with secretions or food and predispose patients to infection. Tracheostomized and ventilator-dependent patients are at additional risk of aspiration because they often have poor airway protection secondary to long-term tracheostomy and cuff inflation.

3. Levine and Niederman (1991) reported the multiple mechanisms that may lead to pneumonia in patients who require endotracheal intubation. These risk factors include endotracheal intubation, prolonged cuff inflation, and mechanical ventilation. Some researchers have reported that, for a hospitalized patient who is receiving mechanical ventilation, the risk of developing pneumonia increases 1% per day while on the ventilator (Fagon et al., 1989). This risk appears most acute during the initial period of intubation and increased greatly after the first 24 hours (Langer, Mosconi, Cigada, & Mandelli, 1989).

Table 4-4. Hazards and Complications of Mechanical Ventilation. (From *Clinical Application of Mechanical Ventilation,* 2nd ed., by D. W. Chang, 2001. Clifton Park, NY: Delmar Learning, p. 196.)

CONDITION	EXAMPLES
Related to positive pressure ventilation	Barotrauma (pneumothorax, mediastinal air leak, subcutaneous air leak)
	Hypotension, decrease in cardiac output
	Arrhythmia
	Oxygen toxicity
	Bronchopleural fistula
	Bronchopulmonary dysplasia (in infants)
	Upper gastrointestinal hemorrhage
Related to patient condition	Infection (due to reduced immunity)
	Physical and psychologic trauma
	Multiple organ failure (may be preexisting)
Related to equipment (ventilator and artificial airway)	Ventilator and alarm malfunction
	Ventilator circuit disconnection
	Accidental extubation
	Main bronchus intubation
	Postintubation stridor
	Endotracheal tube blockage
	Tissue damage
	Atelectasis (due to inadequate tidal volume)
Related to medical professionals	Nosocomial pneumonia (due to cross-contamination)
	Inappropriate ventilator settings
	Misadventures (due to lapses of understanding and communication)

D. Psychosocial

The emotional impact of ventilator dependence can adversely affect patients. The loss of control over so essential a function as breathing can create high levels of anxiety and often dependence on the medical staff and the ventilator itself. This lack of control is heightened by the loss of oral communication, often an initial consequence of ventilator dependence. Options for both oral and non-oral communication will be discussed in Chapters 5 and 6.

Table 4-4 lists some of the above hazards and complications of mechanical ventilation as they relate to condition.

IX. CONSIDERATIONS IN WEANING

There are two major variations in weaning patients from invasive mechanical ventilation. One involves gradual progression through the levels of intermittent mandatory ventilation (IMV). The other variation in weaning technique involves disconnection from mechanical ventilation for progressively longer periods of time.

A. Progression from Controlled Ventilation

The pulmonologist, assisted by the respiratory care practitioner and nurse, makes the primary decisions regarding the timing and progression of the weaning process. A respiratory care driven protocol has also been used successfully in a long-term care setting with a ventilator subacute unit. Fleming, Sobol, and Chua (1997) reported the success of a slow weaning process which emphasized monitoring by respiratory care practitioners and noninvasive assessment techniques (i.e., capnography and oximetry).

1. Weaning with IMV/SIMV

    a. Long-term mechanical ventilation is usually an indication for a slower, more gradual weaning process. If a patient has been receiving mechanical ventilation for several months, there have usually been difficulties maintaining adequate ventilation and blood gas levels. Other factors including infection, renal/cardiac failure, and psychological/emotional status will enter into the decision to begin a gradual weaning process.

    b. This type of weaning protocol attempts to move the patient from full mechanical support to more spontaneous attempts at triggering breaths. For example, patients who are receiving the IMV/SIMV mode of ventilation can be slowly decreased in respiratory rate, thus allowing the patient to assume more of the responsibility of breathing. In other words, the patient will not receive ventilator breaths as frequently and should be thus encouraged to trigger spontaneous breaths. If the number of breaths is set too low, the patient's work of breathing will increase. The patient is carefully assessed to determine how many breaths he or she is capable of triggering before the IMV/SIMV levels are decreased. For example, if the patient is breathing at 8 and the SIMV/IMV setting is at 6, it is clear that the patient is able to spontaneously breathe the 2 additional breaths. The physician and respiratory care practitioner may attempt to reduce the number of controlled breaths. However, a low IMV requires a continuous effort from the patient and does not allow for prolonged rest periods. Fleming and Sobol (1997) reported on successful weaning of 47 patients in an extended care setting, who could not be weaned in the acute care environment, using an SIMV weaning mode.

c.   Once the mechanical support has been withdrawn, a patient might be given a trial of CPAP. This involves totally spontaneous breathing but insures a supply of air via the tracheostomy. The patient also has a mechanism for reconnection if spontaneous breathing stops. At this point the apnea alarm would sound. Another option is the use of oxygen via a T-piece or trach collar for additional support and to eliminate the patient's rebreathing expired air. It is possible that during the weaning process the patient may be off the ventilator during all waking hours, perhaps needing oxygen only via trach collar, but require mechanical ventilation at night. Once a patient no longer is connected to the ventilator, the monitoring functions of the ventilator are then lost.

2. **Weaning by Time off the Ventilator**

a.   Another variation to the weaning protocol that may be utilized for a medically stable patient who demonstrates signs of spontaneous breathing is stopping all ventilatory support for a set period of time. Stopping mechanical ventilatory support is similar to providing the patient with an exercise period. This exercise may be alternated with periods of rest or reconnection to mechanical ventilation. In some cases, the patient may be only briefly disconnected from mechanical ventilation. The patient is closely supervised and monitored with objective monitoring tools during this process. Clinical impressions of patient comfort and discomfort are also necessary. The patient is observed for ability to breathe spontaneously and for any signs of increased work of breathing, or air hunger, known as *dyspnea*. Blood gas analysis follows as a truly objective way of measuring the adequacy of ventilation. Off ventilator time is gradually increased, perhaps alternated with periods of full ventilatory support. Another way to withdraw ventilatory support is to decrease respiratory rate and tidal volume which decreases the amount of alveolar ventilation provided.

b.   It is important to review patient predictors for this type of weaning protocol. In general, the individual who is medically stable (without major cardiac or pulmonary problems), well nourished, and alert will have better success with the process. Sobol, Fleming, Chua, and Leddy (1998) reported age as a predictor of weaning outcome and survival in a long-term care facility.

c.   During this type of weaning, patients may also utilize trach collar, T-piece, or CPAP when off the ventilator to provide oxygen and may be reconnected to mechanical ventilation at night.

3. **Noninvasive Mechanical Ventilation**

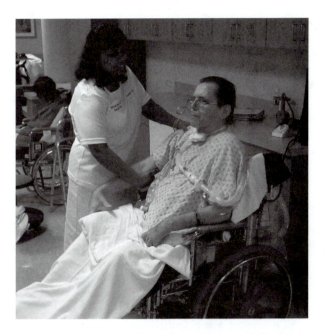

Figure 4-16. Ventilator-dependent patient participating in rehabilitation therapy.

The increased use of noninvasive methods of mechanical ventilation has provided increased options for individuals who require mechanical assistance for breathing but do not necessarily require long-term tracheostomy tube placement. Patients with more stable medical conditions, especially those who can participate in respiratory rehabilitation programs, may move from tracheostomy intermittent positive pressure ventilation to noninvasive methods (Bach & Alba, 1990b).

B. Respiratory Rehabilitation Programs

Respiratory rehabilitation is an important part of weaning. Patients who participate in physical therapy to address mobility and ambulation (as pictured in Figure 4-16), and occupational therapy to assist activities of daily living will reach their overall rehabilitation goals much faster. Portable ventilators enable patients to leave their bedsides and participate in therapeutic and recreational activities. Nursing care can address not only medical needs such as mobilization of secretions, but independence in such tasks as self-suctioning. A true respiratory rehabilitation program incorporates all members of the transdisciplinary team (Kazandjian & Dikeman, 1993).

C. Progression to Decannulation

Removal of a tracheotomy tube is desirable because long-term tracheotomy is associated with numerous complications as discussed in Chapter 3. The decannulation process can be accomplished via several techniques, including down-sizing the tracheotomy tube, using a fenestrated tracheotomy tube, or placing a one-way valve prior to capping the tube.

1. Weaning from Tracheostomy

a. Candidacy issues

Several techniques are used to wean a patient from a tracheostomy tube. Whether the size of the tracheostomy tube is gradually reduced or the tube is occluded for periods of time, the amount of airway resistance the patient experiences when inspiring will increase. This increased resistance occurs when the patient attempts to inspire the same volume of air through a smaller area (i.e., the smaller diameter tracheostomy tube), or perhaps through the upper airway. The ability to tolerate this greater resistance and potential increase in the work of breathing without symptoms of distress or shortness of breath is an indication of readiness to take on more responsibility for breathing. A prerequisite of this tolerance is the presence of a patent airway. Therefore, a patient is usually seen for laryngeal evaluation prior to decannulation especially if there has been a previous history of laryngeal or tracheal obstruction such as stenosis, granuloma, or bilateral vocal fold paralysis.

A patient with a tracheostomy is also considered ready to begin the decannulation process when medical status is stable and the factor precipitating the need for an alternate airway has resolved. Recall that secretion management and the need for pulmonary toilet are factors that may have influenced the decision to place the tracheostomy tube. Therefore, the level of patient consciousness, ability to protect the airway, and need for suctioning are predictors of candidacy for decannulation.

b. Decannulation procedure

The decannulation process can vary from institution to institution. Although procedures may vary, the clinician must consider the status and tolerance of the patient when implementing the steps in weaning.

(1) One technique in decannulation is the gradual reduction of the size of the tracheostomy tube to the smallest tube available. The small-size tube is then capped for a particular time interval, perhaps 72 hours. If the patient does not exhibit difficulties with breathing or secretion management, the tracheostomy tube is then removed, with physician

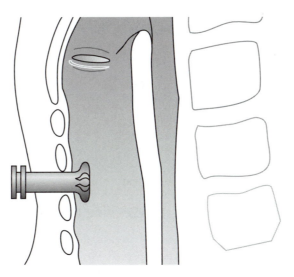

Figure 4-17. Olympic Trach-Button and closure plug. (Courtesy of Olympic Medical Corp.)

order. The development of one-way speaking valves has provided another weaning option. One-way valves introduce a small amount of airway resistance when they are worn. The patient is still able to inspire through the tracheotomy tube with the one-way valve. Le, Aten, Chiang, and Light (1993), in their comparison of the use of capping to the use of one-way valves during weaning, noted that patients reported increased comfort when they were able to breathe at least partially through the tracheostomy tube, as with a one-way valve.

(2) The change from a cuffed to a cuffless tracheostomy tube is often combined with the downsizing process. Because even a deflated cuff takes up some space in the tracheal lumen, its removal provides increased area for airflow and increased use of the upper airway.

(3) The use of a fenestrated tracheostomy tube can be incorporated into the decannulation process. The presence of a fenestration allows more passage of air through the upper airway and facilitates upper airway usage. Either fenestrated inner and outer cannulas can be placed or the nonfenestrated inner cannula can be removed, opening the fenestration of the outer cannula. Removal of the nonfenestrated inner cannula is indicated only when secretion management is not a problem.

(4) Another weaning technique incorporates the use of a tracheal button which serves to maintain an open stoma allowing pulmonary toilet and replacement of a tracheostomy tube in an emergency. This device was discussed in Chapter 3 and is illustrated in Figure 4-17.

Table 4-5. Effects of Undernutrition. (From *Clinical Application of Mechanical Ventilation* [2nd ed.] by D. W. Chang, 2001, p. 354. Clifton Park, NY: Delmar Learning.)

1. Depletion of cellular stores of glycogen and protein
2. Fatigue of respiratory muscles
3. Impaired pulmonary function
4. Decreased cell-mediated immunity
5. Interstitial or pulmonary edema
6. Poor wound healing
7. Decreased surfactant production

D. Issues That Impede the Weaning Process

Before beginning the weaning process, the primary indication necessitating mechanical ventilation must be improved. Weaning the tracheostomized and ventilator-dependent patient is a complicated process that is affected by numerous physical and psychosocial factors. Unstable medical status (e.g., cardiac complications, renal failure) will limit the success of any efforts at weaning. Examples of specific issues that may impede the progression through the weaning process include:

1. Poor Nutritional Status

Nutritional status is integral in the selection of a weaning candidate. Trache-ostomized and ventilator-dependent patients have high caloric demands. Their diets must be adjusted to meet full nutritional needs as well as to compensate for co-existing medical conditions. Protein-calorie malnutrition, often a complicating factor in any critical illness, can have an especially devastating effect on the ventilator-dependent patient during the weaning process. Respiratory muscle strength and function, particularly diaphragm muscle mass, is reduced (Pierce, 1995). However, overfeeding is as dangerous as underfeeding. Chang (2001) noted that high calorie enteral nutrition can increase oxygen consumption and carbon dioxide production. For many ventilator-dependent patients, a low carbohydrate diet with balanced protein and higher fat content is helpful. This diet is designed to maximize energy intake and minimize oxygen utilization and carbon dioxide production. Other factors also influence weaning. To determine if the patient can tolerate the physical stress of weaning, the physician reviews the laboratory results for values such as protein (**albumin**). An albumin that is too low may prevent a ventilator-dependent patient from being weaned. In monitoring and managing these nutritional factors, the registered dietitian is an essential member of the transdisciplinary treatment team (Kazandjian & Dikeman, 1993). Tables 4-5 and 4-6 describe the possible effects of undernutrition and overfeeding.

2. Repeated Aspiration Pneumonia

Pneumonia, especially repeated infections, impacts on ventilatory status and may physically debilitate individuals so that the weaning process is inter-

Table 4-6. Effects of Overfeeding. (From *Clinical Application of Mechanical Ventilation* [2nd ed.] by D. W. Chang, 2001, p. 354. Clifton Park, NY: Delmar Learning.)

1. Increased oxygen consumption
2. Increased carbon dioxide production
3. Increased work of breathing
4. Decreased surfactant production
5. Interstitial or pulmonary edema
6. Fatty degeneration of liver

rupted. The presence of long-term tracheostomy, associated with numerous complications, may predispose patients to colonization of bacteria in the lower respiratory tract (Niederman, Merrill et al., 1984). Tracheostomized individuals with poor nutritional status appear even more susceptible to this type of infection. Oropharyngeal colonization of bacteria is very common in hospitalized patients, with or without tracheostomy, and is linked to recurrent aspiration pneumonia caused by ingestion of oral secretions.

3. Anxiety

Patients who receive mechanical ventilatory support commonly report feelings of anxiety. The inability to control so basic a function as breathing often causes patients to become overly dependent on the ventilator. Attempts to decrease time spent on the ventilator can precipitate a clinical reaction that necessitates a return to full ventilatory support. This can occur even when more objective measures (such as capnography) record that the patient is tolerating less support or even breathing on his or her own. For patients who demonstrate significant anxiety, a gradual transition through the stages of weaning will be necessary. This will allow the patient to realize that, although the ventilator is providing less support, ventilation is nonetheless adequate. All members of the team need to be cognizant of the impact anxiety can have on the weaning process, and provide emotional support. Psychological intervention may be appropriate. Additionally, pain can create heightened anxiety and must be controlled, although overmedication can suppress the patient's respiratory drive.

X. ALTERNATIVES TO MECHANICAL VENTILATION

Some individuals who require continued ventilatory support may be able to use alternatives to mechanical ventilation. Although these techniques cannot replace mechanical ventilation, they may facilitate improved oxygenation and carry additional benefits that contribute to a healthy respiratory system. The following technique may provide maintenance of pulmonary capacity through lung expansion and clearance of secretions that interfere with adequate gas exchange.

A. Glossopharyngeal Breathing

Glossopharyngeal breathing, often referred to as frog breathing, is a method of inflating the lungs. It may be used to increase vocal volume or to produce a cough for clearance of secretions. Glossopharyngeal breathing has also been used to increase vital capacity and to maintain respiratory function. Some individuals, such as those with high spinal cord injuries or postpolio syndrome, have achieved time off the ventilator by utilizing this technique to force air into their lungs (Bach & Alba, 1990b).

1. Glossopharyngeal breathing involves using the tongue, soft palate, pharynx, and larynx to push or gulp air into the lungs, coordinating the injection of air through the lips, stroking movement of the tongue, and opening/closing of the vocal folds. Air enters the lungs with each stroke or gulp. Glossopharyngeal breathing can therefore be considered a substitute method of breathing.

2. Pineda (1984) states that patients can achieve a tidal volume of 500 to 2500 ml using this technique, which actually mimics the physiological function of the normal sigh breath. This expansion of the lungs, which is absent in patients with significant respiratory muscle dysfunction, may help preserve pulmonary compliance. This air is also available for speech, coughing, and clearing of secretions. Alba (1986) provides step-by-step instruction for the training of glossopharyngeal breathing.

XI. ALTERNATIVES TO INVASIVE MECHANICAL VENTILATION

Noninvasive positive pressure ventilation (NPPV) provides ventilation without an artificial airway, reducing or eliminating some of the complications of traditional positive pressure ventilation. There have been recent trends to utilize NPPV in acute care, emergency room settings to avoid respiratory failure secondary to COPD exacerbation or other chronic conditions. Many of these complications, for example, intubation trauma and prolonged tracheostomy which impact upon speech and swallowing, are avoided with noninvasive techniques.

An understanding of respiratory care techniques, including mechanical ventilatory support, is necessary for the clinician who works with this challenging population. This working knowledge provides the clinician with the information needed to proceed with effective intervention for communication and swallowing.

5

Oral Communication Options

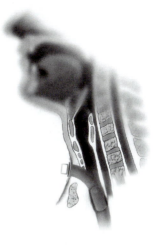

The loss of oral communication can have a devastating effect not only on a patient's communication but also on his or her emotional and psychological well-being. Most tracheostomized and ventilator-dependent individuals will experience at least some period of aphonia during their medical treatment. It is the role of the speech-language pathologist to preserve oral communication when feasible. Many communication options are available to the tracheostomized and/or ventilator-dependent patient. In essence, ventilator dependence and oral communication are not mutually exclusive. An appropriate assessment and treatment process, incorporating most members of the transdisciplinary team, is necessary to establish candidacy for oral communication. The sample protocols provided in this chapter demonstrate that team members may share roles during the assessment and treatment process. However, the speech-language pathologist will direct the effort to restore oral communication.

I. POPULATION

Table 5-1 reviews the etiologies that were discussed in Chapter 1. They include respiratory-specific and vascular conditions, trauma, and degenerative diseases. To provide a helpful framework for initial assessment these conditions and diseases and their presenting symptomatology can be loosely classified as *temporary, static,* and *degenerative.*

A. Temporary Conditions

A temporary medical condition describes the patient who has, in an emergency, been intubated and placed on a ventilator following either a trauma, vascular event, or decline in medical/respiratory status. The temporary classification refers to a patient who may not require either long-term intubation or the more permanent

Table 5-1. Temporary, Static, and Degenerative Disease Populations.

RESPIRATORY-SPECIFIC	VASCULAR	TRAUMA	DEGENERATIVE
COPD	CVA	MVA	ALS
Tracheomalacia	Tumor	GSW	MS
Sleep apnea	Cardiac conditions	SCI	MD
Acute upper airway infections			AIDS
Upper airway obstructions			Guillain-Barré

intervention of a tracheotomy. An example is a patient with emphysema who is admitted to the intensive care unit (ICU) with acute respiratory symptoms secondary to pneumonia. If respiratory status cannot be stabilized, this individual may require intubation and connection to mechanical ventilation. However, the patient may have excellent potential for weaning once the acute infection has been treated and resolved. This patient may require intervention on a temporary basis, during the period of intubation and aphonia. Communication needs will probably be specific to the intensive care environment as the patient, staff, and family interact with one another.

B. Static Conditions

In contrast, a static medical condition refers to a physical status that is not expected to change significantly, even after the initial acute episode has passed. This may include a patient following a vascular or traumatic event that requires long-term tracheostomy and ventilatory support because of permanent respiratory impairment. A patient with a C1–C2 spinal cord injury from a motor vehicle accident would fall into this category. This patient may achieve a stable medical status but will require mechanical ventilatory support with little potential for weaning. Long-term intervention will be required to meet the patient's ongoing communication needs and to adapt to changing communicative settings and partners.

C. Degenerative Conditions

In a degenerative medical condition, the patient's medical status is expected to decline. This includes the degenerative neurological disease processes which commonly impair respiratory function. An individual with amyotrophic lateral sclerosis will often experience a progressive decline in respiratory status. Initially, the patient may present with only reduced breath support but eventually require tracheostomy and 24-hour ventilator dependence. Intervention is a long-term process and must be modified to meet the changing needs of the patient (Kazandjian, Dikeman, & Bach, 1995).

This framework of temporary, static, and degenerative classifications can assist clinicians in the initial communicative assessment of the patient and provide a rationale for the treatment approach.

II. ASSESSMENT

A. Continuum of Disability

The continuum of disability represents not only a range of deterioration from one point to another but a fixed scale on which a patient's status can be described in terms of *physical-motor, speech, cognitive-linguistic abilities,* and *behavior.* Table 5-2 details the components of the continuum of disability.

1. Physical-Motor Status

Physical-motor status includes the patient's medical diagnosis and neurological condition. For that reason it is addressed first during the assessment process. The continuum (see Table 5-2) is read from left to right, beginning with normal upper extremity function with adequate range of motion and good strength and endurance. It continues toward the right, illustrating progressive weakness and limitations in movement. The final point on the scale demonstrates the severest form of physical-motor impairment or *pentaplegia* (paralysis from the head down). Physical-motor impairment may limit the choice of oral communication options by impairing upper extremity function and endurance.

2. Speech and Voice Status

Table 5-3 defines speech, voice, and language disorders. Speech abilities range from normal phonation and articulation to aphonia and severe motor speech weakness, either dysarthria or anarthria. The patient may have involvement of voice only or disruption of both voice and motor speech production. Speech and voice function observed during the initial contact will form the basis for further evaluation and the selection of an oral communication option.

3. Cognitive-Linguistic Status

Cognitive abilities range from intact status, to deficits in orientation, memory, reasoning, and other higher level language functions, to more severe deficits in basic alerting and attentional skills that will limit the patient's ability to initiate and perform volitional tasks. Language abilities may range from mild to severe *aphasia* or actual language impairment. Cognitive and language impairments often limit a patient's ability to benefit from intervention. Cognitive-linguistic impairment often disrupts learning new information and carrying over treatment techniques from session to session. At the most severe end of

Table 5-2. Components of the Continuum of Disability. (Adapted from "Continuum of Disability" by C. Salciccia, 1986. In C. Salciccia, L. Adams, & G. Kapassakis, *Communication Management of Respiratorily-Involved Quadriplegic Adults*. Paper presented at Goldwater Memorial Hospital, New York, NY)

Physical Motor	Normal UE ROM and fine motor. Good endurance.	Adequate UE ROM and fine motor. Fair endurance.	UE Weakness. Gross movement adequate. Limited ROM. Poor endurance.	Significant weakness. Limitations in ROM. Poorly coordinated UE function. Severely limited endurance.	Quadriplegia. No upper/lower extremity function.	Pentaplegia. No movement including head.
Speech/Voice	Phonation with good vocal intensity, Articulation WNL.	Phonation with decreased intensity. Good articulation.	Phonation poorly ordinated with ventilation.	Aphonic with good mouthing. / Aphonia with mild dysarthria.	Aphonia with moderate dysarthria.	Aphonia with severe dysarthria.
Cognitive-Linguistic	No deficits, intact status.	Mild deficits (memory, orientation, reasoning, anomia).		Moderate deficits (impairments in language expression/reception).	Severe deficits.	Profound deficits.
Behavior	Patient indicates concerns, highly motivated for treatment.	Mild anxiety, but can be reassured.		Moderate anxiety, difficulty in transitioning through intervention stages. Treatment is interfered with.		Severe anxiety. No intervention possible.

Note: UE = upper extremity; ROM = range of motion; WNL = within normal limits.

Table 5-3. Speech and Language Disorders.

Dysphonia:	An impairment in voice, usually affecting vocal quality and loudness level.
Aphonia:	An inability to produce voice due to paralyzed vocal folds or lack of subglottic airflow. This can be due to structural airway abnormalities or tracheostomy cuff inflation.
Dysarthria:	An impairment of the speech musculature that affects articulation, resonance, phonation (voicing), and respiration. Speech intelligibility is disrupted.
Anarthria:	The severest form of muscle weakness, rendering the patient unable to move the musculature to produce speech.
Aphasia:	An impairment in linguistic function affecting verbal expression, auditory comprehension, visual language function (reading and writing), and gesture.
Apraxia:	An impairment in the ability to plan volitional movements.

the continuum (see Table 5-2) are the most profoundly impaired individuals who are alert but do not demonstrate purposeful communication.

4. **Behavioral Status**

Behavior can range from the expression of concerns that any medically compromised patient might normally experience, to anxiety that can be alleviated with verbal reassurance, to severe or extreme anxiety that interferes with the ability to accept intervention. It is not uncommon for tracheostomized and/or ventilator-dependent patients to experience periods of anxiety concerning their condition and prognosis.

B. The Patient and the Continuum of Disability

1. **Use of the Continuum**

Assessment of the tracheostomized and/or ventilator-dependent patient, like assessment of any communicatively impaired individual, is an ongoing process. The unique needs and often multiple impairments of the tracheostomized and/or ventilator-dependent individual necessitate a comprehensive evaluation.

a. The Continuum of Disability helps identify the patient's strengths and weaknesses. This will guide the speech-language pathologist to issues relevant to the initial evaluation and assist in the development of a treatment protocol. In other words, the evaluator can use the continuum to identify areas that are integral in beginning communicative intervention. For example, Table 5-4 illustrates a patient with a diagnosis of COPD. The results of a neurological evaluation are essentially within normal limits. The patient demonstrates good upper extremity range of motion and fine motor control on the physical-motor scale. Endurance may be limited. The patient is aphonic secondary to tracheostomy (inflated cuff) and ventilator-dependent with good mouthing. Cognitive-linguistic status is intact. The patient reports and demonstrates mild anxiety, but when rationale for treatment is presented, patient cooperation is high.

b. When this patient is viewed in terms of the temporary, static, and degenerative classification system, his essentially stable medical status places him in the static framework. Although the disease itself is ultimately a degenerative condition, the patient often is stable for long periods of time and maintains consistent function in terms of communication. An exception might be when the patient deteriorates in respiratory capacity and no longer tolerates cuff deflation. If the patient becomes aphonic secondary to cuff inflation, communicative intervention would change to address this loss of function.

III. ORAL COMMUNICATION OPTIONS: CANDIDACY ISSUES

Oral/verbal communication allows a patient to participate in communicative exchanges via speech. Oral communication involves use of the articulators and, with the exception of mouthing, voice. Of all communicative techniques, an oral method should be the preferred intervention as it approximates normal communication. Some patients are candidates for oral communication options during structured treatment paradigms (dysarthria, aphasia), but cannot rely on the oral system as the primary method of communication. It is the role of the speech-language pathologist to identify patients who are candidates for a particular type of intervention and provide a functional communication system.

A. Indicators

Candidates for oral communication options include patients who present with the following:

1. Aphonia

2. Adequate oral motor function

3. Potential for speech and language production (e.g., mild-moderate aphasia or dysarthria)

Table 5-4. The Patient with COPD: Continuum of Disability. (Adapted from "Continuum of Disability" by C. Salciccia, 1986. In C. Salciccia, L. Adams, and G. Kapassakis, *Communication Management of Respiratorily-Involved Quadriplegic Adults*. Paper presented at Goldwater Memorial Hospital, New York, NY)

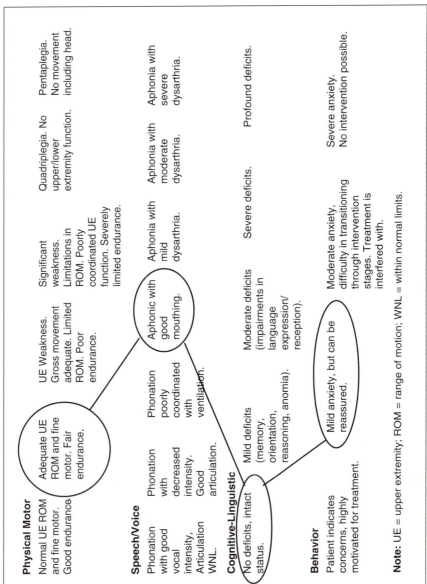

Physical Motor

Normal UE ROM and fine motor. Good endurance.

Adequate UE ROM and fine motor. Fair endurance.

UE Weakness. Gross movement adequate. Limited ROM. Poor endurance.

Significant weakness. Limitations in ROM. Poorly coordinated UE function. Severely limited endurance.

Quadriplegia. No upper/lower extremity function.

Pentaplegia. No movement including head.

Speech/Voice

Phonation with good vocal intensity, Articulation WNL.

Phonation with decreased intensity. Good articulation.

Phonation poorly coordinated with ventilation.

Aphonic with good mouthing.

Aphonia with mild dysarthria.

Aphonia with moderate dysarthria.

Aphonia with severe dysarthria.

Cognitive-Linguistic

No deficits, intact status.

Mild deficits (memory, orientation, reasoning, anomia).

Moderate deficits (impairments in language expression/ reception).

Severe deficits.

Profound deficits.

Behavior

Patient indicates concerns, highly motivated for treatment.

Mild anxiety, but can be reassured.

Moderate anxiety, difficulty in transitioning through intervention stages. Treatment is interfered with.

Severe anxiety. No intervention possible.

Note: UE = upper extremity; ROM = range of motion; WNL = within normal limits.

B. Contraindications

1. Severe dysarthria/anarthria

2. Profound cognitive-linguistic deficits:

   • inability to initiate interaction

   • severe behavioral problems (e.g., severe agitation)

IV. TREATMENT APPROACHES

A. Mouthing

1. Candidacy

Mouthing may be used, with variable success, for patients who have adequate oral motor strength and are aphonic. The patient may be tracheostomized and ventilator-dependent or intubated with a nasotracheal airway. Oral intubation contraindicates the use of mouthing as a viable oral communication option. Other factors also affect the usefulness of mouthing. For example, cognitive-linguistic deficits or extreme anxiety may interfere with effective message transfer. A patient who continues to mouth rapidly with little regard for the listener's comprehension will not be an effective communicator.

2. Procedure

Mouthing is an obvious but effective strategy made even more powerful by the fact that it is often self-generated. The speech-language pathologist may capitalize on an immediately available behavior and provide some modifications to increase functionality. Patients can be instructed to emphasize articulatory movements, decrease speech rate, utilize short phrases, and avoid very complex words. It is important that a patient be responsive to the needs of the communication partner while mouthing.

3. Trouble-Shooting

Although the benefits of mouthing as an immediate method of communication are clear, there are obvious limitations. For example, the patient who is limited to mouthing is unable to call for attention and requires the communication partner to be in the immediate physical area. Additionally, because not all speech sounds are visible on the lips, message interpretation may not be accurate. Because only approximately 30% of consonants are obvious during mouthing, message transfer breakdown is common (Bloodstein, 1979).

a.   Repeated instruction in rate control and articulatory precision and encouraging the patient to monitor for listener comprehension can be helpful in increasing the intelligibility of mouthing.

b.   Denture use facilitates better articulatory contacts and subsequently improves consonant intelligibility. Patient and staff should be reminded to insert dentures whenever possible.

B. Electrolarynges

1. Candidacy

To expand the use of mouthing the speech-language pathologist can provide an alternative vibratory source. This alternative source of phonation eliminates the need for vocal fold vibration or subglottic air pressure. The typical tracheostomized and ventilator-dependent patient is aphonic because air cannot reach the vocal folds. The electrolarynx can be a valuable communication tool for the clinician who is working with an aphonic patient with good oral motor control (Adler & Zeides, 1986). Candidacy may also include, for example, any patient who lacks a vibratory mechanism for voice such as the patient with paralyzed vocal folds. This patient may be a long-term user of an electrolarynx. As with mouthing, contraindications for use include significant cognitive-linguistic deficits or anxiety. Anxiety can interfere with the ability to receive feedback regarding speech intelligibility from a communication partner.

2. Procedure

There are essentially two types of electrolarynges or alternate vibratory sources, hand-held and intra-oral devices. These mechanical devices create sound via electronic vibration. The artificial voice thus created is modulated into speech by the movements of the vocal tract and articulators. Placement of the vibratory source varies by the type of device utilized.

a.   Hand-held (neck type)

The hand-held electrolarynx is the standard device pictured in Figure 5-1. It is usually placed on one side of the neck, under the chin, or on the side of the face (buccal area). It is activated by a switch located on the side of the device. Pitch and volume controls are also available. Either the patient or the communication partner must have adequate hand function and strength to manipulate and position the device. The patient must be instructed in the coordination of articulation with the activation of the device. A slower rate of speech coupled with exaggerated articulatory contacts will usually maximize speech intelligibility.

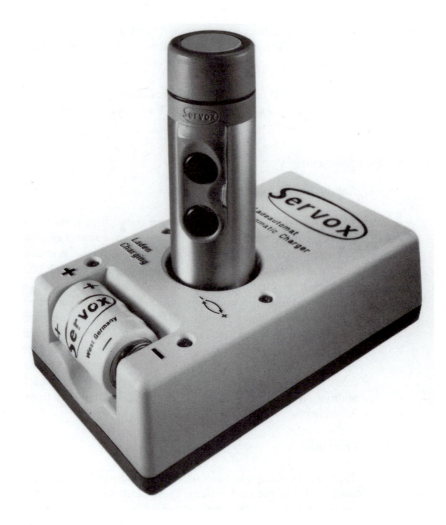

Figure 5-1. A standard hand-held electrolarynx. (Servox Inton photo courtesy of Siemens Hearing Instruments)

b. Intra-oral

The intra-oral electrolarynx produces sound through a plastic tube which is placed into the mouth. Tones are generated and articulated into speech. As with the hand-held device, the intra-oral electrolarynx must be activated by an on-off switch. Volume and pitch controls are provided. The oral device is indicated for patients who would find it difficult to use the hand-held device (e.g., a patient with a spinal cord injury and a special positioning collar for stabilization of the neck). It is also more easily adapted for the quadriplegic patient or individual without sufficient upper extremity function, who cannot manipulate a hand-held device. Through activation of special remote switches, these patients can still be independent users of an electrolarynx. Some facilities will utilize the combined efforts of occupational therapists and rehabilitation engineers to design adapted activation systems for their patients.

3. Trouble-Shooting

The electrolarynx is often a beneficial temporary means of communication. It can be used to quickly restore oral communication, improve interaction with staff and family, and reduce a patient's frustration and anxiety. The immediate restoration of communication is especially helpful in the hospital environment with the acutely ill patient who cannot tolerate modifications of the tracheostomy tube or ventilator. However, the same patient selection criteria discussed regarding mouthing also apply to the electrolarynx user. Individuals who use an artificial larynx must be cognizant of listener reaction and modify their utterances according to listener comprehension. Noisy environments, such as the ICU, may interfere with the listener's ability to perceive the unfamiliar sound of the electrolarynx. Patients with cognitive dysfunction often have particular difficulty receiving this type of feedback and cannot effectively use the compensatory strategies that maximize speech intelligibility. They may also have difficulty with placement of the electrolarynx or coordination of articulation and voice. General instructional techniques for the electrolarynx user that may be helpful include:

a.   Teach staff and patient alternate areas of the neck or cheek where the electrolarynx can be repositioned to maximize intelligibility.

b.   Maintain firm contact against the skin.

c.   Model exaggerated articulatory contacts and a decreased rate of speech.

d.   Insure that patient coordinates activation of the sound source with articulation (i.e., does not continue to press the on switch and produce sound when not speaking).

e.   Encourage patient to provide the listener with opportunities for message clarification by pausing between sentences, maintaining eye contact, and observing conversational turn-taking.

C. Manipulation of the Tracheostomy Tube

Individuals who are able to mouth and/or use the electrolarynx on an immediate or temporary basis must have adequate oral motor function. These individuals can also be eventual candidates for restoration of voicing ability via changes in the type or size of tracheostomy tube. Multiple criteria must be met before patients are considered candidates for restoration of voice.

1. Candidacy: Assessment of Tracheostomized Patients

a. Voice production with tracheal occlusion

Clinical assessment of voice production ability can be accomplished during the initial evaluation. Optimally, the patient will have received a **nasopharyngolaryngoscopy** that carefully evaluated the ability to produce voice, as well as provided an accurate visual image of the vocal folds and airway. However, occlusion of the tracheostomy tube, which redirects air through the upper airway for speech purposes, does provide a gross vehicle for assessment of voice production.

(1) For patients who are tracheostomized, tracheal occlusion can begin the assessment process. One limitation of this bedside approach is that, if a patient is unable to produce voice, it will be difficult to determine if the aphonia relates to vocal fold status or the size of the tracheostomy tube relative to the tracheal lumen. Recall that the first step should always be to deflate the tracheostomy tube cuff, following physician order and after proper suctioning technique, to ensure passage of air through the upper airway. If the patient has an air-filled cuff (as opposed to a foam or sponge cuff), deflation may be either partial or full. Partial cuff deflation involves removing sufficient air from the cuff to allow the patient access to the upper airway. Partial cuff deflation is achieved when the patient begins to produce voice and moves secretions into the upper airway. Full cuff deflation is complete removal of air from the cuff. Table 5-5 provides a sample transdisciplinary protocol for deflation of a tracheostomy tube cuff that involves the physician (MD), respiratory care practitioner (RCP), nurse (RN/LPN), and speech-language pathologist (SLP).

If the cuff has been deflated and the patient is still unable to achieve voice, consider the size of the tracheostomy tube. If the tracheostomy tube completely fills the trachea, airflow cannot pass around the walls of the outer cannula and will be unable to reach the vocal folds. This is depicted in Figure 5-2.

(2) Before modifying tube size, manipulations of the tracheostomy tube itself should be attempted. If the patient has a fenestrated tracheostomy tube with a *nonfenestrated inner cannula* and cannot achieve voice, the inner cannula can be removed and the outer cannula occluded. This should permit airflow to pass up through the fenestration in the outer cannula and reach the vocal folds. A patient with a fenestrated tracheostomy tube with a *fenestrated inner cannula* should have at least some passage of air through the fenestration and upward

Table 5-5. Sample Interdisciplinary Cuff Deflation Protocol for Tracheostomized Patients.

1. MD order obtained for cuff deflation.
2. RCP determines if patient needs preoxygenation or bagging. Patient placed on noninvasive monitoring.
3. Suction the patient using established suctioning procedure through the tracheostomy tube; cuff inflated (RCP/RN/SLP).
4. Allow patient to rest. Reinsert suction catheter into tracheostomy tube. Insert syringe into cuff valve. Apply suction while simultaneously removing air slowly from the cuff, with a syringe. Deflate 2 cc at a time, pausing briefly during the process. Suction as needed.
5. Allow patient time to rest. Suction orally if needed.
6. Insert syringe into cuff valve and *slowly* withdraw air until cuff is fully deflated.
7. Allow patient time to adjust to airflow through the upper airway; SLP encourages voicing and blowing to reestablish use of the upper airway.
8. Assess patient's response via monitoring tools. Assess presence of additional secretions and need for repeated suctioning.
9. Reinflate cuff if needed while staff (MD, RN, SLP, RCP) determine if patient can be maintained with continuous cuff deflation.

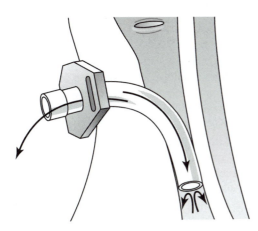

Figure 5-2. A tracheostomy tube filling the entire tracheal lumen.

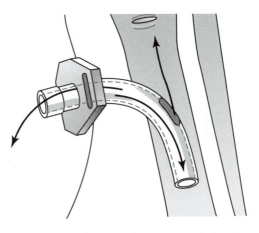

Figure 5-3. A fenestrated outer cannula in relationship to the fenestrated inner cannula.

to the vocal folds, with the inner cannula in place. This is depicted in Figure 5-3.

In some cases, a patient with fenestrated inner and outer cannulas will be able to achieve voice even with the cuff inflated, as shown in Figure

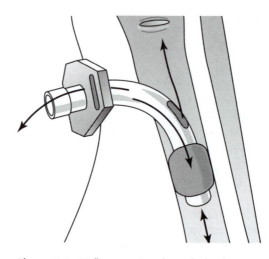

Figure 5-4. Airflow moving through the fenestration of a cuffed fenestrated tracheostomy tube.

5-4. After the speech-language pathologist has attempted the above tracheostomy tube manipulations and tracheal occlusion still does not result in production of voice, vocal fold dysfunction is suspected.

b. Nasopharyngolaryngoscopy

If an evaluation of vocal fold and airway status has not yet been performed, the next step in establishing candidacy for restoration of voice is an assessment of laryngeal function via nasopharyngolaryngoscopy. The procedure utilizes a flexible fiberoptic endoscope as shown in Figure 5-5. This procedure is usually performed by an otolaryngologist (ENT). If adequate vocal fold function for speech purposes is being assessed, a speech-language pathologist often participates. The fiberoptic study will also rule out anatomical abnormalities such as intubation granuloma or laryngeal stenosis which might interfere with airway patency. Essentially, the patient must have adequate vocal fold function for speech purposes. The airway must also be free from significant obstruction to airflow.

(1) Nasopharyngolaryngoscopy is performed transnasally. The lubricated scope is inserted into the nares and passed through the nasal turbinate to allow viewing of the nasal and oral pharynx. The scope is then advanced to the larynx, as depicted in Figure 5-6a. This procedure is effectively performed when the fiberoptic scope is connected to a video camera. To document the examination, the image can be displayed on a monitor and recorded to videotape. Initially the ENT and speech-language pathologist visualize the larynx during respiration, as illustrated in Figure 5-6b. The patient is then

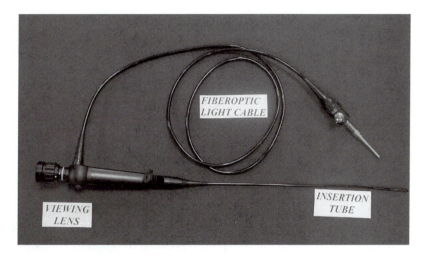

Figure 5-5. A flexible fiberoptic endoscope.

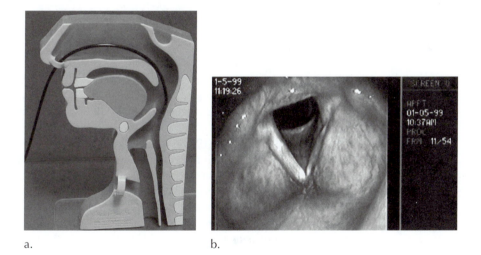

a.

b.

Figure 5-6a. The flexible fiberoptic scope in place for viewing the larynx. **b.** View of the glottis, fully abducted during inspiration.

instructed to produce vowels, consonant-vowel (CV) and consonant-vowel-consonant (CVC) combinations that target particular speech sounds. The patient will also be asked to vary vocal pitch and intensity. To participate in this procedure, a patient with a tracheostomy and inflated cuff must tolerate cuff deflation long enough to allow airflow for vocal fold vibration. Patients who have had long-term cuff inflation may have difficulty producing voice during this examination, even with the cuff deflated. It is important that proper suctioning procedure be followed to ensure that the patient does not aspirate during the period of cuff deflation and efforts to produce voice.

(2) Nasopharyngolaryngoscopy is a valuable tool for direct visualization of the larynx and associated structures. It does not provide the degree of imaging provided by **stroboscopy,** however. Stroboscopy illustrates the finer aspects of laryngeal activity such as abnormalities in the mucosa. It also delineates structural (e.g., carcinoma) as opposed to physiologic irregularities of the larynx not typically detectable to the eye. In contrast, problems that can be diagnosed during nasopharyngolaryngoscopy include more obvious anatomical abnormalities (e.g., vocal fold paralysis, glottic chinks, vocal nodules, polyps or lesions, laryngeal granuloma, and laryngeal stenosis). The procedure can also provide information regarding other components of the speech system, such as velar movement.

2. Procedure

a. Table 5-6 outlines the steps in performing the assessment of voicing ability for patients with tracheostomy tubes.

b. If assessment of the laryngeal mechanism revealed either unilateral or bilateral vocal fold dysfunction, the speech-language pathologist's intervention may begin with direct voice therapy. Hyperfunctional techniques are indicated in cases of vocal fold *paresis* (weakness) or paralysis (Andrews, 1999; Aronson, 1985). These techniques are designed to facilitate vocal fold approximation via forceful adduction exercises. Increased breath support must also be stressed during this period as lack of sufficient airflow impacts upon phonation. *Medical clearance must be obtained prior to introduction of any effortful treatment procedures.* Some cardiac patients, for example, may have contraindications for any technique that could potentially increase blood pressure. Techniques may include:

(1) Pushing or pulling against resistance while phonating. Modifications for the quadriplegic patient involve resistance with the forehead or shoulders instead of the upper extremities.

(2) Forceful coughing, throat clearing, or vocalization (i.e., /ha/-/ha/).

(3) Phonation immediately after a swallow (to utilize the vegetative function of laryngeal closure during swallowing).

(4) Pitch and loudness variation exercises.

c. If laryngeal paresis or paralysis is combined with a dysarthria, oral motor exercises will be indicated for restoration of functional oral communication. A thorough assessment of the peripheral speech mechanism is necessary

Table 5-6. Flow Chart for Assessing Voicing Ability.

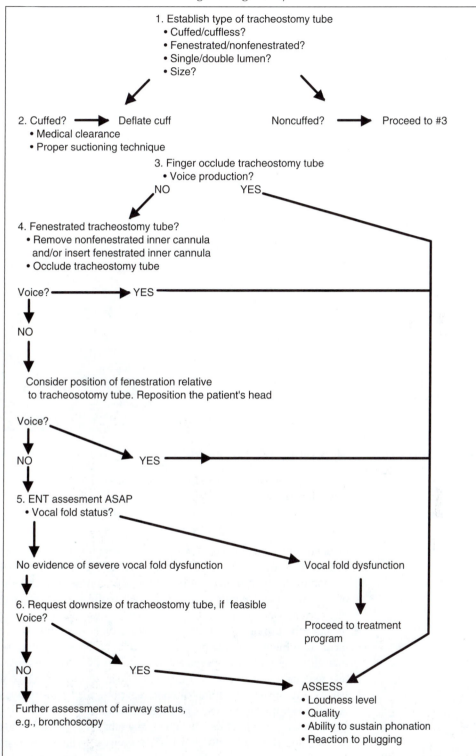

1. Establish type of tracheostomy tube
   - Cuffed/cuffless?
   - Fenestrated/nonfenestrated?
   - Single/double lumen?
   - Size?

2. Cuffed? ⟶ Deflate cuff
   - Medical clearance
   - Proper suctioning technique

   Noncuffed? ⟶ Proceed to #3

3. Finger occlude tracheostomy tube
   - Voice production?

   NO   YES

4. Fenestrated tracheostomy tube?
   - Remove nonfenestrated inner cannula
     and/or insert fenestrated inner cannula
   - Occlude tracheostomy tube

Voice? ⟶ YES

NO

Consider position of fenestration relative
to tracheosotomy tube. Reposition the patient's head

Voice?

NO   YES

5. ENT assesment ASAP
   - Vocal fold status?

No evidence of severe vocal fold dysfunction   Vocal fold dysfunction

6. Request downsize of tracheostomy tube, if feasible
Voice?

NO   YES

Further assessment of airway status,
e.g., bronchoscopy

Proceed to treatment
program

ASSESS
- Loudness level
- Quality
- Ability to sustain phonation
- Reaction to plugging

183

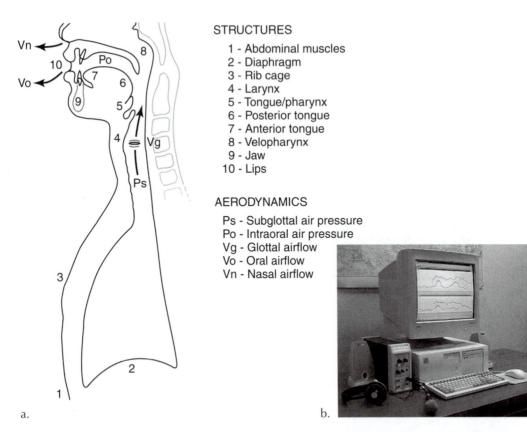

STRUCTURES

1 - Abdominal muscles
2 - Diaphragm
3 - Rib cage
4 - Larynx
5 - Tongue/pharynx
6 - Posterior tongue
7 - Anterior tongue
8 - Velopharynx
9 - Jaw
10 - Lips

AERODYNAMICS

Ps - Subglottal air pressure
Po - Intraoral air pressure
Vg - Glottal airflow
Vo - Oral airflow
Vn - Nasal airflow

a.

b.

Figure 5-7a. The structures and resultant aerodynamics used in speech production. (From *A Neurobiologic View of the Dysarthrias,* by R. Netsell, 1986, p. 3. San Diego, CA: College-Hill Press, Inc. Copyright 1986 by R. Netsell. Reprinted with permission). **b.** An example of a speech instrumentation system. (Visipitch 3900 photo courtesy of Kay Elemetrics Corp.)

to identify the components of the speech system that must be targeted in treatment (Netsell, 1986). The reader is referred to Netsell's (1986) discussion of the adult motor control system that considers the relationship of airflow to the structure of the vocal tract as illustrated in Figure 5-7a. The current state of the art in the treatment of dysarthria and dysphonia includes the use of speech instrumentation, such as the instrumentation pictured in Figure 5-7b, to provide objective feedback regarding physiological function of each speech subsystem. It is beyond the scope of this text to detail all available instrumentation. The reader is referred to Appendix A to obtain further information regarding speech instrumentation. A general outline of treatment procedures includes:

(1) *Articulation:* direct lingual, labial, mandibular, and facial strengthening and range of motion (ROM) exercises. Syllable-word-phrase-sentence production in repetition, oral reading, and spontaneous speech output.

(2) *Resonance:* exercises as above but targeted to stress velar function. Prosthetic devices such as *palatal lifts* may also be evaluated.

(3) *Phonation:* see above.

(4) *Respiration:* exercises to improve diaphragmatic strength (consult with physical therapist). Incentive spirometry. Compensatory techniques in the form of phrasing and reduced speech rate. Prosthetic devices such as *abdominal binders* may also be helpful.

3. Trouble-Shooting

During the assessment of voicing function, trouble-shooting involves moving through the steps outlined above and determining where dysfunction exists in the respiratory/phonatory system. In some cases, manipulation of the tracheostomy tube alone will lead to restoration of voice and oral communication. However, intervention will always not be so straightforward, and it will be necessary to make referrals to other team members, such as the ENT, for careful assessment of the airway. The flow chart shown in Table 5-6 is designed to assist the speech-language pathologist through the trouble-shooting process.

D. Manipulation of the Tracheostomy Tube and Ventilator

For patients who are ventilator dependent, restoration of voice may involve both manipulation of the tracheostomy tube *and* modifications of the ventilator. Some of the steps outlined above are applicable to the ventilator-dependent patient. For example, it would be helpful to have a report detailing vocal fold function and airway status prior to assessing voicing potential. However, if the speech-language pathologist's assessment precedes the laryngeal examination and the patient is unable to achieve voice, the nasopharyngolaryngoscopy evaluation can be recommended as part of the trouble-shooting process. Assessment of the ventilator-dependent patient is, in general, more complex and will usually require the assistance of the respiratory care practitioner.

1. Candidacy: Assessment of the Ventilator-Dependent Patient

a. Voice production while on a ventilator

The initial step in the assessment of the ventilator-dependent patient involves identifying the presence of a tracheostomy tube cuff and noting the degree of inflation. Some individuals will achieve a small degree of voice from the leak that is created by a partially deflated tracheostomy tube cuff. If the tracheostomy tube cuff is fully inflated and the patient is aphonic (as are most ventilator-dependent patients), team members must evaluate the patient's potential for cuff deflation. *Medical clearance by the physician is mandatory before any attempts at cuff deflation.* Some patients are not candidates for cuff deflation secondary to unstable medical status, difficulty maintaining adequate ventilation, and/or high risk of aspiration. If the patient can tolerate even brief cuff deflation and can produce voice, the procedure for allowing oral communication can be implemented. For some ventilator-dependent patients, cuff deflation may not result in voice production due to an insufficient air leak from the ventilator. In most cases, the patient achieves the greatest amount of voice production during the inspiratory cycle of the ventilator. As air is delivered from the ventilator during inspiration, it leaks upward through the vocal folds and allows voice production. Modifications of some ventilator settings are typically necessary to create increased airflow for audible voice production. Aphonia that persists after these multiple manipulations of the tracheostomy tube and ventilator will require initiation of the troubleshooting process.

2. Procedure

a. Obtaining a *baseline measure of the patient's ventilatory status* is necessary before proceeding with any modifications to the ventilator. This is a joint assessment procedure, usually performed with the respiratory care practitioner. It establishes a patient's readiness to tolerate changes in ventilation.

(1) **Oxygen saturation,** as measured by pulse oximetry, should typically be at a level of 95% and above. *Carbon dioxide* levels, as measured by capnography, should be between 35 and 45 mm Hg. Some patients with diseased lungs will present with higher CO_2 levels as the norm; therefore, it is important to obtain baseline status for comparison to post-intervention measures. Blood gases can certainly be obtained prior to beginning intervention and will provide the most accurate picture of the patient's status. However, this is an invasive procedure which provides a picture of the patient's status only at a given moment and it does not assess trends over time, unless repeated. ABGs also do not give clinicians the immediate feedback provided by the noninvasive tools. Physicians often request repeated ABGs to document change in patient status.

(2) **Spirometry,** used with an oral adapter, is utilized to estimate the amount of air that passes through the upper airway, such as with the leak created by cuff deflation. The patient exhales into the spirometer through an oral adapter. A reading indicates the amount of air that is now passing from the lower airway to the mouth. Additional ventilator air is used to compensate for this leak.

b. Once baseline measures are obtained and are judged to be relatively stable, the team may proceed with the treatment protocol. If there are no contraindications, *cuff deflation* may proceed. Prior to any attempts at cuff deflation, proper suctioning technique is necessary. The air should be removed gradually from the cuff, perhaps 2 cc at a time, with the syringe attached firmly to the cuff inflation line. It is especially important to remove air slowly if the patient has a long-term tracheostomy and cuff inflation. Gradual deflation will allow the patient to adjust to the change in ventilation and redirection in airflow. Abrupt removal of air from the tracheostomy tube cuff can result in laryngospasm, a hypersensitive reaction of the larynx due to the change in airflow (Zenner, 1992). During the initial trials, once the patient achieves audible voice, is comfortable and displays adequate monitoring signs, the cuff can be left partially deflated. This may assist the patient in adjusting to the new sensation of airflow through the upper airway.

c. Concurrently with cuff deflation, *changes of the ventilator* that will compensate for the loss of volume through the upper airway must be made. Because a ventilator is usually set to provide optimal ventilation to a patient with an *inflated* cuff, the following parameters are typically adjusted by the respiratory care practitioner when cuff deflation creates a leak in the system:

(1) *Volume:* Tidal volume is usually the first parameter adjusted. Because of the leak created by cuff deflation, the patient does not receive the amount of air that was preset on the ventilator. The respiratory care practitioner must compensate for the leak by increasing the tidal volume setting of the ventilator. For example, if the patient was receiving a tidal volume of 800 milliliters (ml) and the cuff is deflated, the exhaled or return volume will decrease to possibly 600 ml. The ventilator will indicate this loss of tidal volume via the tidal volume setting on the ventilator. The respiratory care practitioner must compensate for this loss via increasing the tidal volume from 800 ml to 1000 ml. This 200 ml increase should counteract the loss of air from the leak. Spirometry would be helpful in providing an estimate of the increase in tidal volume. Spirometry measures the amount of air that the patient can exhale through the upper airway when the cuff is deflated.

Bach and Alba (1990a) reported on the use of cuff deflation with long-term tracheostomy intermittent positive pressure ventilation (IPPV). The authors discussed the conversion of 91 (out of 104) patients from IPPV with an inflated cuff to either a deflated cuff or no cuff. Invasive and noninvasive monitoring tools were utilized to assess patient status. The authors stated that "in advancing the patient to cuff deflation or removal it is always necessary to maintain the same ventilatory pressures and blood gases and therefore the same supported ventilation that existed when the cuff was inflated" (Bach & Alba, 1990a, p. 680).

In some cases, in order to maintain adequate ventilation with a deflated cuff, the size of the tracheostomy tube is increased. Again, the size of the tracheostomy tube relative to the tracheal lumen is first considered. If the amount of leakage is so great that ventilation cannot be maintained even after an increase in tidal volume, an increase in the size of the tracheostomy tube may be indicated. With a larger size tube, and a partial leak of air, the patient may achieve voice. Tidal volume levels will not become excessively high. Placement of a larger sized tracheostomy tube is usually utilized in patients who are poor candidates for eventual weaning and/or decannulation (Kazandjian, Dikeman, & Adams, 1991).

In increasing ventilatory volumes to compensate for the leak created by cuff deflation, it is important to realize that excessive tidal volume can lead to barotrauma. This is especially true for patients who present with higher airway pressures at the onset of the procedure. It is therefore imperative that increases in tidal volume be applied slowly, high pressure alarms on the ventilator are monitored, and clinical assessment of the patient is ongoing. During this process, noninvasive monitoring tools also supply valuable information regarding the patient's status. In some cases, patients with severe lung disease cannot tolerate the loss of volume even after ventilatory modifications. They will demonstrate clinical signs of discomfort and changes in baseline status, such as increased heart rate caused by the increased work of breathing. In these cases, it may be possible to gradually deflate the cuff only for short periods of time with close monitoring. Patients with interstitial lung disease are at high risk for retention of air volumes and barotrauma due to the loss of lung compliance.

(2) *Respiratory Rate/I:E Ratio:* Commonly during modifications of volume settings, ventilatory rate is also evaluated. Normal breathing ranges between 8 and 16 breaths per minute and is set within this range for the ventilator-dependent patient. When the tracheostomy tube cuff is deflated, an air leak is created and is available for speech, primarily on the inspiratory cycle. Inspiration is the phase in which the ventilator delivers air. If the respiratory rate is rapid, the patient may have difficulty coordinating phonation with the brief delivery of air from the ventilator. Because volume has been increased, it may be possible to decrease the respiratory rate slightly while maintaining alveolar ventilation. This decrease in volume is often coordinated with a slight change in the inspiratory/expiratory ratio.

The I:E ratio is affected by the inspiratory flow rate, which determines the length of inspiration. Recall, the I:E ratio is the relationship of the inspiratory/expiratory phases of the ventilator. Generally, the expiratory cycle is 1.5 times longer than the inspiratory cycle

(Eubanks & Bone, 1990). If the inspiratory time is lengthened by lowering (or slowing) the inspiratory flow rate, the patient should have more time to phonate. The respiratory care practitioner must determine whether the patient can tolerate these changes and carefully review the status of the I:E ratio. The desired result of these ventilatory setting changes is to allow the patient time to coordinate voice with the cycles of the ventilator.

d. If the patient is unable to achieve voice following these ventilator modifications, the steps outlined above for use with tracheostomized patients are applicable. Size of the tube and status of the vocal folds should receive first consideration. The type of tracheostomy tube is also assessed. Ventilator-dependent patients may have fenestrated tracheostomy tubes, although this is less common because the continuous leak from the fenestration would interfere with the delivery of ventilator air. If a fenestration is in place and is tolerated, it can offer additional airflow over what is created with cuff deflation. To allow connection to mechanical ventilation, a 15-mm hub, whether on the outer or inner cannula, must be in place.

e. Instruction in **glottic control** is one technique that can assist in compensating for air leakage during cuff deflation. Glottic control is the use of the vocal folds to regulate airflow through the upper airway. The patient is taught to stop airflow by volitionally adducting the vocal folds during the periods of cuff deflation. This action of stopping the airflow mimics the action of the inflated cuff. The patient is able to eliminate the constant flow of air out of the mouth, either using the trapped air to speak or blowing it periodically from the mouth. Adequate oral motor and vocal fold function are prerequisites of this technique. Tippett and Siebens (1991) described the use of deflated cuffs with ventilator-dependent patients who used glottic control to regulate the amount of airflow delivered from the ventilator to the lungs. They stated that volitional control of the glottis allows a patient to participate in establishing adequate ventilation.

f. Some researchers have investigated a patient's ability to maintain adequate ventilation during sleep, despite cuff deflation (Weller, Siebens, & Marshall, et al., 1995). This appears to relate to changes in the cross-sectional shape of the airway in supine, which narrows the pharynx. In supine, the velum and tongue "fall" toward the posterior pharyngeal wall (Tippett & Vogelman, 2000). The narrowing created by this change in position corresponds to a higher airway resistance. Tippett and Vogelman concluded that such findings further support the use of cuff deflation in ventilator-dependent patients.

Table 5-7 outlines a sample transdisciplinary protocol for cuff deflation to be used while establishing voicing candidacy for the patient who is ventilator-dependent.

Table 5-7. Sample Interdisciplinary Cuff Deflation Protocol for Ventilator-Dependent Patients.

1. MD order obtained for cuff deflation and ventilator modifications.
2. RCP determines if patient needs preoxygenation or bagging. Patient placed on noninvasive monitoring.
3. Suction the patient using established suctioning procedure, through the tracheostomy tube; cuff inflated (RCP/RN/SLP).
4. Allow patient to rest. Reinsert suction catheter into tracheostomy tube. Insert syringe into cuff valve. Apply suction while slowly removing air from the cuff with the syringe. Suction as needed.
5. Reinflate cuff to baseline. Allow patient time to rest. Suction orally if needed.
6. Insert syringe into cuff valve and *slowly* withdraw air until cuff is fully deflated, 2 cc at a time.
7. Begin ventilator modifications. After assessing airway pressures, increase *tidal volume* (e.g., from 0.8 liters to 1.0 liters) (RCP).
8. SLP assesses patient's ability to voice with the newly created leak by encouraging vocalization, initially during inspiration. Reestablish use of the upper airway by having patient vocalize an extended /a/ or blow gently.
9. Reassure patient and monitor readings on pulse oximetry and capnography. If patient expresses discomfort, increase oxygenation level (e.g., from 30% to 35% O_2) (RCP). Watch for signs of air trapping in the lungs related to the increased volume. This may include patient complaints of a tight chest or an upward trend in CO_2 via capnography.
10. If patient is unable to voice adequately, review other settings of the ventilator. Decrease *respiratory rate* (e.g., from 12 to 10 bpm); decrease *inspiratory flow rate* (e.g., from 60 bpm to 40) (RCP).
11. Reassess patient's voicing ability and comfort. The team looks for both clinical and more objective signs of increased work of breathing, such as decreases in O_2 saturation. Engage patient in more extended conversation and determine maximum number of syllables that can be produced on each ventilator breath.
12. Staff determine if patient can be adequately ventilated with cuff deflation for periods of time (e.g., for 30–60 minutes during family visits) after analyzing trends via monitoring devices (MD/RCP/RN/SLP).
13. Orders for specific periods of cuff deflation and ventilator modifications added to patient's treatment sheet (MD).

E. One-Way Tracheostomy Speaking Valves

Tracheostomy speaking valves are another oral communication option. There are several different types of speaking valves. Each differs in design. The function of a **one-way speaking valve** is illustrated in Figure 5-8. Several types of one-way valves are pictured in Figures 5-9a–g. These are also discussed in detail in Table 5-8.

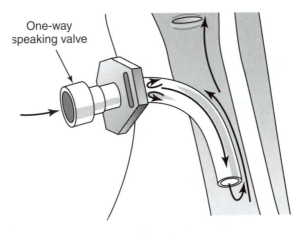

One-way
speaking valve

Figure 5-8. A one-way speaking valve in place on a tracheostomy tube illustrating redirection of airflow. Air enters the valve on inspiration only.

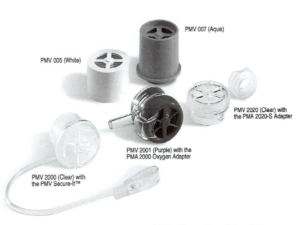

PMV 007 (Aqua)

PMV 005 (White)

PMV 2020 (Clear) with
the PMA 2020-S Adapter

PMV 2001 (Purple) with the
PMA 2000 Oxygen Adapter

PMV 2000 (Clear) with
the PMV Secure-It™

Passy-Muir Tracheostomy and Ventilator Speaking Valves

Figure 5-9a. Passy-Muir tracheostomy and ventilator speaking valves. (Photo courtesy of Passy-Muir, Inc.)

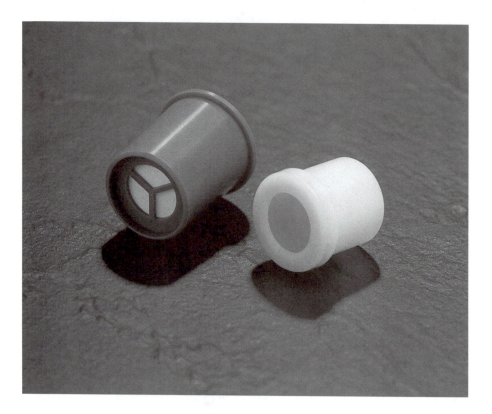

Figure 5-9b. Montgomery speaking valve and Vent-Trach speaking valve. (Photo courtesy of Boston Medical Products)

Generally, one-way valves are placed onto the 15-mm hub of the tracheostomy tube and eliminate the need for finger occlusion in order to produce voice. Note that the Tracoe combines a speaking valve and an inner cannula. One-way valves serve to redirect airflow through the upper airway by allowing air to enter the tracheostomy tube on inspiration. During expiration the valve is closed so that air is directed into the trachea and upward to the vocal folds, as pictured in Figure 5-8. Air is then available for airway clearance and for speech.

The use of one-way speaking valves with the tracheostomized and ventilator-dependent population has received increasing attention in the literature (Britton, Jones-Redmend & Kasper, 2001; Bell, 1996; Fornataro-Clerici & Zajac, 1993; Le et al., 1993; Leder, 1994; Manzano, Lubillo, Henriquez, Martin, Perez, & Wilson, 1993). Before attempting clinical use, the speech-language pathologist must have a good understanding of the function of each valve. The following section provides not only a guide for clinical use but assists the clinician in the problem solving process and in selecting appropriate candidates for speaking valve use.

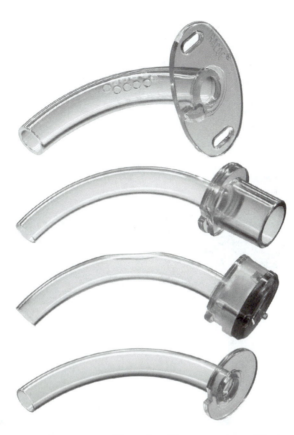

Figure 5-9c. Tracoe speaking tube. (Photo courtesy of Boston Medical Products)

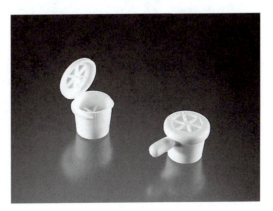

Figure 5-9d. Shiley Phonate tracheostomy speaking valve. (Photo reprinted by permission of Nellcor Puritan Bennett Inc., Pleasanton, CA)

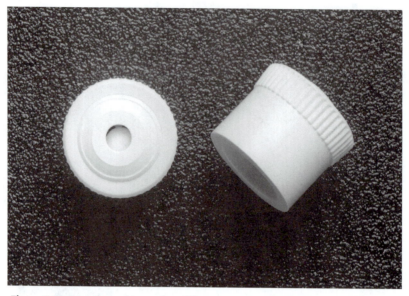

Figure 5-9e. Hood speaking valve. (Photo courtesy of Hood Laboratories)

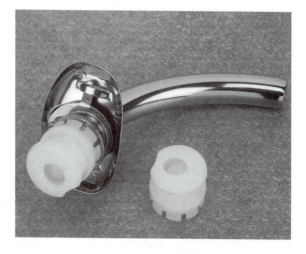

Figure 5-9f. Shikani-French speaking valve. (Photo courtesy of Pilling Surgical)

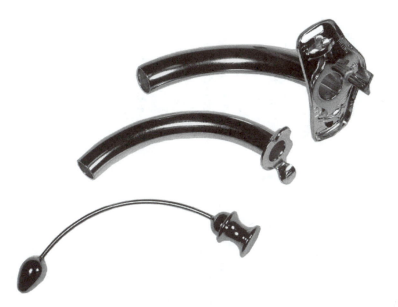

Figure 5-9g. Tucker tube. (Photo courtesy of Pilling Surgical)

1. Candidacy: Indications for Speaking Valves

The candidate for a speaking valve is aphonic secondary to tracheostomy, and may also be ventilator dependent. Indications for use include:

a. Tolerance of cuff deflation

The issue of cuff deflation is encountered more often with ventilator-dependent patients who may rely on the inflated cuff to maintain settings of the ventilator. The inflated tracheostomy tube cuff prevents air from traveling through the upper airway. If a one-way valve is placed on the tracheostomy tube of a patient with an inflated cuff, air will not be able to escape either through the airway or back through the tracheostomy tube. The airway pressures will increase significantly with subsequent heightened airway resistance and accumulation of back pressures. This issue is especially critical for the ventilator-dependent patient because the ventilator continues to cycle and push air into the ventilator. Barotrauma may result quickly. With the tracheostomy tube cuff deflated, air escapes through the upper airway (out the mouth and nose) from the lungs. *A speaking valve cannot be placed unless the tracheostomy tube cuff is fully deflated.* Figure 5-10 illustrates the trapping of air below the level of the cuff secondary to blockage of both the tracheostomy tube and the upper airway.

Table 5-8. Characteristics of One-way Speaking Valves.

VALVE	TYPE	ATTACHMENTS TO TRACHEA	VALVE CHARACTERISTICS
Passy-Muir speaking valve #2000, 2001, 005, 007 (Passy-Muir, Inc.)	One-way valve for tracheostomy and ventilator use.	Fits on standard 15-mm hub or can be placed in-line with ventilator tubing. 2020 fits on Jackson improved metal tracheostomy tube.	One-way silicone membrane with based *closed* position. Valve opens on inspiration. Creates positive closure feature. Available with Secure-It and O_2 adapter.
Montgomery Vent-Trach Montgomery Speaking Valve (Boston Medical Products, Inc.)	One-way valve for ventilator use. One-way valve for tracheostomy use.	Fits on standard 15-mm hub or Boston cannula system.	Open position valve. Special cough release feature (tracheostomy speaking valve only).
Tracoe (Boston Medical Products, Inc.)	Two types of fenestrated inner cannulas, which contain hinged valves for tracheostomy use.	Tracheostomy tube with attachment occludes inner cannula of tube. Two designs.	Open position. Tracheostomy tube is modified by the placement of an inner cannula, which contains a one-way valve.
Shikani-French speaking valve (Pilling Surgical)	One-way valve for tracheostomy use.	Fits on 15-mm hub (metal or plastic) or can be sized to fit Jackson improved metal tracheostomy tube.	Open position design. Ball valve moves with inspiration and exhalation to block opening of inner cannula.
Hood (Hood Laboratories)	One-way valve for tracheostomy use.	Fits on standard 15-mm hub.	Open position valve. Valve contains a ball, which moves, opening upon inspiration and closing upon exhalation.
Shiley Phonate (Nellcor, Puritan & Bennett Inc.)	One-way valve for tracheostomy use.	Fits on standard 15-mm hub.	Open position valve. Has cough release feature. Oxygen port available.
Tucker Tube (Pilling Surgical)	Hinged valve built into Pilling Surgical Tucker tracheostomy tube.	Special tracheostomy tube	Open position design. Hinged valve (leaflet) opens upon inhalation and closes upon exhalation.

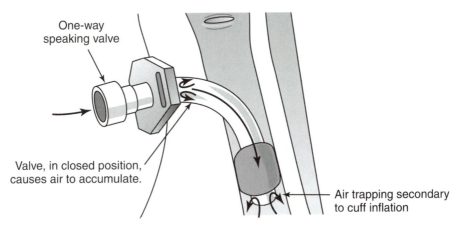

One-way
speaking valve

Valve, in closed position,
causes air to accumulate.

Air trapping secondary
to cuff inflation

Figure 5-10. Speaking valve used in the presence of an inflated cuff.

b. **Proper size of the tracheostomy tube relative to the tracheal lumen**

The size of the tracheostomy tube should also be considered when assessing the patient's airway for speaking valve use. A patient may achieve enough leakage around the sides of the tracheostomy tube to achieve voice. Placement of a one-way valve on the tracheostomy tube will create some resistance to airflow, and this resistance will vary among manufacturer devices (Fornataro-Clerici & Zajac, 1993). Downsizing of the tracheostomy tube may be necessary to compensate for the increased work of breathing that occurs when the valve is placed. Recall that in general the tracheostomy tube should fill no more than two thirds to three quarters of the tracheal lumen (Simmons, 1990). Speaking valve candidates may need additional consideration of the sizing issue before they can tolerate the device.

c. **Maintenance of acceptable baseline respiratory status**

Noninvasive monitoring devices should be used prior to and during the placement of a speaking valve to assess the patient's response to the change in airflow. Candidates should present with a stable respiratory status prior to intervention. The team must immediately intervene when decreases in O_2 saturation or increases in CO_2 levels occur with the speaking valve in place. For decreased O_2 saturation, modifications of the ventilator may include increasing FIO_2 or the addition of pressure support. A patient with upward trending exhaled CO_2 should be instructed to "blow out" air quickly to determine if the trend can be reversed. It is important to combine pulse oximetry and capnography to assess the trend in both oxygen and carbon dioxide levels. The clinician should monitor baseline changes in O_2 and CO_2 levels and any clinical symptoms of patient distress. Although the team should be prepared to transition the patient through the initial wearing process, *when in doubt*, the speaking valve should be removed.

Valves can be used for patients using oxygen or humidified air, as with trach-collar. Respiratory treatments or medication is not administered during valve use. These substances may cause the membrane or hinge on the valve to stick. Patients should continue to receive O_2 or humidification to insure patient comfort and tolerance of the valve.

2. **Candidacy Issues: Contraindications for Speaking Valve Use**

Most of the exclusion criteria for use of a speaking valve will involve airway issues that interfere with a patient's ability to tolerate the additional resistance to airflow caused by a one-way valve or any occlusion of the tracheostomy tube. The following potential contraindications are often identified in conjunction with otolaryngology, pulmonary medicine, and respiratory therapy.

a. **Severe tracheal/laryngeal stenosis**

b. **Airway obstruction**

These airway issues will affect airflow through the upper airway, even when the tracheostomy tube size has been adjusted and the cuff deflated. The result can be increased work of breathing, secondary to the difficulty obtaining oxygen, and gradual retention of CO_2, secondary to difficulty expelling air through the upper airway. Patients utilizing tracheostomy tubes with sponge cuffs should not utilize speaking valves. The large sponge cuff cannot be fully deflated. It retains its bulky size and shape in the airway, creating a large amount of airway resistance and placing a patient at risk of air trapping.

c. **Inability to tolerate full cuff deflation**

d. **Endstage pulmonary disease**

Some individuals, usually those with diseased lungs, will have difficulty tolerating cuff deflation and increased air volumes due to their tendency to retain air in the lungs.

e. **Unstable medical/pulmonary status**

Individuals with unstable medical conditions may not tolerate the changes in ventilatory settings that create physiological stresses (increased blood pressure or cardiac fluctuations) or which increase the work of breathing.

f. **Anarthria**

g. **Laryngectomy**

Individuals who cannot produce speech or who are not able to phonate are not candidates for this type of intervention. For severely *dysarthric* individuals, cuff deflation can be used to work toward voice production during speech treatment. Laryngectomized patients use tracheostoma valves that have a different application than tracheostomy speaking valves. However, cuff deflation during mechanical ventilation *may* still be used to decrease the risk of laryngeal trauma or as part of the weaning protocol for anarthric or laryngectomized individuals who are not candidates for oral communication.

h.   Severe anxiety and/or severe cognitive dysfunction

Some individuals become so anxious that they cannot tolerate any changes in the ventilator settings. They create their own physiological stresses and report keen sensations of discomfort even when monitoring tools provide satisfactory feedback (i.e., even when blood gas levels indicate adequate ventilation). Repeated reassurance from the clinician and reference to objective devices, such as capnography, may be helpful. Patients may adjust gradually to the different sensations that result from cuff deflation and can be moved slowly from partial to full cuff deflation. Psychological services and judicious use of anti-anxiety medications are often indicated. It is usually the patient who demonstrates anxiety out of proportion to the situation, perhaps one who has developed an extreme reliance on the ventilator, who cannot tolerate the process of cuff deflation.

Individuals with severe cognitive dysfunction may be unable to cooperate with the cuff deflation protocol. They often have significant difficulty reestablishing use of the upper airway. If oral communication appears at all feasible, that is, if oral motor function and airway/vocal fold status are adequate, these individuals should be assessed for cuff deflation. Reliance on objective monitoring tools (e.g., blood gases, oximetry, capnography) may be greater than for the intact individual who can provide an ongoing report of comfort level. Severely impaired individuals who are alert but noncommunicative may use cuff deflation only during trial weaning attempts. There is anecdotal use of the valve with comatose individuals for the purposes of coma stimulation. At Silvercrest Extended Care Facility, the authors use one-way speaking valves on tracheostomized individuals with traumatic brain injury for sensory stimulation (taste and smell) and weaning.

3. Procedure: Tracheostomized Patients

The transdisciplinary team approach was demonstrated above during the cuff deflation protocol. Placement of a speaking valve demands the participation of the speech-language pathologist, respiratory care practitioner, nurse, and physician. The entire team should be aware of the purpose and use of the speaking valve so that communication can be normalized across a variety of situations.

a. Cuff deflation

The protocol outlined above detailed the procedure for cuff deflation with the tracheostomized patient. That procedure should be followed prior to placement of any type of speaking valve. First, the speech-language pathologist optimally assesses airway status in conjunction with the oto-laryngologist. The flow chart (see Table 5-6) that detailed the assessment of voicing ability reviews the steps in problem solving tracheostomy and airway issues.

b. Trial valve placement

For the patient who tolerates full cuff deflation and produces voice with tracheal occlusion, the procedure continues with placement of the speaking valve. Initial speaking valve placement for the tracheostomized patient with a deflated cuff is again attempted in conjunction with the respiratory care practitioner. Because a valve does offer some resistance to inspired air, the patient's response to the valve must be closely monitored. Pulse oximetry and capnography provide the necessary feedback regarding tolerance of the valve and adequacy of ventilation. Table 5-9 details a sample transdisciplinary protocol for speaking valve placement with patients who are tracheostomized.

4. Benefits of Speaking Valve Use for Tracheostomized Patients

Placement of a speaking valve provides a number of benefits to the tracheostomized patient. Benefits include:

a. Elimination of finger occlusion

b. Normalization of airflow

c. Facilitation of voicing

Passy-Muir, Inc., manufacturers of the Passy-Muir Speaking Valve, list other associated benefits of their speaking valve (Passy-Muir, Inc.). Their literature reports clinical accounts of improved olfaction, taste, and reduced secretions (as a result of normalized airflow); enhanced airway protection (as a result of air passage through the vocal folds); and assistance in decannulation. The use of a Passy-Muir valve in decannulation attempts with 12 patients with long-term tracheostomies was reported by Le et al. (1993). They reported a comparison between use of the Passy-Muir speaking valve and conventional capping, and compared length of time needed to achieve decannulation. Ten patients in all were successfully decannulated, 5 in each group. The patients

Table 5-9. Sample Interdisciplinary Speaking Valve Placement Protocol for Tracheostomized Patients.

1. Follow cuff deflation protocol ensuring that cuff is completely deflated.
2. Place the speaking valve on the 15-mm hub of the tracheostomy tube (RCP/RN/SLP).
3. If applicable, reconnect T-piece or trach collar (RCP/RN/SLP).
4. Instruct patient to breathe through the upper airway by blowing out the mouth and nose.
5. Begin trial attempts at phonation. SLP encourages patient to vocalize /ah/, count 1–5, or sing a song (automatic speech tasks are especially helpful for cognitively impaired patients.)
6. Simultaneously, monitor trending O_2 saturation *and* CO_2 levels via oximetry and capnography (RCP/RN).
7. Look for symptoms of increased work of breathing or clinical symptoms/complaints of discomfort.
8. If voice is minimal or strained, reassess breathing pattern and provide instruction in coordination of phonation with the *expiratory* phase of respiration (e.g., additional phonatory tasks such as counting and extended vowel productions coupled with assistance in diaphragmatic support) (SLP). Remember that patients may have difficulty adjusting to more normalized airflow.
9. Team will determine extent of wear time based on results of noninvasive and invasive (i.e., blood gases) monitoring and patient's clinical response to the speaking valve (MD/RN/RCP/SLP).
10. Orders for speaking valve use added to patient's treatment sheet (MD).

who used the speaking valve were decannulated in 18 days; the patients who were capped were decannulated in 23 days. This difference did not reach statistical significance; however, patients were able to tolerate the Passy-Muir with less expression of discomfort during the weaning period. The authors concluded, "in this small group of patients, neither method appeared to be superior, although subjective observation suggested that patients appeared to be more comfortable with the one-way valve" (Le et al., 1993, p. 1166).

Leder (1994) evaluated four different one-way speaking valves in the areas of "perceptual speech quality rankings, mechanical functioning, and maintenance of respiration as measured by oxygen saturation" (p. 1308). The subject pool consisted of five patients. Differences were reported in speech quality and "clinically relevant mechanical problems" (Leder, 1994, p. 1308). Maintenance of respiration was not found to be affected by the valves studied. This study is one of the few that has attempted to quantify differences among speaking valves for clinical purposes. Fornataro-Clerici and Zajac (1993) reported the various aerodynamic, airway resistance characteristics of four one-way tracheostomy speaking valves.

In essence, one-way valves assist in restoring more normalized physiology to the tracheostomized patient. The redirection of airflow up through the vocal folds and upper airway can avoid many of the problems associated with longer term placement of a tracheostomy tube. The restoration of oral communication is a primary benefit of one-way valve use, and assists in improving the tracheostomized patient's quality of life.

5. Procedure: Ventilator-dependent Patients

The need for interdisciplinary team involvement is clearly illustrated through the placement of a speaking valve with a ventilator-dependent patient. The team members including the respiratory care practitioner, speech-language pathologist, nurse, and perhaps physician work together at the patient's side during this procedure. Presently, two speaking valves are FDA approved for use with a ventilator. These are the Passy-Muir Speaking Valves (Passy-Muir, Inc.) and the Vent-Trach (Boston Medical Products). However, the Passy-Muir closed-position speaking valve has been used most extensively with ventilator-dependent individuals, with applications for communication, weaning, and swallowing reported through the literature (Bell, 1996; Manzano et al., 1993).

a. Open versus closed position valves

As noted in Table 5-8, one-way speaking valves can be separated into open-position valves or closed-position valves. Open-position valves, as the name implies, maintain an open posture and open further upon the "push" of inspired air during inspiration. The Passy-Muir speaking valves are currently the only closed-position valves on the market. The closed-position valve creates a phenomenon described by the company as "positive closure." Positive closure is created because the silastic membrane of the speaking valve maintains a based closed position at all times *except* during inspiration. In other words, the membrane rests against the front of the valve and opens only when inspiratory pressures are sufficient. Immediately after inspiration, the pliable membrane resumes its closed position. Therefore, when air is supplied from the ventilator, the valve will open, closing when the inspiratory flow ceases. Air accumulates in the tracheostomy tube and airway. There is no loss of air from the valve on either inspiration or expiration, so that no additional air leakage occurs in the ventilatory system. Air escapes only via the upper airway. The benefit of this feature is that air is available for both speaking and airway clearance throughout the ventilatory cycle. However, this feature can also increase the possibility of *air trapping* in the system, as air can build up behind the valve, in the tracheostomy tube, the trachea, and the lungs. It is essential that the upper airway be free from obstruction, whether mechanical (tracheostomy tube cuff) or anatomic (severe stenosis), to ensure that adequate airflow occurs. Air trapping is also more common in the patient with diseased lungs that are stiff and do not easily allow exhalation of inspired air, such as in patients with COPD. The risk of air trapping can be diminished by monitoring tidal volume and high pressure ventilator settings, insuring that the tracheostomy tube cuff is completely deflated and that the airway is free from obstruction, and instructing the patient to exhale out the upper airway. Figure 5-11a depicts the effects of positive closure with a Passy-Muir speaking valve in place.

(1) The Passy-Muir is available for ventilator-dependent patients in the specially designed, aqua-colored #007 size. This valve is colored for enhanced visibility and sized for easy placement in the disposable ventilatory tubing. However use of the 2000/2001 valve is not contraindicated for ventilator-dependent patients. Figure 5-11b pictures a ventilator-dependent patient using the #007 speaking valve in line with the ventilator circuitry.

b. Preliminary considerations in valve placement

Placement of a speaking valve in the ventilatory tubing demands an understanding of respiratory physiology, the fundamentals of the ventilator, and the effects of a one-way valve in the ventilatory circuitry. In the usual ventilatory system, air is provided to the patient, returning to the ventilator on passive exhalation. The amount of air in the system is regulated partly by the exhalation valve, which is located in the tubing. The exhalation valve, described in Chapter 4, is also a type of one-way valve. It allows excess air to escape to the atmosphere, maintaining appropriate pressure in the tubing. When the speaking valve is placed in the ventilatory circuit, air is delivered to the patient in the usual way; however, *air cannot return to the ventilator. Air can escape from the patient only by passing through the upper airway. It is therefore imperative that the upper airway is free of obstruction and that the ventilator settings are adjusted to reflect the presence of the valve in the circuit. Failure to do so could result in serious complications, which may include:*

(1) Barotrauma.
(2) Carbon dioxide retention.
(3) Hypoxemia.
(4) Increased work of breathing leading to cardiac symptoms.

c. Cuff deflation and ventilator modifications

Any speaking valve cannot be used unless the tracheostomy tube cuff is deflated. The cuff is deflated by following the protocol outlined in Table 5-7.

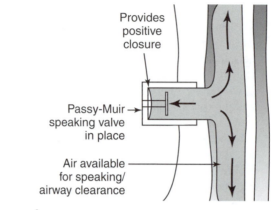

a.

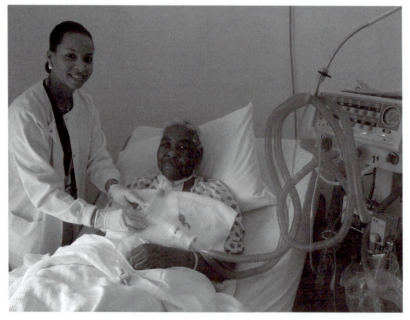

b.

Figure 5-11a. Positive closure with a Passy-Muir speaking valve. **b.** A ventilator-dependent patient using the #007 Passy-Muir speaking valve.

The issues faced by the team will involve maintaining ventilation with the cuff deflated, especially for individuals with diseased lungs. The deflation of the cuff, loss of air volume, and introduction of even a small amount of resistance to inspired air via the speaking valve can increase the work of breathing and lead to clinical symptoms of discomfort. However, ventilator adjustments can effectively compensate for these changes and quickly alleviate the patient's symptoms. The Passy-Muir speaking valve can be used with all modes of ventilation.

(1) *Increasing the tidal volume* provided by the ventilator is the first modification that may occur during in-line placement of the Passy-Muir speaking valve. The increase in tidal volume compensates for the significant loss of air that occurs when the cuff is deflated. Without this increase in tidal volume the patient often cannot be adequately ventilated, as he is receiving only a portion of the air that is actually set on the ventilator. The procedure for increasing tidal volume is the same as that detailed during the cuff deflation process described previously. The respiratory care practitioner will carefully monitor the high pressure settings of the ventilator during this process to ensure that acceptable tidal volume limits are not exceeded. The placement of the valve in line with the ventilator will increase the possibility of air trapping or retention of air within the lungs. It is often helpful to estimate the necessary increase in tidal volume via a spirometer, with the tracheostomy tube cuff deflated, before the valve is placed. This will measure the amount of air that is leaking around the cuff, past the tracheostomy tube, and through the mouth.

One scenario when tidal volume should not be automatically increased is in the presence of high peak airway pressures represented by numbers reaching above 30–40 cm H_2O. This level is obtained on the ventilator via the peak inspiratory pressure reading. High pressure readings usually exist because of airway obstruction or noncompliant lungs. Airway obstruction should have been ruled out during the valve assessment process; therefore persistent increased airway pressure usually relates to the status of the lungs. In the presence of high airway pressures, it obviously is not advisable to introduce more air into the ventilatory system. If all other indicators are favorable, the patient can sometimes be deflated and the valve placed without changing the tidal volume. The patient's response to the valve placement should therefore be monitored prior to making significant changes to the ventilatory settings.

(2) An increase in the oxygen setting, at least in the initial stages of valve placement, may assist in maintaining oxygen settings in the blood. The loss of air from the ventilator due to cuff deflation may serve to temporarily decrease oxygen saturation in the blood. This change is usually slight and can be reflected by the use of pulse oximetry during the speaking valve protocol. An increase in the overall FIO_2 setting of the ventilator serves to compensate for this loss of supplied oxygen. Since a patient may report feelings of discomfort and show clinical signs of decreased oxygenation, the monitoring of O_2 levels is very important. Over time, use of a Passy-Muir speaking valve in line with the ventilator may serve to actually improve oxygenation levels. This appears to relate to the auto-PEEP feature of the valve associated with positive closure.

(3) PEEP, or positive end expiratory pressure, refers to the amount of air that remains in the lungs after a patient has passively exhaled. PEEP is important in promoting healthy lungs which are well oxygenated, and avoiding lung collapse. PEEP is supplied from the ventilator for certain patients who are at danger of atelectasis. Because of the positive closure feature of the Passy-Muir speaking valve, physiologic or auto-PEEP is created by the air trapped in the upper airway and lungs. This may have positive implications for some patients who require the PEEP setting and are being weaned from mechanical ventilation. Use of a Passy-Muir speaking valve creates approximately 2 cm of PEEP (Mason, Watkins, & Romey, 1992b). This must be taken into account when setting ventilator PEEP levels. For example, if the pulmonologist has designated a maximum PEEP level of 5 and a Passy-Muir speaking valve is introduced, the PEEP level may actually reach over 7. This may place some patients with more delicate lungs tissues at risk of barotrauma. Therefore, Passy-Muir, Inc., recommends that PEEP settings of 5 or above be reassessed prior to valve use.

(4) Providing pressure support via the ventilator may enhance patient comfort and tolerance of the speaking valve. Recall that pressure support is a mode of ventilation that assists patients in reducing the work of breathing. For patients utilizing the speaking valve in line, it can provide the additional pressure and subsequently higher amounts of tidal volume to overcome the resistance created by the speaking valve and the increase in the work of breathing created by cuff deflation.

(5) Altering the sensitivity setting of the ventilator can also be helpful for a patient's adjustment to speaking valve placement. For mechanically ventilated patients on control mode ventilation, the ventilator will provide each inspiratory breath regardless of patient effort. However, the spontaneously breathing patient who is on the assist mode of ventilation must now inspire against the resistance provided by the valve membrane. The patient's respiratory effort may increase. Therefore, the patient may gradually fatigue due to the increased inspiratory effort. If the sensitivity at which a breath will be triggered from the ventilator is decreased, the patient will receive a breath after less inspiratory effort. This may have the effect of reducing the work of breathing.

The hallmark of successful valve placement for the ventilator-dependent patient is the ongoing interaction of the team members during the process, continuously monitoring and evaluating the patient's responses. The above guidelines discuss many of the potential changes, but a patient-specific approach is mandatory.

d. **Trial speaking valve placement**

(1) Following complete cuff deflation, the speaking valve is placed in line with the ventilatory circuitry. It is advantageous for the patient to have acclimated to cuff deflation prior to the initial placement of the speaking valve. To increase the chances of a successful valve placement, it is helpful to observe patient tolerance of cuff deflation, at least long enough to observe trends illustrated via capnography/oximetry. Speaking valve placement is performed jointly with respiratory therapy. The respiratory care practitioner assists in fitting the valve within the tubing as well as modifying ventilatory settings according to the patient's response. All team members participate in monitoring the patient. The respiratory care practitioner, however, makes the ongoing judgment of patient's tolerance during these initial trials, and will make the ultimate decision to continue or stop the procedure. This decision will be based on the ventilator settings, noninvasive monitoring tools, and the patient's clinical responses (e.g., work of breathing, sensation of adequate ventilation, complaint of chest tightness). After initial valve placements, a wearing schedule will be ordered by the physician and developed in conjunction with nursing and respiratory staff. Table 5-10 illustrates a sample transdisciplinary Passy-Muir speaking valve placement protocol for ventilator-dependent patients.

(2) The actual placement of the speaking valve in the ventilatory tubing will vary depending on the particular circuitry. For example, some facilities consistently use swivel adapters to connect the ventilatory circuitry with the tracheostomy tube. The swivel adapter is utilized to reduce pulling on the tracheostomy tube, facilitate easier connection or disconnection, and therefore enhance patient comfort. If there is a swivel adapter on the tracheostomy tube, the speaking valve is usually placed on the bottom of the adapter, at the point of connection between the swivel and the ventilatory tubing, as pictured in Figure 5-12. If there is no swivel adapter present, the speaking valve is placed directly onto the hub of the tracheostomy tube. It will now be necessary to use an adapter, such as a small section of disposable tubing, to attach the valve to the circuitry. Figure 5-13 shows Passy-Muir #005 and #007 speaking valves in-line with nondisposable and disposable ventilator tubing.

e. **Speaking valve placement and ventilator alarms**

(1) The literature distributed by Passy-Muir, Inc., indicates that all ventilator alarms with the *exception* of the exhaled return tidal volume alarm are operable (Passy-Muir, Inc.). The return tidal volume alarm cannot be used because the patient no longer exhales into the ventilatory circuitry. The one-way valve, which is closed at all times other than inspiration, prevents passage of air back through the

Table 5-10. Sample Interdisciplinary Speaking Valve Placement Protocol for Ventilator-Dependent Patients.

1. Begin with the suctioning and cuff deflation protocol (MD/RCP/RN/SLP).
2. Ensure total cuff deflation with appropriate ventilator modifications (e.g., increase tidal volume setting) (RCP). Monitor closely while allowing for "leak speech."
3. Take the ventilator speaking valve. Disconnect the patient from the ventilator and place the valve on the hub of the patient's tracheostomy tube. The speaking valve can then be connected to a section of disposable tubing which attaches to the ventilatory tubing (RCP/RN/SLP). (Recall that the need for an additional section of tubing to be used as an adapter will depend on individual setup and where the valve is being placed in the circuitry. The valve may also be placed upon the swivel adapter of the ventilator.)
4. Readjust the exhaled tidal volume alarm (RCP).
5. Watch the response of the ventilator and monitoring tools after introduction of the valve. Observe the peak inspiratory pressure, respiratory rate, heart rate, oxygen saturation, and carbon dioxide levels (RCP/RN). Readjust ventilator settings (e.g., increase or decrease tidal volume) as needed (RCP).
6. SLP instructs patient in usage of the upper airway via "blowing out" air through vocalization, singing, counting, or conversation. Use of bedside spirometry may also facilitate relearning upper airway usage. Remind patient that talking is possible *throughout* the ventilator cycle.
7. Utilize additional ventilator modifications as needed: pressure support, increased FIO_2, respiratory rate, sensitivity setting (RCP). As long as patient is not in distress, explore these changes to enhance patient's voice and comfort.
8. Determine if patient can tolerate a consistent wear schedule. Assign team members responsibilities for valve use according to facility policy and procedure.
9. At end of valve use, detach valve from tracheostomy tube hub and reconnect swivel adapter in-line. Readjust ventilator settings and alarms to previous levels (RCP). Reinflate cuff if patient has not been tolerating long-term cuff deflation.
10. Team assesses patient's ability to tolerate cuff deflation and speaking valve usage (MD/RCP/RN/SLP).
11. Orders for speaking valve use placed on patient's treatment sheet (MD).

tracheostomy tube and ventilatory system. Instead exhalation now takes place through the upper airway. Therefore, this alarm must be temporarily ignored and turned off by the respiratory care practitioner when possible. Some acute care ventilators do not allow this alarm to be bypassed; therefore, patients are often switched to portable ventilators as soon as possible. If the patient cannot be placed on a portable ventilator, the sensitivity of the alarm can be reduced. However, on some ventilators this alarm will remain audible and may be a distraction for the patient and the staff.

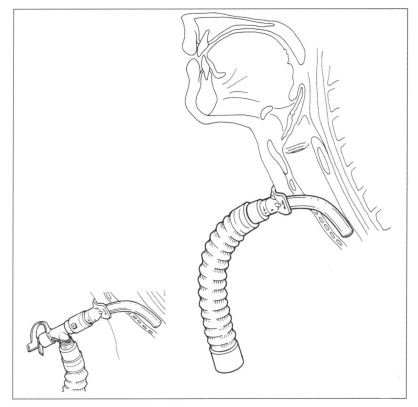

Figure 5-12. Passy-Muir speaking valve on a swivel adapter for in-line ventilator use. (Photo courtesy of Passy-Muir, Inc.)

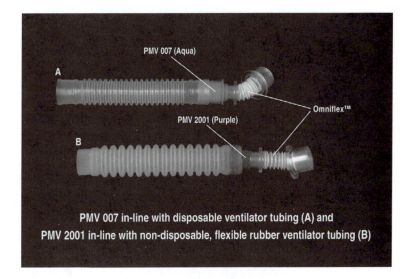

PMV 007 (Aqua)

A

Omniflex™

PMV 2001 (Purple)

B

PMV 007 in-line with disposable ventilator tubing (A) and
PMV 2001 in-line with non-disposable, flexible rubber ventilator tubing (B)

Figure 5-13. Passy-Muir valves in-line with respiratory tubing. (Photo courtesy of Passy-Muir, Inc.)

(2) Pressure alarms (high and low pressure levels) may need adjustments to compensate for the changes in airflow and resistance created by the placement of a one-way valve in the system. It may be necessary to decrease the sensitivity of the high pressure alarm if the ventilator settings indicate that the pressure limits are within acceptable levels, yet the alarm is sounding. The alarm may be responding to the intermittent accumulation of pressure that may occur when the patient is not exhaling air or talking. In other words, the positive closure feature of the one-way valve results in an increase of air in the system that is available for phonation or airway clearance. This increased air pressure may also be sensed by the ventilator and at times can trigger the high pressure alarm. If the patient has been instructed in techniques to control airflow and exhale appropriately, and volume settings have been correctly adjusted, pressures should not exceed acceptable limits. Of course, high pressure settings must be carefully monitored at all times, in order to avoid barotrauma. Tidal volume can be decreased if pressure settings are approaching their set limits.

The timing or apneic interval of the low pressure alarm may need to be increased. The low pressure alarm is designed to activate when the machine senses a decrease in air pressure (e.g., below 10 cm H_2O) for a particular time period (e.g., 10 seconds). The increase in tidal volume should help the ventilator to sense that there is an adequate connection between the machine and the patient.

f. Benefits of speaking valve use for ventilator-dependent patients
(1) Restoration of oral communication.
(2) Improved ability to phonate uninterrupted utterances regardless of the ventilator cycle.
(3) Use of the upper airway via cuff deflation and normalized airflow.

Manzano et al. (1993) reported that ventilator-dependent patients achieved improved communication abilities while using a Passy-Muir speaking valve. The authors found that the patients could be adequately ventilated with the cuff deflated and the valve placed in-line with the ventilatory circuitry. They also reported "that other advantages were the decrease in tracheobronchial and pharyngeal secretions, improved cough effectiveness, and the reestablishment of the ability to smell" (p. 516). Passy-Muir, Inc., also discusses the benefits of their speaking valves in their literature. The valve's use as an aid to weaning has been credited to the creation of auto-PEEP, which is theorized to improve oxygenation levels in the blood (Mason, Watkins, & Romey, 1992a).

Clinically, these authors have noted that some individuals can tolerate cuff deflation and valve use more easily than cuff deflation alone.
This may be related to the improved oxygenation discussed above.
Additionally, although both cuff deflation and valve placement can
increase the patient's work of breathing, cuff deflation alone may
particularly stress the patient's system. The leak created by cuff deflation may be too great for a patient to tolerate. Again, it is careful
clinical assessment by the respiratory care practitioner and speech-
language pathologist that will determine the individual needs of the
patient during valve use.

Britton, Jones-Redmond, and Kasper (2001) reviewed commercially
available speaking valves and summarized some of the literature
regarding benefits for swallowing and weaning. These authors concluded that valves may positively impact functional vocal communication and airway clearance and provide assistance to tracheostomized individuals who must learn specific breathing strategies.
Benefits for reduction of aspiration and weaning were reported as
variable. Britton et al. promote transition to a cuffless tracheostomy
tube prior to speaking valve use.

6. Trouble-Shooting: Problems and Responses

a. Patient unable to tolerate cuff deflation

This difficulty can eliminate a patient as a potential valve user. It is a
more common concern with the ventilator-dependent patient. If issues
such as aspiration have been addressed, the most common problem is an
inability to maintain adequate ventilation in the presence of cuff deflation. This type of patient experiences increased work of breathing with
concomitant signs of clinical distress. Monitoring tools show that oxygen
saturation, CO_2 levels, and respiratory/pulse rates are unsatisfactory.

(1) For the tracheostomized patient, the provision of supplemental oxygen may be helpful during the initial attempts at cuff deflation. For
the ventilator-dependent patient, modifications of the ventilator that
compensate for the patient's responses should be attempted. These
include increasing tidal volume (unless peak airway pressures are
high), increasing FIO_2, increasing number of back-up breaths (for
patients on assist mode), providing pressure support, or adjusting the
ventilator sensitivity settings. In most cases, a patient's inability to
tolerate cuff deflation is related to the inability to safely compensate
for the amount of leakage created. For example, a patient may be losing 300 ml of volume, but a comparable increase in tidal volume
would cause airway pressures to rise beyond acceptable levels. This

occurs more often with patients who have a diagnosis of diseased lungs. In some cases, these patients *may* be able to maintain cuff deflation when a speaking valve is placed in-line with the ventilator. The valve can reduce the amount of leakage because of its positive closure, air trapping feature, reducing the need for large increases in tidal volume. The clinical decision to proceed with valve placement will be made by the team members (pulmonologist, respiratory care practitioner, nurse, speech-language pathologist). The following case vignette briefly describes a patient who could not tolerate cuff deflation but was a successful Passy-Muir speaking valve user.

(2) The maintenance of cuff deflation in the presence of mechanical ventilation is still somewhat controversial, especially in acute care settings, and preliminary discussions with physicians and respiratory care practitioner may be necessary before attempting either cuff deflation or valve placement. The benefits of the team approach to treatment of this population quickly become evident when a forum for the exchange of clinical information is available. The benefits of cuff deflation for some patients can be shared, potential problems discussed, and appropriate candidates for intervention selected by the entire team.

(3) There will be individuals who are not candidates for cuff deflation, despite the attempts at compensations and modifications of the ventilatory system. These patients may be candidates for other oral communication approaches, such as a talking tracheostomy tube. Talking tracheostomy tubes will be discussed in the next section.

b. Patient unable to tolerate valve placement

If a patient shows an unfavorable response to valve placement, the troubleshooting response should explore what can be provided, either clinically or from the ventilator, to ease the adjustment process. Problems typically encountered include patient discomfort secondary to air trapping and retained CO_2 and increased work of breathing with oxygen desaturation. Air trapping has been discussed in depth as a potential complication of speaking valve use on a ventilator. Air trapping, with consequent CO_2 retention, is usually described by the patient as a feeling of "tightness" in the chest. Clinically, restricted chest wall movement may be seen. The valve should be removed immediately in these cases. A chief cause of air trapping for both tracheostomized and ventilator-dependent individuals includes an inhibited exhalation pattern that may relate either to the patient's unfamiliarity with the upper airway or to upper airway obstruction. The need for a normalized airflow pattern should be explained to the patient (see also the response to problem "d" below). The upper airway should be reassessed in terms of the patient's ability to clear exhaled air around the tracheostomy tube and out the mouth and nose. There may be

CASE VIGNETTE: FRITZ

Fritz, a 57-year-old male with a diagnosis of COPD, was admitted to an extended care facility on full mechanical ventilatory support of assist-control, rate of 16, FIO_2 of 40% and a tidal volume of 800. Fritz communicated primarily via mouthing and writing. He was considered an excellent candidate for oral communication. However, any changes to the tracheostomy tube and ventilator prompted increased anxiety from the patient. Baseline monitoring via capnography and oximetry revealed a CO_2 of 45, an oxygen saturation level of 97, and a pulse rate of 85. Fritz's cuff was slowly deflated with tidal volume increased 200 ml to compensate for the leak. This allowed him to produce clear, audible voice. He was instructed to wait and use the airflow to speak. Within 2 to 3 minutes Fritz began to report that, "it's getting hard to breathe." His O_2 saturation decreased to 90% and his pulse rate began to rise. Clinically he became diaphoretic. Fritz requested that the cuff be reinflated.

The next day Fritz's cuff was deflated again. However, once it was fully deflated a Passy-Muir speaking valve was placed in-line with the ventilatory circuitry. Fritz was monitored with capnography and pulse oximetry and demonstrated no change in O_2 saturation while the valve was in-line. He reported feeling more comfortable and clinical symptoms revealed no significant increase in the work of breathing. He was able to tolerate full cuff deflation with the speaking valve in-line for 30 minutes on this initial trial.

Three months later, Fritz used the speaking valve for 2-hour periods throughout the day. He independently deflated the cuff and placed the valve in-line to communicate orally. He was maintained on a portable ventilator (room air) on assist control, rate of 10, a tidal volume of 800, and room air (21% FIO_2). Until his death, from unrelated causes, Fritz used his Passy-Muir speaking valve in-line with the ventilator during all waking hours.

a need for a decrease in tracheostomy tube size which was not obvious during cuff deflation alone. Consider all the ways air could be trapped in the system and address them one by one. Patients with end-stage pulmonary diseases usually experience the most significant air trapping due to their loss of lung elasticity, small airway collapse, and their difficulty exhaling passively.

(1) Another cause of air trapping could be excessive tidal volume. With the introduction of the one-way valve, the tidal volume initially provided when the cuff was deflated can often be adjusted, usually decreased. Airway pressure readings should be monitored for this information.

(2) Oxygen desaturation may be related to the increased work of breathing that occurs with the introduction of a leak to the ventilatory system, and to the resistance to inspired air. The ventilator compensations described above are often useful for these cases. An increase in FIO_2, for example, may result in normalization of O_2 saturation. To further decrease patient effort, adjustment of back-up breaths or sensitivity levels and addition of pressure support to open up the airway are often useful. These changes should be individualized to patient needs, not applied in a cookbook method.

(3) Just as some patients cannot tolerate cuff deflation alone, but can use a speaking valve, others will be able to maintain cuff deflation but evidence discomfort with a valve. Although oral communication is clearly enhanced with successful valve placement, cuff deflation alone often can provide a patient enough leak speech to convey daily needs and concerns. Again, the team must decide what is optimal for each patient and adjust the management plan accordingly.

c. **Patient expresses fear regarding modifications of ventilator/valve usage**

Anxiety can prevent successful valve placement and use and must be addressed as early as possible. Many patients will react to the mere suggestion that the ventilator will be adjusted from its usual settings. Hyperventilation can result from increased anxiety which will demonstrate itself in objective measures (i.e., increased respiratory and pulse rates and decreased CO_2). Patient education and reassurance are crucial. If a patient possesses adequate cognitive skills, a basic explanation of normal and disordered respiratory anatomy and physiology and the rationale for valve placement is helpful. The Passy-Muir company has suggested supplying patients with its educational materials, including videotaped excerpts of other successful valve users (this may also be helpful for family members). If a patient can understand the use of the noninvasive monitoring tools, they can be used to provide ongoing reassurance at the bedside. Our more difficult speaking valve placements have been with patients who were cognitively intact enough to become anxious, but had difficulty understanding the purpose of our intervention. For these individuals, and for all patients, repeated verbal reassurance was given. To reduce anxiety, valve wear time can be slowly increased.

d. **Patient has difficulty adapting to more normalized exhalation pattern**

Tracheostomized patients (non-ventilator-dependent) may experience problems adapting a normalized exhalation pattern. This problem occurs more frequently when there are concomitant language or cognitive deficits. The patient appears unable to voluntarily coordinate phonation with exhalation. This problem may resolve with time, as the patient continues to use the upper airway for speech. Once the normal pattern is reestablished, both tracheostomized and ventilator-dependent patients may complain of an irritating sensation associated with the airflow through the upper airway. They may also report increased salivation. Reassurance that this breathing pattern is a normal pattern, disrupted by tracheostomy tube placement, often is enough to help the user move throughout the initial adjustment period.

(1) Patients who wear speaking valves in-line with the ventilator may initially complain that air constantly escapes out their mouth and nose, even when they do not want to talk. Intermittent glottic control is helpful in controlling this airflow, if patients can be taught to periodically exhale as appropriate.

(2) Adequate exhalation is vital to any valve user in order to avoid air trapping. Again, patients with more advanced cognitive abilities may benefit from explanations of airflow directions, use of a spirometer, and extended practice in conversation to adjust to the new airflow patterns. Patients who are cognitively limited benefit from visual presentations of airflow, such as during blowing, or more automatic speech tasks.

e. **Patient continuously coughs off the speaking valve**

This is of special concern for patients who cannot replace the valve. Coughing off speaking valves is usually related to high airway pressure such as that generated during coughing. Tracheostomized patients (not ventilator-dependent) can be assessed with a speaking valve that contains a cough release valve (e.g., Montgomery speaking valve, Boston Medical Products) that opens at excessive pressures and can be reset without removing the valve. Ventilator-dependent patients should be reassessed regarding tidal volume settings if the valve is frequently coughed off. One simple but valuable approach is to ensure that patient and staff are comfortable with proper valve placement on the tracheostomy tube hub.

f. **Using valves with metal tracheostomy tubes**

Speaking valves can be used with metal tracheostomy tubes when a 15-mm adapter is used. However, Passy-Muir has also developed a new low-profile PMV 2020 valve to fit the Pilling-Weck Jackson improved metal tube, sizes 4–6, which is attached with the new PMV 2020 adapter.

F. Talking Tracheostomy Tubes

Talking tracheostomy tubes are used primarily for ventilator-dependent patients who are candidates for oral communication but cannot tolerate cuff deflation.

There are no medical contraindications for use of a talking tracheostomy tube with a tracheostomized (non-ventilator-dependent) patient; however, because an outside air source (e.g., air tank) is used with this device, patient mobility can be restricted. A talking tracheostomy tube is a variation of the standard cuffed tracheostomy tube. A separate, external air tube is connected to an outside source of air. Through this additional tube, air passes into the trachea above the level of the cuff and is available to reach the vocal folds. With a talking tracheostomy tube, ventilation and phonation are separated due to their distinct air sources. The designs of talking tracheostomy tubes vary slightly. For example, the talking tracheostomy tube available through Portex, Inc./Bivona contains a foam cuff for use with patients with airway abnormalities (e.g., tracheomalacia). Figures 5-14a and b picture two types of talking tracheostomy tubes.

With a talking tracheostomy tube, the patient is breathing on air supplied by the ventilator and is talking with air supplied by the external air source. The airflow from the air source is regulated by the external port pictured in Figure 5-15. When this port is covered, air flows through the tube and into the trachea above the level of the cuff. When the port is open, this additional air for speaking escapes into the atmosphere. Talking tracheostomy tubes provide a source of air for phonation for patients who are unable to tolerate attempts at normalizing the upper airway through cuff deflation.

1. Candidacy Issues: Indications for Use

a. Aphonia secondary to tracheostomy and ventilator dependence

Candidates for talking tracheostomy tubes are unable to produce voice due to tracheostomy (inflated cuff) and ventilator dependence.

b. Inability to tolerate cuff deflation

The primary indication for a talking tracheostomy tube is the inability to tolerate cuff deflation due to ventilatory needs and/or chronic, severe aspiration. During our previous discussions of speaking valve use, cuff deflation was identified as the initial stage of the speaking valve protocol. When all attempts at cuff deflation are unsuccessful, talking tracheostomy tubes should be considered as an alternate option in the restoration of oral communication. Talking tracheostomy tubes may be an effective option for patients with end-stage pulmonary diseases or more fragile medical status, who do not adjust well to the ventilator modifications that accompany cuff deflation.

c. Adequate oromotor/vocal fold function

As with all types of oral communication, articulatory skills must be at least adequate for the production of intelligible speech. In addition, vocal

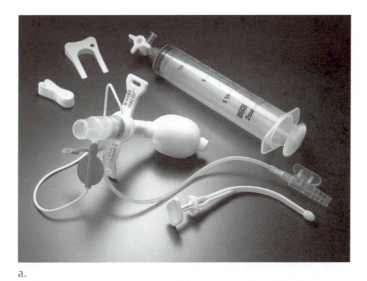

a.

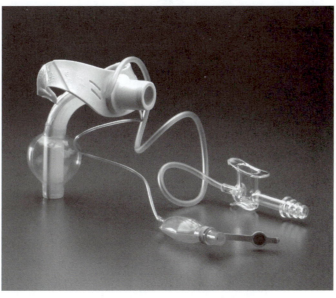

b.

Figure 5-14a. The Bivona Fome-Cuf® with talk attachment. (Photo courtesy of Portex, Inc./Bivona). **b.** The Portex "Trach-Talk" tracheostomy tube. (Photo courtesy of Portex, Inc./Bivona)

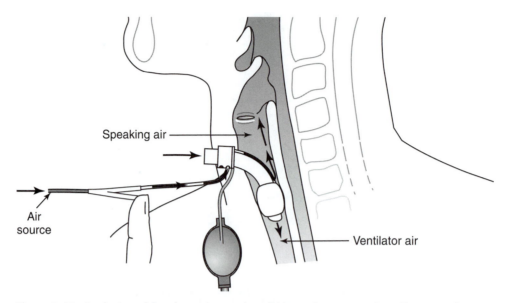

Figure 5-15. Occlusion of the external port of a talking tracheostomy tube, allowing redirection of airflow for speaking.

fold movement must also be adequate. The talking tracheostomy tube provides only a source of external air that can be used for phonation. The patient provides the vibratory mechanism via the vocal folds and articulatory mechanism via the mouth.

2. **Candidacy Issues: Contraindications**

   a. **Bilateral vocal fold paralysis**

   A patient who is unable to modulate the airstream supplied by the external source of air will not be able to produce effective voice. In the case of true bilateral vocal fold paralysis, the patient will remain aphonic even with the airflow provided by the talking tracheostomy tube. In the case of partial vocal fold paresis, the airflow supplied to the patient may assist in mobilizing any residual vocal fold function especially during voice therapy.

   b. **Copious pulmonary secretions**

   Large amounts of secretions can interfere with the ability to phonate by clogging the directional airflow ports of the talking tracheostomy tube or by occluding the opening of the external tubing. If clogging occurs often, it may not be practical to constantly clear secretions before the patient wishes to speak.

c. **Severe dysarthria**

d. **Decreased alertness level**

e. **Cognitive-linguistic impairment**

f. **Severe anxiety**

Impaired cognition, language skills, and severe anxiety are factors that potentially can limit the success of the talking tracheostomy tube. There is a degree of cooperation that must be expected with the use of the device. Additionally, when voice is achieved and verbal output consists chiefly of jargon, communication obviously will not be enhanced. However, this may provide the means for implementing a speech-language treatment program as a patient can now respond verbally. Anxiety can significantly affect the patient's acceptance of changes of the tracheostomy tube. If the patient perceives the talking tracheostomy tube as a modification of existing ventilatory status, the psychological and possible physiological reaction may interfere with the adjustment to the device. For example, airflow rate may need to be repeatedly modified in order to improve voice quality. This creates varying sensations for the patient who must be able to tolerate these adjustments.

Leder (1991) discussed prognostic indicators for the use of the talking tracheostomy tube and notes that seven factors appeared to relate to successful use of the device. These issues included stable medical status, a daily rehabilitation program, proper adjustment of airflow, adequate oromotor and vocal fold function, user motivation, and staff and family support.

3. **Procedure**

Once a potential candidate is identified, the patient can be scheduled for placement of the device. Placement of the talking tracheostomy tube is another arena for the interdisciplinary approach. Respiratory therapy, nursing, speech pathology, and perhaps pulmonary medicine will collaborate in the initial trials to achieve voice. The talking tracheostomy tube is usually placed by the team member responsible for tracheostomy changes in that particular facility, the otolaryngologist, physician, or respiratory care practitioner. Table 5-11 provides a sample transdisciplinary protocol for talking tracheostomy tube use.

a. An oromotor evaluation and brief assessment of voicing ability precede placement of the tube, as this is an important step in establishing candidacy.

b. Even individuals who cannot tolerate cuff deflation for any significant amount of time can usually participate in a brief trial of cuff deflation for

Table 5-11. Sample Interdisciplinary Talking Tracheostomy Tube Placement Protocol.

1. Placement of the talking tracheostomy tube is accomplished with the members of the interdisciplinary team as during routine tracheostomy tube change (MD/RCP/RN). It is optimal to wait 24 hours to allow any edema to subside before attempting voice production.
2. Suction the patient following established suctioning procedure to lessen the chance of pooled secretions blocking the airflow outlets (RCP/RN/SLP).
3. Determine what source of external air will be used. Attach the external airflow line to the external air source. Connect a source of humidification (RCP).
4. Regulate airflow as the patient is encouraged to vocalize. Begin with approximately 6 liters/min and adjust airflow as needed, in 1 liter increments. Airflow should not exceed 15 liters. Clinical judgment and patient comfort will guide this setting.
5. Continue trial attempts at phonation, incorporating longer utterances as voice is achieved. Provide patient with directions to maximize speech intelligibility, such as decreasing speech rate and using overarticulation (SLP).
6. Provide in-service training to patient, staff, and family in use and maintenance of the device.
7. Incorporate problem solving methods if voice is not achieved.
8. Set a schedule for daily usage as per patient need and tolerance.
9. Order for use of a talking tracheostomy tube placed on patient's treatment sheet.

assessment of voicing potential. Any attempts at cuff deflation are contingent on medical status and patient response. The sole purpose is to assess the patient's ability to produce voice using the upper airway. If the patient has failed to achieve voice during trial phonatory attempts, ENT assessment can be conducted at this time.

c. After candidacy is demonstrated, the talking tracheostomy tube is placed using the procedure for routine tracheostomy tube changes. It is helpful to place the talking tracheostomy tube 24 hours prior to any attempts at phonation to allow any edema or bleeding to subside.

d. Once the tracheostomy tube is placed, an external air source must be obtained and connected. Air sources may include tanks of oxygen or compressed air or oxygen from central sources such as in room connection. The air source should be humidified to prevent drying of mucosal tissue that can occur with continuous airflow. Via oxygen tubing, the air source connects to the external air line of the tracheostomy tube as pictured in Figure 5-16. This is most commonly the role of respiratory therapy.

e. When the air source is turned on and the port of the external line is occluded, the air flows through the tubing and begins to circulate above the level of the cuff. The airflow must be adjusted to a level which will allow

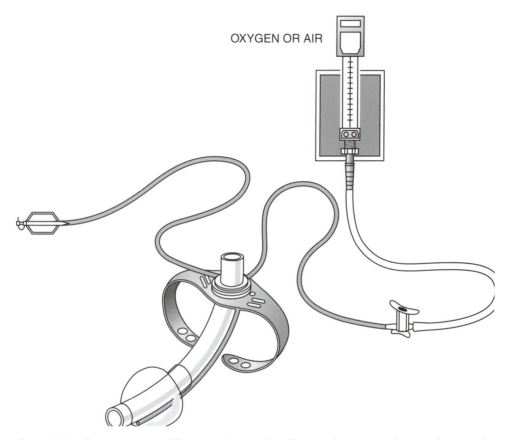

OXYGEN OR AIR

Figure 5-16. The connection of the external port of a talking tracheostomy tube to airflow supply. (Courtesy of Portex, Inc.)

for audible, intelligible phonation. There is no standard setting; Leder (1991) notes that successful flow rates have ranged from 3 liters/min to 15 liters/min. Initially, an airflow setting of approximately 6 liters per minute is suggested, because at this level the majority of patients begin to achieve some phonation. A gradual progression, in 1 liter amounts, is then begun until a balance is reached between optimal vocal quality and intensity and the patient's comfort level. Inability to achieve this balance is one of the major reasons the talking tracheostomy tube may be unsuccessful, so the process should not be hurried. Depending on the patient's tolerance level, adjustments may be made over several sessions.

f. Patients will respond to the sensation of air flowing through the system with varying reactions. If voice can be achieved fairly quickly, the patient can begin directing the airflow for speech purposes and can more easily tolerate the novel sensation. Trial attempts at phonation should begin immediately as this is an integral part of the airflow adjustment process. Vowel and syllable production, automatic speech tasks, and social greetings that do not tax the patient's communication abilities are suggested to reduce distractions. At this time, flow rates can be increased or decreased by one team member, such as the respiratory care practitioner, while the speech-language pathologist and nurse encourage the patient to vocalize. The voice achieved will not be of normal quality even under the best circumstances. Speech production obtained with a talking tracheostomy tube is often described as hoarse or harsh (Leder, 1990; Leder & Traquina, 1989) but should nonetheless be intelligible.

g.   Patient, staff, and family in-service training is integral to the success of the device. Optimally, patients should be taught to intermittently occlude the airflow port on their own talking tracheostomy tube whenever they wish to speak. This reduces patient frustration at not having control over communication and helps regulate the duration of airflow through the system. Consistently occluding the port, which is sometimes done to make sure that the airflow is always available, can lead to dry mucosal and oral tissues and increased patient discomfort. If patients cannot self-occlude the airflow port themselves, due to emotional, cognitive, or physical restrictions, family and staff members may take this role. Activation systems for quadriplegic patients have also been described by some authors (Levine, Koester, & Kett, 1987) and may be attempted for patients who have achieved successful communication with the talking tracheostomy tube.

4. Trouble-Shooting: Problems and Responses

a.   Airflow outlets clog with secretions

(1)   Secretions can easily occlude areas that are designed as outlets to airflow, preventing effective phonation. Frequent oral suctioning may help decrease the amount of material that accumulates on the cuff. The airflow line itself should be periodically detached from the external air source and fastened to a suction catheter as illustrated in Figure 5-17. Secretions can be carefully removed from above the cuff in this manner. If copious secretions continuously clog the airflow ports, suction can be used as the source of airflow. With this technique, secretions are constantly removed from the airway. In other words, air is drawn in through the oral cavity, upper airway, and vocal folds, reversing the standard airflow pattern. The use of suction to achieve voice is described by Portex, Inc. in its literature and by King (1994). Disadvantages include difficulty in adjusting airflow rates, drying of mucosa, and patient complaints regarding the continuous sensation associated with suctioning.

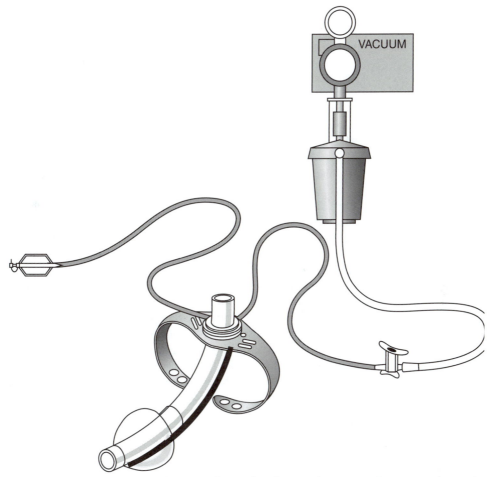

Figure 5-17. The connection of the external port of a talking tracheostomy tube to a suction supply. (Courtesy of Portex, Inc.)

(2) A clogged airflow outlet can also be cleared by briefly increasing airflow, in short bursts of 15 liters/min, for 2–3 seconds. Coughing and clearing of material are possible. Secretions can then be removed via oral suctioning. This technique can also dislodge drier secretions so they are available for suctioning via the airflow line. To avoid damage to delicate mucosa, the airflow cannot be increased indiscriminately. Also, patients may react poorly to this type of secretion removal, especially if they have sensitivity to airflow variations.

(3) Intermittently, respiratory or nursing staff deflate the inflated cuff to thoroughly suction the airway and remove pooled secretions above

the level of the cuff. This decreases the incidence of bacterial colonization in the airway. It also serves to remove material that might potentially clog the airflow outlets of the talking tracheostomy tube. A patient's tolerance of and need for this procedure vary, and it cannot be used constantly during the communication process. Instead, this method may be helpful at the beginning of a communicative session using the talking tracheostomy tube.

b.   Air leakage around the stoma site

Failure to achieve adequate voice may result from inadequate amounts of air reaching the vocal folds despite increases in airflow rates. Leakage around the stoma site may be responsible. Significant leaks may be evidenced by the presence of secretions and air bubbles escaping around the tracheostomy tube. Less obvious leaks may be detected by placing a gloved hand around the tracheostomy tube next to the stoma and applying a gentle pressure. If the patient begins to achieve audible voice at this time, a leak may be present. Proper sizing is a concern. Because talking tracheostomy tube sizes vary among manufacturers, devices should be ordered by inner and outer diameter measurement and comparing them to the tracheostomy tube presently in place. This should lessen the chance of a poor fit. One immediate response to a leak around the stoma site should also be to check the tie strings on the tracheostomy tube to ensure that they have not stretched. Inflating the cuff will not help prevent a leak since the airflow of concern is above the level of the cuff. The use of a talking tracheostomy tube with an additional cuff placed high on the shaft behind the flange of the tracheostomy tube, such as the Stoma-Seal™ manufactured by Portex, Inc./Bivona, may also be an option (Figure 5-18).

c.   Poor speech intelligibility

Users of a talking tracheostomy tube will not achieve a normal voice. Voice quality is usually breathy but should be intelligible.

(1) Patients should be rated as to the effectiveness of their speech production. If patients are attempting to speak rapidly, are mildly dysarthric, or have poor awareness of their listener, they may need additional intervention and training. Leder (1991) noted that one of the seven prognostic indicators of successful use of a talking tracheostomy tube was a daily rehabilitation program by a speech-language pathologist, as well as ongoing staff and family education. In other words, once the device is placed, ongoing attention and continued training are necessary.

(2) If speech is not intelligible, adjustment of airflow rates should be considered. If the patient can achieve sound but speech is poorly

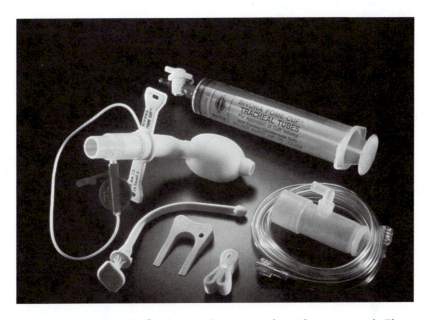

Figure 5-18. A Fome-Cuf® talking tracheostomy tube with a stoma seal. (Photo courtesy of Portex, Inc./Bivona)

understood, airflow rates might need further adjustment. To ensure that airflow is sufficient for speech production, a variety of settings should be attempted.

A variety of methods can be used to restore oral communication. Each patient must receive a careful assessment to determine his or her candidacy for a particular technique. Most importantly, transdisciplinary team members must work together to ensure successful and safe usage.

6

Nonoral Communication

The abrupt cessation of voice is characteristic of tracheostomy and ventilator dependence, regardless of the underlying disease process. Although this loss of oral communication may be temporary, nonoral communication techniques are often required. Intervention incorporates a wide range of options that allow the nonoral individual to communicate in a variety of settings. It is the role of the speech-language pathologist to facilitate communication in each communicative setting and ensure that the nonoral patient, who is tracheostomized and/or ventilator-dependent, can always communicate his or her needs. This chapter will provide a framework for assessment and intervention, allowing the clinician to respond to the changing needs of the tracheostomized and ventilator-dependent patient. The term *nonoral* will be utilized to refer to the patient who is unable to communicate functionally through speech and/or voice.

I. NONORAL COMMUNICATION OPTIONS: CANDIDACY ISSUES

Nonoral communication allows a patient to participate in communicative exchanges via methods other than speech. Nonoral communication involves use of alternative techniques that range from use of yes/no systems to sophisticated, computerized speech output systems. Nonoral systems may also supplement oral communication efforts. The speech-language pathologist is instrumental in identifying candidates for a particular intervention method and in providing a functional communication system.

A. Continuum of Disability: Speech/Voice

Table 6-1 reviews the speech/voice subsystem of the continuum of disability. Patients who are candidates for nonoral communication will fall somewhere on the right side of the continuum. Oral communication may be only temporarily interrupted.

227

Table 6-1. Continuum of Disability: Speech-Voice Subsytem. (Adapted from "Continuum of Disability" by C. Salciccia, 1986. In C. Salciccia, L. Adams, & G. Kapassakis, *Communication Management of Respiratorily-Involved Quadriplegic Adults.* Paper presented at Goldwater Memorial Hospital, New York, NY.)

Speech/Voice						
Phonation with good vocal intensity. Articulation WNL.	Phonation with decreased intensity. Good articulation.	Phonation poorly coordinated with ventilation.	Aphonic with good mouthing.	Aphonia with mild dysarthria.	Aphonia with moderate dysarthria.	Aphonia with severe dysarthria.

Note: WNL = within normal limits.

An example is an individual who is aphonic secondary to cuff inflation and presents with good mouthing. Anarthric individuals are more often long-term or permanent nonoral candidates. Tracheostomized and ventilator-dependent patients may move through the continuum in either direction. Nonoral techniques will change to match their status.

Candidates for nonoral communication options include patients who present with some or all of the following:

- Motivation to communicate but inability to make needs known.
- Failure to successfully utilize oral communication techniques.
- Inadequate oral motor function.
- Medical instability.

Options for oral communication were detailed in Chapter 5. Oral communication options should be considered first during the problem-solving process, because they most closely approximate normal communicative interactions. However, when oral communication is not feasible, it is essential to provide the patient with a functional method of message transfer.

II. POPULATION

Recall the population classification described in Chapter 5. Classifications of temporary, static, and degenerative conditions and diseases assist the clinician during the selection of appropriate nonoral communication techniques.

A. Temporary Conditions

During the temporary, acute stages of an illness or traumatic event, a period of non-oral communication may be warranted. A fragile medical status may not support normal message transfer. For example, a patient recently placed on mechanical ventilation may present with pulmonary and cardiac complications. Modifications of the tracheostomy tube and ventilator that would allow phonation are contraindicated. The patient must, however, have an immediate method of communication, at least a means of calling for help and a consistent, reliable yes/no system. For patients who fall into this temporary category, nonoral communication methods are usually required over a limited period of time. Ultimately, the patient is expected to return to oral methods. The provision of nonoral communication options is designed to meet the acute needs of this patient.

B. Static Conditions

The resumption of speech function can be difficult for patients with a more static medical status. These patients typically present with chronic medical conditions that warrant nonoral communication over an extended period of time. An example is an individual with a high spinal cord injury who has 24-hour ventilatory needs that preclude frequent cuff deflation. Long-term communication needs must also be addressed in many communicative settings with various partners. Intervention now involves provision of a more sophisticated method of nonoral communication. Patients in the static category may or may not regain speech/voice production. Therefore, nonoral communication may be required to supplement or replace oral attempts.

C. Degenerative Conditions

Diseases and conditions that are degenerative in nature, such as ALS, require intervention that changes to match the patient's declining medical and physical status. Patients initially may be successful oral communicators. However, as dysarthria worsens and speech intelligibility deteriorates, oral communication must eventually be supplemented or replaced by nonoral techniques. Patients with degenerative diseases often utilize sophisticated electronic systems which allow multiple methods of access and permit communication even when severe physical disability exists.

III. COMMUNICATIVE SETTINGS

The clinician must carefully assess the tracheotomized and ventilator-dependent patient's overall needs and medical status in a variety of communicative settings. The role each interdisciplinary team member plays in meeting the needs of the patient is guided by the constraints of each communicative setting. Communicative settings include acute care medical, rehabilitative care, long-term care, and home care settings.

A. Acute Care Medical

The acute care setting includes the ICU units as well as general medical and pulmonary units of the hospital. Patients in these settings may have either a temporary inability to communicate verbally or require communication systems for long-term use. Inherent in an acute care setting are issues such as the often tenuous medical status of the patient, multiple IV lines, oxygen tubing, nonportable ventilator equipment, numerous communication partners, and a busy medical staff. Communication often takes a backseat when more life-threatening issues arise. Staff must resort to fast and easy methods of message transfer to allow the patient to convey immediate needs. Nonetheless, the acutely ill but alert ventilator-dependent patient needs a communication system that allows for the efficient transmission of questions and comments. This is a high priority for the patient, family, and medical personnel. Providing a practical and reliable communication system will not only enhance service delivery but will assist the patient in making adjustments to an often frightening and unfamiliar environment.

B. Rehabilitative Care

In the rehabilitative setting the patient is past the critically ill stages of recovery but still requires medical intervention. Patients on the rehabilitation unit of the hospital or trauma center receive intensive intervention from a variety of disciplines. This includes the traditional rehabilitation services of physical therapy, occupational therapy, and speech-language pathology. In this setting, each team member has the opportunity to work more intensively with the patient, allowing for the provision of more sophisticated communication systems. Tracheostomized and ventilator-dependent patients may begin the weaning process at this time but still rely on nonoral methods of communication to reliably transfer daily messages.

C. Long-term Care

Tracheostomized and ventilator-dependent patients in long-term care facilities have achieved a generally stable medical status and require extended care to assist in ventilatory needs. These patients will receive intervention from each interdisciplinary team member on a less intensive basis. Placement in an extended care facility allows the clinician the time to fully evaluate the needs of the individual and determine the most appropriate communication system for long-term use. For appropriate candidates, it is often in this setting that a sophisticated electronic communication system is provided to meet a broad range of communicative needs. Because daily medical care is routine, recreational/vocational activities and family involvement can be emphasized. Care plans are directed toward maximizing the patient's quality of life while increasing independence and communication abilities.

D. Home Care

For some tracheostomized and ventilator-dependent patients, medical needs can be met in the home environment. Interdisciplinary team involvement changes as daily needs are met by the family or nurse/nurse aide who functions as the caregiver. Rehabilitative visits may continue; however, intervention is often dictated by agency support or financial constraints. Treatment by the respiratory care practitioner is typically maintenance oriented. The patient's ventilatory status is monitored and proper functioning of ventilatory equipment ensured. Nonoral communication methods can be designed to meet a variety of communicative needs. Vocational needs can be examined in detail to facilitate continued employment, if possible.

IV. ASSESSMENT: COMMUNICATIVE NEEDS

Appropriate selection of a communication system should not take place without a thorough understanding of the patient's physical-motor, cognitive-linguistic status, behavior, environmental settings, and communicative partners. Unfortunately, there is no formalized test that provides all of this information. The diagnostic process must be modified to meet the special needs of the tracheostomized and ventilator-dependent patient (Adams & Connolly, 1993). The speech-language pathologist must rely on all of the members of the team as well as the information provided by the patient and caregivers, allowing for a comprehensive view. Direct observation of the patient's interactive style, assertiveness, independence, rate of message transfer, and desire to communicate is essential in developing a plan for a communication system (Fishman, 1987).

A. Needs Assessment

Beukelman, Yorkston, and Dowden (1985) outline the areas required for a complete assessment of communicative needs. The Communication Needs Assessment located in Appendix B assists the speech-language pathologist in prioritizing the patient's needs in the selection of a nonoral communication system. Information is obtained through observation and direct interview with the patient, family, and caregivers. The authors report that

> the needs assessment serves several purposes. It encourages the staff and those they serve to develop specific, mutually agreed upon goals. Second, it encourages early consideration of how the system is to be used so that systems are selected with the greatest potential to meet the individual's actual needs. Third, it acquaints the clients and their communication partners with communication possibilities that they may have not considered. (p. 9)

1. The Communication Needs Assessment outlines patient needs related to positioning, partners, and settings. The patient begins to delineate locations and communicative settings by identifying the environments in which communication takes place. The patient, with the assistance of significant others, will also

name the various important communicative partners who will act as message receivers. Finally, types of message needs are included, such as greeting people, making requests, and so on. With this information, the clinician is ready to begin the process of identifying the most appropriate communication system for the tracheostomized and ventilator-dependent patient. The following case examples highlight the identification of needs during the assessment process.

B. Continuum of Disability: Physical-Motor, Cognitive-Linguistic, and Behavior

Table 6-2 illustrates the remaining components of the continuum of disability. The patient is placed on the continuum according to his or her presenting status at the time of the evaluation. The continuum allows the clinician to assess the areas that will directly affect the selection of a communication system. For example, a patient with head injury and quadriplegia has physical motor restrictions combined with cognitive impairment. This patient has a limited amount of commercially available communication systems from which to choose.

C. Case Vignettes: Assessment

The following section presents case vignettes illustrating the information obtained during the assessment process. Intervention techniques for Cases 1–4 will be discussed later in this chapter.

1. Acute Care Medical Setting: Howard

Howard was a 68-year-old man who presented with multiple trauma secondary to a pedestrian–motor vehicle accident. He was in respiratory and cardiac arrest when the paramedics arrived at the scene. Howard was immediately intubated and full life support measures were utilized to revive him enroute to the hospital. On admission to the emergency room the patient was in a coma, neurologically unresponsive to verbal and noxious stimuli. Howard was scheduled for emergency surgery to address multiple internal injuries. Along with multiple fractures of the thorax/ribs, arms and legs, the patient sustained a severed spinal cord at a C1–C2 level. A cervical collar was placed to immobilize his head and neck. Howard's physical motor assessment revealed no motor control below his chin, rendering him pentaplegic. He was positioned exclusively on his back on a special mattress which continuously altered the pressure exerted on his skin and delivered percussion regularly.

This physician made a referral to the speech-language pathology service for a communicative assessment. Initial contact indicated that Howard's cognitive status had slightly improved from his admission. However, he was extremely lethargic and had a limited attention span to verbal and visual stimuli. He was also anxious and had difficulty focusing on verbal instructions. Howard

Table 6-2. Continuum of Disability: Physical-Motor, Cognitive-Linguistic, and Behavior Subsystems. (Adapted from "Continuum of Disability" by C. Salciccia, 1986. In C. Salciccia, L. Adams, & G. Kapassakis, *Communication Management of Respiratorily-Involved Quadriplegic Adults*. Paper presented at Goldwater Memorial Hospital, New York, NY.)

Physical Motor					
Normal UE ROM and fine motor. Good endurance.	Adequate UE ROM and fine motor. Fair endurance.	UE Weakness. Gross movement adequate. Limited ROM. Poor endurance.	Significant weakness. Limitations in ROM. Poorly coordinated UE function. Severely limited endurance.	Quadriplegia. No upper/lower extremity function.	Pentaplegia. No movement including head.
Cognitive-Linguistic					
No deficits, intact status.	Mild deficits (memory, orientation, reasoning, anomia).	Moderate deficits (impairments in language expression/ reception).		Severe deficits.	Profound deficits.
Behavior					
Patient indicates concerns, highly motivated for treatment.	Mild anxiety, but can be reassured.	Moderate anxiety, difficulty in transitioning through intervention stages. Treatment is interfered with.		Severe anxiety. No intervention possible.	

Note: UE = upper extremity; ROM = range of motion.

233

required a nonfatiguing method of transferring short, personally relevant messages that could assist the medical staff in providing daily care.

A tracheotomy was performed. A few days later Howard began to mouth words. Mild oral weakness was noted. Voice production was not possible due to the fully inflated cuff. Cuff deflation was not an option due to his tenuous medical condition. The medical staff had difficulty stabilizing Howard's blood pressure and cardiac condition. As Howard's cognitive-linguistic status improved, more unpredictable message needs arose. He began to request detailed information from his physicians regarding his medical care. Howard had a doctoral degree in philosophy and spoke five foreign languages. He communicated his fears and anxiety in losing his independence and decision-making capacity. Howard's communicative partners included numerous medical personnel and his immediate family.

2. Rehabilitative Care Setting: Kenny

Kenny was a 26-year-old man who sustained a C1–C2 fracture from a motorcycle accident. He was initially sent to a trauma center in the rural area where he lived. Prior to his accident Kenny worked in a factory. He had a high school education. Following stabilization of his medical condition, he was transferred to a specialized rehabilitation hospital in another state. On admission to this rehabilitation facility, Kenny was quadriplegic, tracheostomized, and ventilator dependent. His mode of ventilation was assist control, rate of 12, tidal volume of 800 ml and FIO_2 of 45%. He had a fully inflated tracheostomy tube cuff. Initial speech, voice, and swallowing assessment indicated that prolonged cuff deflation was not feasible due to a paralyzed vocal fold and severe risk for aspiration. Kenny presented with both aphonia and a moderate dysarthria, which affected his ability to mouth words functionally. Language testing procedures were adapted to meet Kenny's special needs. Because he was quadriplegic and unable to verbally indicate his responses, items were placed on a board and the patient was instructed to "look" at the correct answer. Cognitive-linguistic abilities were judged to be within normal limits. Audiological testing revealed adequate hearing for daily needs. Although he reported depression related to his condition, Kenny was motivated to participate in any program that would assist in restoring communication. He was particularly interested in oral options.

Unfortunately, initial attempts at oral communication were not successful. However, Kenny had immediate communication needs. He was primarily positioned in bed but tolerated 2 to 3 hours daily in a wheelchair. Kenny was dependent on others to transport him around the hospital in his wheelchair. He traveled daily to physical and occupational therapy and speech pathology appointments. Because his family lived out of state, communication was necessary not only on the phone but via letters. His immediate communication partners included his nurses, therapists, and doctors. Kenny also needed to communicate with people unfamiliar with his communication system such as other patients in the hospital. Kenny's message needs included medical concerns, such as frequent suctioning and repositioning, expressing anxieties about his treatment program to therapists, and socializing with patients and staff.

3. Long-term Care Setting: Tom

Tom was a 72-year-old man with a diagnosis of left brainstem CVA. He was admitted to the tracheostomy and ventilatory unit of an extended care facility for long-term care. Tom was a retired machinist and had a high school diploma. On initial evaluation, he was tracheostomized with a fully inflated cuff and 24-hour ventilator dependent. His mode of ventilation was assist control, rate of 12. His ventilatory settings were FIO_2 of 30%, and TV of 800.

Tom presented with right-sided hemiplegia with mild-moderate limb apraxia. Oral motor weakness was evident. Significant labial and lingual weakness interfered with the intelligibility of mouthing. Assessment of cognitive-linguistic abilities revealed moderate-severe deficits in verbal expression and visual language. Tom could identify his name and the names of family members from written choices. Reading of functional single words was accurate approximately 60% of the time. Visual-perceptual deficits were evidenced with inattention to visual stimuli presented on the right. Impairments in attention, concentration, and memory made task completion difficult. Tom could answer simple, personally relevant questions by nodding or shaking his head. However, Tom inaccurately answered more complex questions that were not contextually supported, leaving family and staff frustrated and confused. Hearing was intact. Attempts at oral communication options failed secondary to ventilatory needs and severe aspiration risk. Use of an electrolarynx was not functional due to the severe impairments in his verbal expression and motor speech.

Tom's needs changed as his medical and ventilatory status improved. Tom was changed from a nonportable to a portable ventilator, allowing him an increased variety of communication interactions and settings. For example, he was able to go outside of the facility with staff and family members. He was slowly being weaned and could tolerate an SIMV of 4, FIO_2 of 21% (room air) and a PSV of 20. Communicative partners were varied. They included other residents with hearing and visual impairments, unfamiliar personnel, unit nurses, doctors, therapists, his young grandchildren, other family members, and friends. Primarily, Tom's daily care needs were anticipated due to his lack of communicative initiation. When he occasionally initiated a message, he used gross gestures such as pointing to an object in his view. For example, he spontaneously requested his oral suction catheter and TV remote control from the nurse by pointing to the items before she left the room.

4. Home Care Setting: Ted

Ted was a 69-year-old male who was referred for communication and swallowing intervention secondary to his diagnosis of amyotrophic lateral sclerosis. Ted was a practicing psychotherapist. On initial speech-language evaluation, Ted was dysphonic with a mild dysarthria. His vocal volume was slightly reduced with articulatory accuracy compromised during periods of fatigue. Ted's cognitive-linguistic status was within normal limits. Physical-motor abilities were characterized by significant limitations in range of motion. He had severely limited endurance. Over a 2-year course Ted's disease progressed, and his speech and voice impairment worsened. He presented with reduced breath support for speech purposes and low vocal volume, hypernasality, and moderate to severe impairment in articulatory accuracy. Speech intelligibility was considered to be fair to poor with communication breakdown occurring frequently. Physical-motor function deteriorated and was eventually limited to essential quadriplegia. Adaptations from a rehabilitation engineer and occupational therapist allowed minor movements of the index finger of the right hand to be utilized for environmental control set-up.

Throughout the course of the disease Ted continued to practice as a psychotherapist in his home office despite being wheelchair-bound and dysarthric. He had gradually become dependent on noninvasive mechanical ventilation (BiPAP™ delivered via a mask) throughout portions of the day and all night. Ted had to communicate throughout his home, while in bed, and over the telephone as well as during occasional visits to the ALS clinic at an area medical center. Message transfer was also necessary at night, in the dark and while the BiPAP™ mask was in place. Communication partners included his live-in caregiver, family, therapists, doctors, and clients. Ted had special needs for message transfer in his psychotherapy practice. He saw his patients in his home office while seated in his motorized wheelchair. He was required to carry on extended conversations over at least 45-minute intervals and during that time make inquiries, express emotion, and provide novel suggestions and solutions.

V. AUGMENTATIVE/ALTERNATIVE INTERVENTION

Intervention begins following the completion of the communication needs assessment (Adams & Kazandjian, 2001). At this point the clinician must have a good understanding of the difference between augmentative and alternative intervention. **Augmentative communication** techniques can be introduced when oral communication is not considered a primary method of functional message transfer. Augmentation or supplementation of oral/verbal communication may include providing the patient with a letter board as a speech supplementation approach. This technique utilizes a standard letter board paired with verbal output. The patient points to the first letter of each word as it is ver-

Table 6-3. Sample Directions for Yes/No Communication System.

How to Communicate with Eddie
1. Eddie uses his eyes to say "yes" or "no."
2. Make sure you ask your question so Eddie can answer "yes" or "no."
3. Eddie looks **up** for "yes."
4. Eddie blinks his eyes **twice** for "no."

---

bally produced. This approach not only provides the listener with a cue as to the word that is being produced, but also serves to separate each word in the string of an extended utterance. This augmentative communication technique introduces an **alternative communication** method without replacing speech as the primary mode of communication. For patients who have regained oral communication but remain severely physically disabled, augmentation often takes the form of computer-assisted techniques used essentially for writing. When oral communication is not possible, intervention moves from augmenting speech to providing alternative communication techniques. Alternative communication techniques range from simple, quick approaches to sophisticated computer-based systems. However, all systems must include a consistent, reliable and understandable yes/no system. This system may consist of a body movement such as a head nod/shake, thumb up/down, or eye gaze up/down. In the absence of these motor movements, yes/no responses can include looking at yes/no cards mounted in an easy to read place or activation of a buzzer, one time for "yes" and two times or "no." This basic communication intervention is needed to prevent constant communication breakdown. Table 6-3 provides sample directions for using a yes/no communication system.

A. Intervention Techniques

Intervention techniques for both augmenting communication and providing alternative communication methods may be immediate, short-term, or long-term. (Kazandjian and Dikeman, 1998).

1. Immediate

Immediate intervention techniques include providing the tracheostomized and ventilator-dependent patient with an alerting signal and a yes/no response system. Establishing a method of alerting a listener, either for initiating communication or for emergency purposes, is the essential first step in the intervention process. An alerting signal is especially important for the aphonic individual who is unable to call out for assistance. This will provide the patient, nursing staff, and family with a sense of security in the event the patient must signal in an emergency. A yes/no response system is equally important for the nonspeaking tracheostomized and/or ventilator-dependent patient to ensure the transfer of important messages. In the acute care medical/ICU setting, with its accompanying restraints, the clinician may initially provide only these immediate intervention techniques.

2. Short-term

Short-term intervention involves expanding communication to allow for the initiation of more lengthy utterances and questions. These systems incorporate simple, nonelectronic solutions that are easy for the patient and others to learn and use. These systems include magnetic or dry erase boards for writing, alphabet boards with which the patient spells spontaneous messages, and phrase boards for communicating predictable medical and positioning needs. Fried-Oken, Howard, and Stewart (1991) discussed the effectiveness of augmentative and alternative communication systems through interviews conducted with patients in acute care settings. Their results support the use of simple, low-tech solutions to provide easy-to-learn, patient-specific methods that maximize communication.

3. Long-term

Once immediate and short-term communication needs are met, the speech-language pathologist can focus on the issue of whether and to what degree long-term augmentation will be needed. Intervention will address verbal and written forms of communication. The patient who needs an augmentative or alternative system for long-term message transfer will require more extensive training, for the patient as well as for others, and continued follow-up.

B. Utilizing Residual Physical Motor Function

The intervention process begins with the profile of the patient that was obtained during the assessment process, using the continuum of disability. The clinician must now determine what residual function can be utilized for a nonoral communication method. For example, the clinician finds that a patient who was placed on the physical motor scale of the continuum with quadriplegia and no upper extremity function has some residual motor movement of his cheek. This residual movement is now examined for consistency and functionality. When examining motor function, the speech-language pathologist may require the assistance of the occupational therapist or rehabilitation engineer. These professionals provide valuable insight into body positioning and use of adaptive devices that will assist the speech-language pathologist in providing an appropriate nonoral communication method.

1. Emergency Call Systems

Once residual motor function has been identified, the clinician can utilize this movement for an emergency call system. As stated previously, call systems or

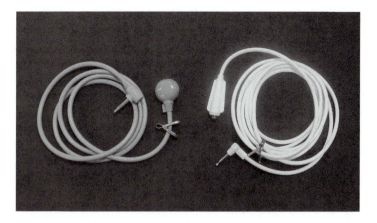

Figure 6-1. Standard call buzzers.

alerting signals are essential when managing a nonoral communicator. Emergency call systems must be considered first in the intervention process. Standard nursing call buzzers, as pictured in Figure 6-1, are typically provided to patients in acute care, rehabilitation, and long-term care settings. However, physical motor impairments often interfere with the patient's ability to access these call systems. The standard variety buzzers must be adapted to meet the needs of more severely disabled patients. Modifications typically substitute a specialized *switch* for the standard round-ball or cylindrical call buzzer available in hospitals. If the specialized or modified switch cannot be directly connected to the nursing call system, it can be attached to a buzzer. To be readily heard by staff, this buzzer can then be amplified. The occupational therapist often assists in evaluating motor function and positioning to determine the most appropriate switch for a particular patient. All medical staff must be inserviced in the use of this new call system, so that they respond to the patient in a timely manner.

C. Access Methods

Access methods are determined by the patient's reliable and consistent physical motor movements. Based on the information regarding physical-motor function, a method of access can be identified. The term access refers to the method by which the patient will operate a communication system. There are various methods of accessing nonelectronic or electronic communication systems. Each must be considered when devising a communication system. For some patients, access methods may begin with simple writing of messages with pen and paper, and progress to other less motorically complex movements, such as scanning. Alternatively, patients who present with limited physical motor impairment initially but improve over time may move from scanning or encoding to writing or direct selection techniques.

1. Handwriting

Patients who have movement of the upper extremities and are able to perform the fine motor movement necessary for manipulating a pen or pencil may utilize writing as a quick method of message transfer. The patient can be provided with a simple pad of paper or notebook and pen. Magnetic boards such as the Magic Slate toy are available. With this item, messages can be quickly written and easily erased by lifting up the top sheet. The patient's positioning is maximized through use of slings, lapboards, or bedside tables. Adaptive devices such as pen grips are provided as necessary. The occupational therapist is consulted to assess the patient for positioning needs and adaptive devices.

2. Direct Selection

Direct selection is another access method which refers to the ability to point to a letter, word, or symbol. It is used when motor movement is too limited for writing. Direct selection can utilize any motor movement, including movement of the eyes. For example, direct selection is performed with the use of the fingers during typing, with a mouth/head stick or light beam when pointing, and with the eyes during eye gaze.

Communication boards range from standard alphabet boards to word/phrase boards that contain frequently occurring messages. Communication boards can be accessed via any direct selection technique (e.g., pointing with a finger, eye, or mouthstick). Examples of simple communication boards are shown in Figure 6-2.

Eye gaze is an effective method of using direct selection. Figure 6-3 illustrates the use of an Eye-Link (Drinker & Krupoff, 1981) to directly select the letters necessary to spell a message. Messages can be transferred from literate individuals who are completely paralyzed but are able to move the eyes in upward, downward, and lateral positions. As the patient gazes through a transparent sheet of plastic at a selected letter, the communication partner moves the Eye-Link until the message sender (patient) and message receiver (communication partner) "link" eyes. Movement of the extremities is required only from the communication partner. The target letter is identified aloud by the receiver and the process begins again. The Eye-Link is a rapid direct selection method available to patients with minimal existing motor capacity, who might otherwise be limited to a slower mode of access. For more detailed instructions in use of the Eye-Link, the reader is referred to the Communication Independence for the Neurologically Impaired (CINI) website at www.cini.org.

For patients who can use eye gaze as a method of direct access but are unable to spell, photos or pictures can be placed on a board. The patient can then select

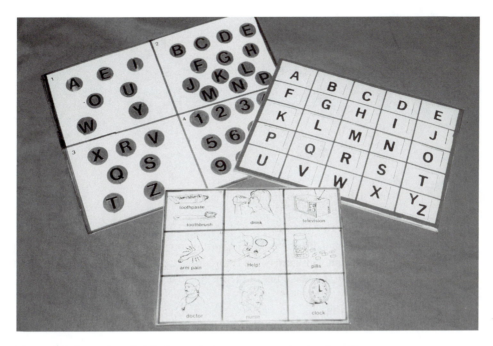

Figure 6-2. Examples of alphabet and picture communication boards.

1. Hold sheet in front of the patient
2. Have patient focus on the first letter of the word desired
3. Move sheet until your eyes "link" with the patient's through the desired letter
4. Check with the patient to see if you are correct
5. Continue the process until you get the message

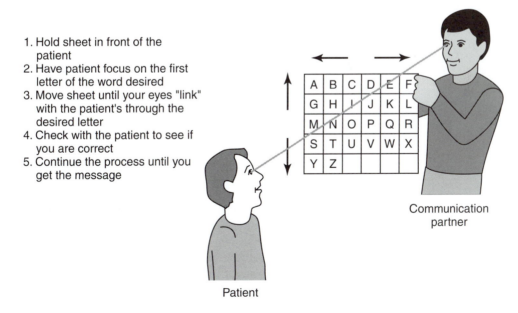

Figure 6-3. Instructions for use of an Eye-Link.

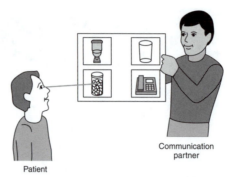

Communication
partner

Patient

Figure 6-4. Direct selection through eye gaze.

the intended item by looking at the corresponding picture. For example, the individual in Figure 6-4 is communicating a need for more pain medication by pointing to the picture of the medicine bottle using eye gaze.

3. Scanning

Scanning, another access method, is useful for patients who have limited physical motor movements. It involves presenting items or letters until the patient uses a predetermined signal to indicate that the target has been reached. The signal must be a consistent and reliable motor movement that can be triggered by a movement of the body (e.g., head nod) or by activation of a switch. For example, the communication partner asks the patient a string of questions that can be answered with either a "yes" or a "no" response. The patient raises his or her eyebrows to indicate a response. The process continues until the information is obtained.

a. Switches

Switches can be utilized to assist the patient in accessing the communication system. Switches range in size, shape, color, texture, method of access, and sensitivity. The patient's residual physical motor function will determine the type of switch prescribed. Figure 6-5 provides examples of switches including a pillow switch, an infra-red switch and pneumatic sip and puff switch. Depending on patient muscle movement and a strength, these switches can be accessed with various areas of the body. The speech-language pathologist, often in conjunction with the occupational therapist and rehabilitation engineer, will select the particular switch to meet the unique communication needs of the nonspeaking tracheostomized and/or ventilator-dependent patient. In some settings, the rehabilitation engineer is called on to fabricate special switches and devices, not commercially available, to meet the individual needs of the patient.

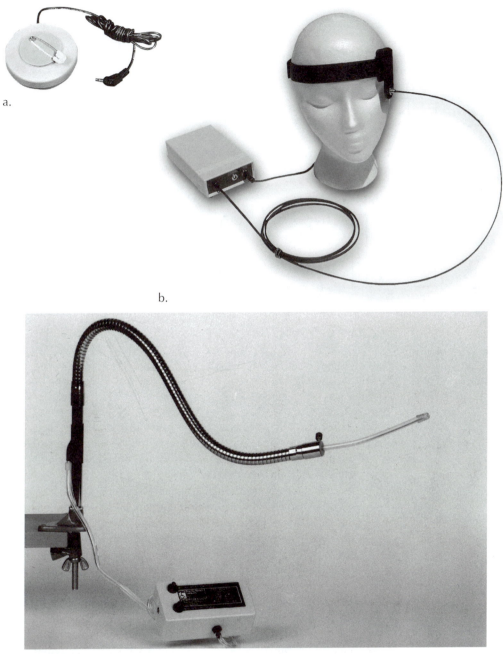

a.

b.

c.

Figure 6-5a. A pillow switch. (Photo courtesy of Crestwood Communication Aids, Inc.). **b.** An infra-red switch mounted for use with an eye blink. (Photo courtesy of Empowering Resources, Inc.). **c.** A pneumatic sip and puff switch. (Photo courtesy of Prentke-Romich Company)

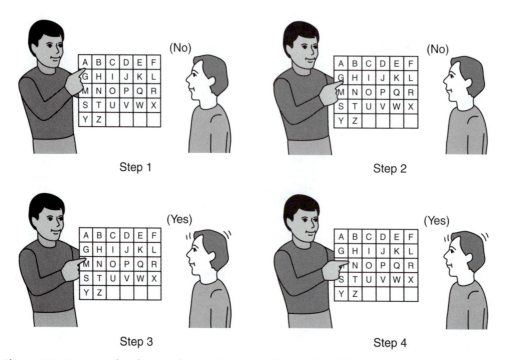

Figure 6-6. An example of row-column visual scanning. (Adapted from *Electronic Communication Aids, Selection and Use,* by I. Fishman, 1987, p. 71. San Diego, CA: College-Hill Press. Copyright by I. Fishman)

(1) Various scanning patterns can be used to transfer messages. The most common pattern is referred to as *row-column scanning.* Row-column scanning utilizes a *group scanning technique,* as it allows the individual to first indicate the group or row where the target item is located before going through each individual item. This technique is useful in reducing the number of items that must be presented before the target is reached. Items can be presented visually or auditorily. During *visual scanning* for example, the patient is presented with the first row of letters and proceeds downward until the desired row (which contains the target letter) is presented. The patient signals a "yes," and the communication partner then proceeds by pointing to each letter along the column until the desired letter is reached. Once the letter is selected, the process begins again until the message has been transferred. Visual scanning is illustrated in Figure 6-6.

(2) *Auditory scanning* is useful for patients who are visually impaired. Items are presented aloud. For example, the communication partner asks: "What is the first letter?" "Is it in letters A through F?" "G through L?" The patient waits until the target group has been presented before signaling a response. Once a group has been selected,

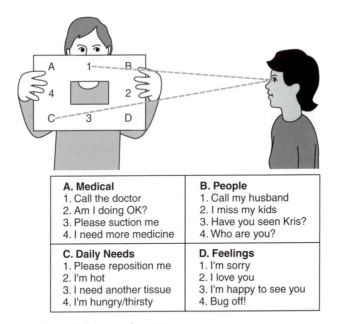

A. Medical	B. People
1. Call the doctor	1. Call my husband
2. Am I doing OK?	2. I miss my kids
3. Please suction me	3. Have you seen Kris?
4. I need more medicine	4. Who are you?
C. Daily Needs	**D. Feelings**
1. Please reposition me	1. I'm sorry
2. I'm hot	2. I love you
3. I need another tissue	3. I'm happy to see you
4. I'm hungry/thirsty	4. Bug off!

Figure 6-7. Encoding through the use of an E-Tran.

the communication partner continues with: "Is it G?" "H?" "I?" and so on, and the patient again signals for the target. Although scanning is considered the slowest method of access, patients who have quick and reliable signals can scan effectively and rapidly. In the interest of time, patients who demonstrate intact cognitive-linguistic status may combine scanning with another method, encoding. Patients scan to communicate novel messages and convey more predictable, recurrent messages via encoding.

4. Encoding

Encoding is another example of an access method used with either direct selection or scanning. It is used to communicate detailed messages when motor control is not sufficient to directly select each item. In encoding, the patient uses a small number of items (or a code) to represent a larger number of messages. An *E-Tran* can be used to communicate messages via encoding. It is a plastic frame with the center removed for direct visualization of the message sender. Although similar to an Eye-Link, the E-Tran is used in combination with an encoding system. Figure 6-7 demonstrates the use of an E-Tran. The patient learns that when he indicates the item C-1 via direct selection eye gaze, this will transfer the message "please reposition me." This message can be displayed on a communication board for reference so that all communication partners are aware of the coded system. To increase the speed of message transfer, a patient can also utilize an encoded system combined with scanning. For example, an encoded system can represent 10 lengthy messages with the numbers 1–10. It will require less time to select a number code, through scanning, and convey a fairly lengthy message, than to scan through the entire alphabet in order to spell each word.

a.   *Morse code* is an example of an encoding system that is accessed with single or dual switches. The Morse code alphabet is the traditional alphabet where each letter and punctuation mark has a corresponding code or combination of dots and dashes. The patient indicates the target letter by activating the switch(es) for a particular length of time. The switch beeps to signify dots or dashes, determining the letter. Figure 6-8 illustrates the Morse code system and an example of an iconic system for easy recall of the code (Romney, 1987). Patients who use Morse code as an access method often utilize a computerized communication system that deciphers the code and produces the corresponding letter. Morse code is utilized as a long-term communication technique as this method of access requires adequate linguistic and cognitive abilities as well as sufficient time for training. Vanderheiden (as cited in Fishman, 1987) reported, "Morse code can greatly increase rate of communication for those individuals with limited physical control by reducing the range of motion required over direct selection and decreasing the time from that required by scanning" (p. 85).

D. Nonelectronic Communication Systems

Nonelectronic communication systems are essential for all nonspeaking tracheostomized and/or ventilator-dependent patients, even when these patients also use electronic systems. For electronic users, the nonelectronic system can be considered a backup when the sophisticated electronic communication system is not functional, unavailable, or when a communication partner is unfamiliar with the electronic system. Nonelectronic communication systems range from simple pen and paper techniques or picture/word boards to more complex encoded systems.

1.   Nonelectronic communication systems offer several benefits. They are

- easily fabricated,
- personalized,
- portable,
- replaceable,
- low cost,
- resistant to breakage,

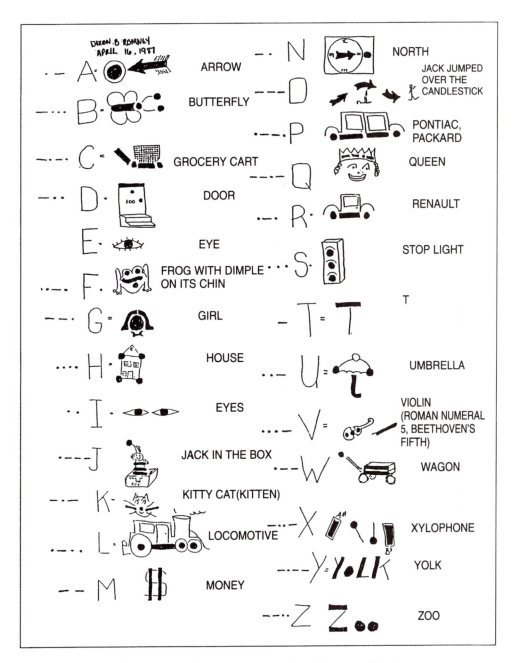

Figure 6-8. Morse code system with iconic representation. (Courtesy of D. Romney)

- often require less training than computerized systems,
- easily modified,
- motorically require less accuracy, range of motion, and degree of pressure (Fishman, 1987).

2. Although nonelectronic solutions have many advantages for nonspeaking patients across communicative settings, there are several drawbacks if the patient is limited solely to the nonelectronic communication system. Non-electronic systems

   - require cooperation and time from communication partners,
   - require communication partners to be present,
   - decrease patient independence,
   - cannot save messages to print (except handwriting),
   - cannot be used on the phone.

3. The patient and clinician will determine which nonelectronic system meets as many of the communication needs identified during the assessment process as possible. However, when particular needs cannot be met solely by the nonelectronic low-tech solutions, introduction to electronics may be indicated.

E. Electronic Communication Systems

Electronic or high-tech communication systems provide more sophisticated options to the nonspeaking, tracheostomized and/or ventilator-dependent patient. Electronic communication systems can be referred to as either *dedicated* or *integrated* communication systems. A dedicated system refers to a device that is used solely for communication purposes. This contrasts with the integrated system, which not only allows for communication, but additionally relies on the use of a commercially available laptop or desktop computer. Electronic communication systems provide increased independence. Message transfer and delivery can be accomplished without the direct assistance of a communication partner. Electronic communication systems also offer the flexibility necessary to communicate novel messages in all communicative settings. Each system contains specific characteristics which must be considered prior to selection of a device. Features of electronic communication systems include:

1. Voice Output (Synthesized or Digitized)

Electronic communication systems often provide the nonspeaking patient with a synthetic voice feature. This synthesized voice is produced artificially via computer programming. Technological advances have improved the quality of synthesized voice to include varying pitch, quality, and rate. Voices can even be selected to sound like a female or male, adult or child. The Multi-voice speech synthesizer (Institute on Applied Technology) offers 12 voices from which the user can select. Voice output immediately increases patient independence. Communication partners must no longer be in close proximity to the communication system, but can be seated across from the patient or even located in another room. For the ventilator-dependent patient with limited mobility, the additional comfort of being able to communicate over the telephone reduces isolation and increases security (F. Christopher, personal communication, 1994). Digitized voice is another example of voice output. Digitized voice is similar to a tape recorder. Prerecorded voices are played back to communicate messages. Such a system has obvious advantages for some patients, such as those with degenerative diseases, who can prerecord messages for later use. Digitized voice does require a significant amount of memory and can be more costly than synthesized voice. Some electronic communication systems offer both synthesized and digitized voice output options.

2. Visual Display

Visual displays provide the nonspeaking patient with visual feedback or "soft copy" during message construction (Fishman, 1987). Visual feedback is especially helpful for the patient who presents with cognitive-linguistic impairment such as memory loss. A visual display allows the patient to create a detailed message and make changes or edit before saving it to hard copy or print. Additionally, visual displays allow the patient to communicate with partners who are hearing impaired. Visual displays vary in:

a. Screen size

Full screen options are available with standard computer monitors. They contrast to single or multiple line displays, which are common to dedicated communication devices. Figure 6-9 pictures single and multiple line displays. With single or multiple line visual displays, the patient may be able to see only a portion of the message at one time. Comparatively longer messages may be viewed on full screen displays. Most electronic communication systems provide one visual display. However, dual visual displays are available. They allow face-to-face communicative exchanges and provide more normalized communicative interactions. Using a dual display, communication partners can face each other during their conversation.

b. Character size

The size of each letter varies among systems and must be considered, especially when the patient presents with difficulties in visual acuity and perception.

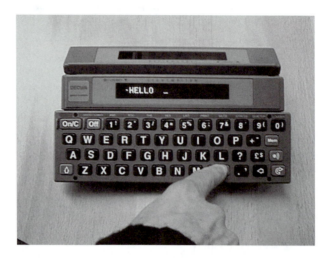

Figure 6-9a. Single line visual display. This system also allows face-to-face communication via its dual visual display. (Photo courtesy of Zygo Industries, Inc.).

c.   Display quality

The quality of the visual display will also differ among dedicated and integrated systems. The quality of the screen on a laptop computer, for example, can affect the patient's ability to see the screen in a variety of contrasting environments, such as inside the house versus outside in the bright sun. Some displays have bright fluorescent print to maximize intelligibility.

3. Printed Output

Print or hard copy output allows the patient to self-generate important messages without face-to-face communicative exchanges. The availability of print can offer the nonspeaking patient in the acute or extended care settings control over the environment. The patient can prepare questions and comments in advance before a busy member of the medical staff is summoned. For some, written output additionally allows continued employment and facilitates communication with individuals out of the immediate physical environment, such as family members living out of state. The print option allows the patient to independently transcribe work without the direct assistance of a communication partner. Print options also vary with the system being used. Single or multiple line versus full page printout is available.

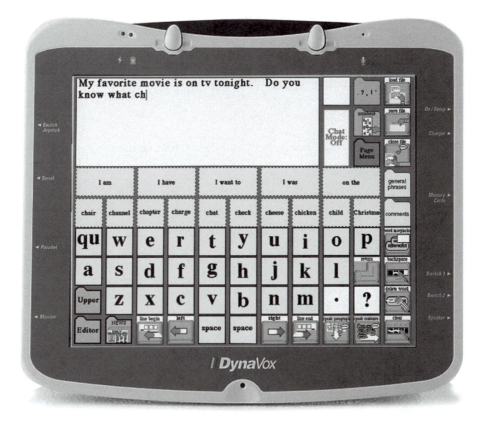

Figure 6-9b. Multiple line visual display. (Photo courtesy of Dynavox Systems LLC)

4. Word Prediction, Abbreviation Expansion, or Other Rate-Enhancing Spelling Options

Electronic communication systems can offer options to increase the speed of message generation and transfer through rate-enhancing features referred to as word prediction, word completion, or abbreviation-expansion.

a. Word prediction

The feature of communication software which provides the next word in a semantic/syntactic construction is referred to as word prediction. In other words, the patient will increase the speed of message transfer when offered a series of possible words which could potentially follow the last word typed. This technique, along with other rate-enhancing features, is designed to reduce the number of keystrokes necessary for the message sender to use and therefore increases the rate of message transfer. Some sophisticated electronic systems offer an option within word prediction which functions to *learn* previously spelled words and word combinations. With this feature, words and word combinations the patient has used frequently will be offered first.

b. Word completion

Word completion is similar to word prediction as it attempts to predict the target word that is being spelled. However, word completion does not allow for semantic/syntactic consideration. It functions solely to *complete* a given target word that is being spelled. For example, if the word "want" has been spelled, the computer may offer "wants, wanting, wanted" as possible selections for completion.

c. Abbreviation-expansion

Abbreviation-expansion is the use of a designated code or abbreviation to create a completely spelled utterance. This feature facilitates quick production of a word or phrase. The patient selects a designated combination of letters which immediately is expanded into the programmed message. For example, the patient who needs to quickly alert the nurse that he or she requires suction types "SMN," which has been previously programmed to indicate "Please suction me now."

5. Memory for Vocabulary Development

Electronics can also allow the patient to select commonly spelled words from dictionaries or vocabulary lists that have been created specifically for the patient. The patient can begin the message and move to the vocabulary list in an effort to quickly retrieve a word that would require multiple keystrokes. For example, if the patient is writing a sentence and begins the next word with the letter D, he or she may access the vocabulary pages containing D words to select the target word. This list may include 50 polysyllabic words beginning with the letter D. This option also can facilitate a more rapid message transfer as the patient saves time by selecting a previously spelled word.

6. Multiple Access Options

Some electronic communication systems provide the clinician with multiple access options. This is especially important for patients with degenerative diseases who are expected to lose motor function over time and therefore may not be able to use their hands throughout the course of the disease. These systems can be operated via different access methods including direct selection, scanning, and encoding. Switches can be connected for single or multiple switch access. Multiple switches, for example, for use with dual switch Morse code, may increase the speed of letter or target selection.

7. Environmental Control Units (ECU)

Independence is greatly increased when the electronic system allows both communication and environmental control. Through the communication software, electronic systems can permit the patient to access common household appliances. This is true even when motor movement is severely restricted. For example, a patient can control the light or the television or dial the telephone via the action of a switch integrated through the communication system.

8. Modem Communication for E-Mail or Electronic Bulletin Boards

The use of telephone or cable lines expands the number of communication partners available to a patient. Computer-based communication systems allow communication through a modem for electronic bulletin board access or electronic mail.

a. *Electronic bulletin boards* are organized resource forums where people exchange ideas or gather information electronically via a modem and a telephone line. Patients with physical disabilities can access these forums through the adaptations that allow computer access. Several electronic bulletin boards offer topic-specific discussions so that a patient can communicate with other individuals around the world who share a common interest. This communication option can expand the world of the homebound tracheostomized and ventilator-dependent patient.

b. *Electronic mail* allows the patient to communicate detailed messages through a software package, modem, and telephone line. Communication over the telephone is often the most difficult scenario for the nonspeaking patient who is tracheostomized and ventilator dependent. Even when voice synthesizers are utilized, message transfer can be long and tiring. E-mail allows the patient to create a message and send it without the pressure of having the communication partner waiting for an immediate response.

F. Using Nonelectronic and Electronic Communication Systems

As stated previously, electronic communication systems must have a nonelectronic system available as a backup. Utilizing a multimodality approach is also suggested to maximize communication for the patient who is tracheostomized and/or ventilator dependent. In other words, both nonelectronic *and* electronic systems are important in meeting the communication needs of the patient. For example, the nonelectronic system may be designated for use in particular environments such as while in bed. In contrast, the electronic communication system is utilized for writing messages to doctors, caregivers, and so on. The clinician and patient must attempt to develop a comprehensive communication system that meets the many needs of a nonspeaking individual, especially one who is tracheostomized and ventilator dependent.

G. Case Vignettes: Intervention

The following cases detail the intervention process that occurred after completion of the Communication Needs Assessment. These cases were initially discussed during the description of the assessment process in Section IV, C.

1. Acute Care Setting: Howard

Several communication techniques were utilized during Howard's treatment course. They included:

a. Call buzzer

During Howard's initial time in the ICU, his attempts at communication were limited to poorly intelligible mouthing and inconsistent yes/no responses via eye blinks. Both Howard and the nursing staff were anxious because he did not have a way of calling for assistance. The first step in the intervention process was the provision of a call buzzer. An alerting signal was essential for Howard to call the nurses when he became uncomfortable. Because his physical-motor function was severely limited but his oromotor function was fair, a pneumatic or sip and puff switch was connected to the nursing call system. Staff was instructed to place the call buzzer in front of Howard's mouth for easy activation. A brief instruction period was required to teach the patient to accumulate intraoral pressure by sucking a small amount of air into the oral cavity, closing the lips, and then blowing into the switch. This alerting system decreased Howard's anxiety and allowed him to concentrate on his rehabilitative treatment.

b. Yes/no system

The medical staff needed pertinent information from Howard to obtain informed consent for daily medical procedures and feedback regarding his medical status. Communication was insured via a reliable and consistent yes/no system. Initially, the patient was presented with yes and no cards mounted on plexiglass. Howard was instructed to use eye gaze to confirm his yes/no responses. This graphic system was effective during the initial stages of recovery. As his physical and cognitive status improved, this system was changed to more normalized head shakes and nods.

c. Eye-gaze system/word-phrase communication board

As attentional skills and endurance increased, the patient began to tolerate longer periods of intervention. An Eye-Link was used to spell novel messages and questions. Initially, if spelling more than a few words, Howard's eye gaze became unreliable. Therefore, a more efficient word/phrase board was developed with the assistance of his family. Words pertinent to his medical care were included to reduce the overall amount of spelling required. Howard dictated a living will, healthcare proxy, and specific instructions with his nonelectronic communication systems. Howard's communication needs were immediate and often revolved around life and death issues. An electronic communication system was not appropriate due to environmental restraints and the limitations of Howard's cognitive and medical status. Additionally, time for training with an electronic system was not available during his stay in this acute care environment.

2. Rehabilitative Setting: Kenny

Communication approaches utilized during Kenny's treatment course included:

a. Call buzzer

Kenny's severe physical-motor impairments precluded his ability to access the standard nursing call buzzer that was provided on the rehabilitation unit. A pillow switch was adapted to the nursing call buzzer system and placed for Kenny to access when in bed (Crestwood Company). Kenny demonstrated lateral movement of the head when in the supine position. The sensitivity of the switch allowed him to activate the call signal with a slight head movement.

b. Eye-gaze system/nonelectronic abbreviation-expansion

Kenny was very depressed and was followed routinely by psychology and psychiatry. Initially, he was not interested in using nonoral communication methods and wanted treatment to address oral options only. However, his dysarthria and poor secretion management interfered with functional oral communication. Only limited intervals of cuff deflation were possible, chiefly during treatment sessions. Kenny needed a communication system that was easy to learn and use secondary to fatigue and depression-related lack of motivation. The rehabilitation staff was skilled in eye gaze communication systems and easily utilized the Eye-Link to obtain messages from Kenny. Messages were transferred quickly and reinforced Kenny's efforts to communicate. Additionally, Kenny used abbreviations via the Eye-Link to rapidly communicate common daily needs.

For example, if he needed suction he spelled "SM" which translated into "suction me now." These coded messages were written on a chart above his bed and on his wheelchair for any unfamiliar communication partner.

c. Single switch access/electronic communication system

Abbreviation-expansion was easily integrated into an electronic communication system. Kenny wrote letters to his family and messages to the medical team. A switch similar to his call buzzer was provided for access to the electronic system. It was mounted to his pillow and accessed with Kenny's lateral head movement. Kenny was instructed in single switch use for electronic scanning. He activated the switch when the target letter was illuminated on the dedicated communication system. Since he was already familiar with the concept of abbreviation-expansion, the transition to an electronic system using this strategy was not difficult. Kenny used abbreviation-expansion as a rate-enhancing technique to facilitate quick access to preprogrammed language and message transfer. For example, "SM" was also preprogrammed into the system to spell out "suction me now." The dedicated communication system also provided synthesized speech which allowed Kenny to communicate short messages to his family. He preprogrammed phrases and short paragraphs detailing recent events and then played these messages over the telephone.

3. Long-term Care Setting: Tom

Communication approaches utilized during Tom's treatment course included:

a. Call buzzer

During the initial stages of intervention, Tom demonstrated the motoric ability to activate the nursing call buzzer with his left hand. However, due to his aphasia and cognitive-linguistic deficits, Tom demonstrated difficulty comprehending the cause and effect relationship between bell activation and obtaining help from the nursing staff. Treatment goals initially focused on instructing the patient to use the buzzer whenever he required attention. The nursing staff was made aware of the importance of quickly entering the patient's room when he activated the buzzer to reinforce the concept.

b. Yes/no response system

Tom's dysarthria affected his mouthing ability. Intervention addressed the oral motor weakness and the development of a nonoral communication system. Establishing a reliable yes/no response system was necessary. Tom often responded inaccurately, especially in the afternoons when he was fatigued. This frustrated his family and afternoon nurses as they would receive reports from the morning staff regarding his accurate responses and progress. Yes/no cards were placed on a communication board. Tom's communication partners were instructed to point to the words on the board for visual cuing when asking a yes or no question. For example, his nurse would ask, "Tom, do you want to be brought outside, yes or no?" while pointing to the corresponding word. Tom began to increase his response accuracy over time, which allowed the speech-language pathologist to develop a more detailed communication system.

c. Picture/word communication board

As Tom began to demonstrate his ability to read some functional single words, visual language skills were addressed further. A list of pertinent words with corresponding pictures was generated with the assistance of the medical team and family. Words and pictures were strategically arranged on a board to ensure that his right-sided inattention would not interfere. Target items were larger and brighter on the right side of the page. This appeared to facilitate better attention to that side. Tom eventually was able to identify each word and picture accurately. However, he rarely initiated use of the board. Conversational topics that his family identified as items of interest prior to his stroke were included. Specific topic boards were created in an attempt to facilitate comments and questions during various activities on the unit and in the facility. When Tom made attempts to communicate, especially spontaneous attempts, he was reinforced by all conversational partners. Communication via gesture and pointing was also reinforced and expanded to increase message transfer.

d. Paper and pen writing

As Tom's limb apraxia and cognitive-linguistic status improved, treatment addressed handwriting and written message generation. Tom began to write single words to indicate items that he wanted from home. "Shaver," "robe," and "sunglasses" were legibly written and quickly provided by the patient's family. Tom developed an increased awareness of his communication abilities and attempted to initiate communication more often. He continued to make progress in his linguistic recovery, approximately 5 years following his admission to the extended care facility. He expired thereafter due to complications from his multiple medical problems.

4. Home Care Setting: Ted

Communication approaches utilized during Ted's treatment course included:

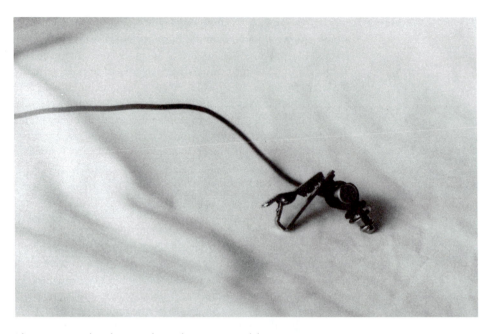

Figure 6-10. A lapel microphone for voice amplification.

a. Speech supplementation approach

During the initial stages of intervention, Ted was provided with a small alphabet board which allowed him to use a speech supplementation approach. Ted was instructed to use exaggerated, slow speech during conversation while pointing to the initial letter of each word in the string. This was a helpful cue to the listener who occasionally needed initial letter cuing to comprehend the message. An amplifier with a lapel microphone, depicted in Figure 6-10, was also provided to increase his vocal volume, especially during his psychotherapy sessions with his clients. Speech supplementation paired with the vocal amplifier was useful in preserving oral communication for approximately 6 months until his physical-motor and speech function deteriorated. Even though oral communication was still considered functional at this time, nonoral approaches were being explored.

b. Integrated electronic communication system

Although Ted initially refused to use electronic communication for message transfer, he agreed to try a system that would provide written communication. As Ted's physical motor function deteriorated, he became quadriplegic and could no longer use his IBM computer for work.

With the assistance of a rehabilitation engineer and occupational therapist, a positioning device (i.e., a sling suspending his right hand) was prescribed and constructed. The sling allowed Ted to access a small mouse and later a single switch. In this manner, he operated his computer. Software was purchased that provided word prediction and abbreviation-expansion to increase the speed of his hard copy computer work. Other software (e.g., a daily planner) was purchased to assist Ted in managing his work-related responsibilities and personal affairs.

c. Eye-gaze system

Oral communication became increasingly difficult for Ted, especially when he was in bed. An Eye-Link was provided to assist Ted in spelling messages to his wife and caregivers while in a supine position. Ted began to experience more episodes of communication breakdown and slowly became more open to the concept of synthesized speech output. A number of synthesizers were demonstrated so that Ted could assess their various voice output qualities. Ted selected a voice synthesizer which he felt was most intelligible to his current clients and other unfamiliar communication partners. His electronic communication system was easily adapted to meet his oral needs. He programmed common phrases, words, and paragraphs into the device to facilitate rapid message transfer. Ted continues to utilize his nonelectronic and electronic communication systems to meet his communicative needs for professional and personal functions.

The use of nonoral communication options, in a variety of communicative settings, is often necessary to meet the changing needs of the patient who is tracheostomized and ventilator dependent. Whether for temporary or more long-term purposes, the clinician must determine the patient's individual communication needs and develop an appropriate nonelectronic and/or electronic communication system.

7

Pathophysiology: Interrelationship of Tracheostomy, Ventilator Dependence, and Swallowing

Management of dysphagia in the tracheostomized and ventilator-dependent patient will challenge all of the members of the interdisciplinary team. If the complex interrelation between deglutition and respiration is disrupted, significant impairment can result. Additionally, due to the shared functions of the hypopharynx and larynx, the impact of dysphagia is often heightened for the individual with respiratory compromise. This chapter will briefly review normal swallowing, discuss the relationship between respiration and swallowing and explore the potential impact of tracheostomy and ventilator dependence on the swallowing process. It will provide a basis for the assessment and treatment protocols to follow in Chapter 8.

I. THE NORMAL SWALLOWING SEQUENCE: A BRIEF REVIEW

The normal swallowing sequence is illustrated in Figure 7-1. The oral, pharyngeal, and esophageal phases are normally identified in tracking the movements of the bolus from the mouth through to the esophagus.

A. Oral Stage

1. The oral stage begins with the entry of food or liquid into the oral cavity and ends with the initiation of the pharyngeal swallow. The oral phase is subdivided into oral preparation, which is distinct from oral transit. Oral preparation is not always needed, as with successive liquid swallows. *Oral preparation* begins the process of readying a bolus for passage through the pharynx

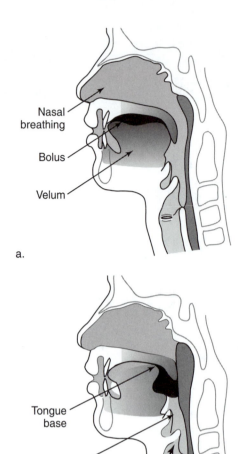

a.

b.

c.

d.

e.

f.

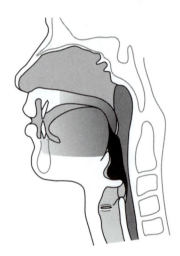

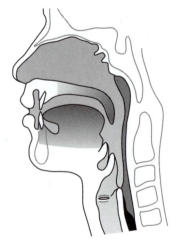

and esophagus. After accepting either a food or liquid bolus, the lips are usually closed to maintain a seal and prevent loss of the material from the oral cavity. If necessary, the tongue and mandible function to move a solid bolus laterally, onto the teeth, for mastication. Saliva, which contains special digestive enzymes, is mixed with the food to assist in softening and moistening the bolus, beginning the digestive process and preparing the bolus for easy passage through the pharynx. Saliva is also a precursor to the sensation of taste. It must be present in adequate amounts to keep the oral cavity moist and well lubricated. Saliva functions both as an **emollient,** to soften, and a **demulcent,** to reduce irritation (Zemlin, 1981). During oral preparation, the velum serves to help keep food in the mouth by resting against the base of the tongue and sealing off the nasal cavity. Typically, breathing during this period is nasal and continues throughout the preparation of the bolus.

2. The oral preparatory stage adapts to the needs of the individual. For example, Martin and Robbins (1995) note that the muscles recruited during oral preparation vary with the consistency and size of the bolus, age of the patient, patterns of eating, and dentition. After oral preparation the bolus is ready for propulsion through the oral cavity. During oral transit the tongue serves to squeeze the food bolus against the hard palate and move it posteriorly toward the hypopharynx. The action of the base of the tongue is integral to this movement and in the propulsion of the bolus into the pharynx. The tongue's role as a mobile agent in the swallow serves to begin the oral-pharyngeal propulsive pump. *Oral transit,* the propulsion of the bolus in an anterior to posterior direction over the tongue and through the faucial arches, is a prerequisite for a successful second stage of the swallow, the *pharyngeal stage.*

B. Pharyngeal Stage

1. The *pharyngeal stage* begins as the bolus passes through the faucial arches and as the pharyngeal swallow is elicited. During this time, the velum elevates to contact the posterior pharyngeal wall and close off the nasal cavity. Once the pharyngeal swallow is elicited, the essential functions of airway protection occur as the larynx moves in an anterior and superior position, pulled by the hyoid bone. As the larynx is pulled upward, the epiglottis is displaced downward to deflect food over the airway. The *epiglottis* is the cartilage which

Figure 7-1. (opposite) The oral, pharyngeal, and esophageal phases of swallowing. The bolus is propelled in a posterior direction **(a)** as the tongue base retracts and the velum elevates **(b, c).** The larynx begins to elevate **(c, d)** as the bolus descends into the pharynx. As the bolus passes through the upper esophageal sphincter **(e),** the bolus moves fully into and through the esophagus **(f).** The oral and pharyngeal phases last approximately 1 second each. The esophageal phase varies from approximately 8 to 20 seconds.

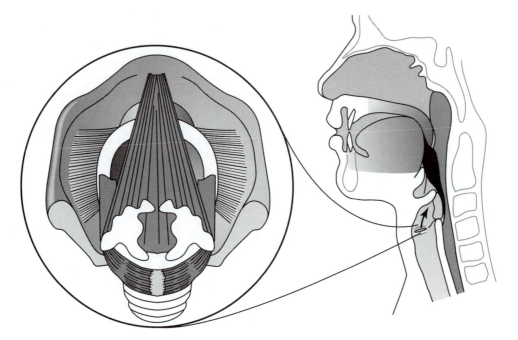

Figure 7-2. Airway closure pictured in lateral (showing laryngeal elevation) and superior (showing vocal fold adduction) views.

normally tips down over the larynx during swallowing of a bolus. It is moved chiefly by the descending bolus, but also by the action of the elevated larynx. Closure of the laryngeal valving system, from the aryepiglottic folds through the false and true vocal folds, occurs at the same time. The **laryngeal vestibule** is therefore protected from entry of foreign material. Closure occurs from the true cords upward, which serves to expel any material that has entered the laryngeal vestibule into the pharynx. Laryngeal closure is contingent on the action of the intrinsic laryngeal muscles (Adran & Kemp, 1952). The intrinsic musculature can function to close the true cords even if laryngeal elevation does not occur. However, for complete airway closure to occur, all components of the laryngeal valving system must function. Respiration ceases briefly during this period of airway closure. This is referred to as **apnea.** When respiration begins again, it normally resumes with exhalation. Figure 7-2 identifies the components of laryngeal closure.

2. The bolus moves over the closed airway and passes into the esophagus through the *pharyngoesophageal (PE) segment,* by way of the *cricopharyngeal sphincter,* located at the top of the digestive tract. This area, also commonly known as the *upper esophageal sphincter (UES),* is composed partly of

the *cricopharyngeus muscle.* It normally maintains a closed position. It is a zone of high pressure that closes off the entrance to the esophagus. The mechanical lift of the elevating larynx, in conjunction with the relaxation of the cricopharyngeus muscle, opens the PE segment and allows the passage of food or liquid into the esophagus. The sphincter must remain closed at all other times to prevent the entry of air into the stomach and the reflux of material from the esophagus into the hypopharynx. The distal end of the esophagus also consists of a sphincter at the *gastroesophageal junction,* known as the *lower esophageal sphincter.*

3. The movement of the bolus is partly dependent on the muscular contractions of the pharynx, but to a large extent, it is the changes in pharyngeal pressures that move the bolus efficiently. The pharynx generates high pressures over a short time period. Several characteristic pressure waves (in the mouth, pharynx, and esophagus) have been identified, and occur in a carefully timed fashion. The initial portion of one wave, the T wave, has been identified as the tongue driving force and is responsible for pushing the bolus (McConnel, Cerenko, & Mendelsohn, 1988). McConnel et al. (1988) write that "the mechanism of . . . oropharyngeal pressure generation has been compared to a pump, with the tongue base being the plunger and the pharyngeal walls being the chamber" (p. 629). Sufficient pressures must accumulate in the pharynx for the generation of these waves and driving forces.

C. Esophageal Phase

With the passage of the bolus through the cricopharyngeal sphincter, the esophageal phase begins. The bolus is propelled on the *primary* and *secondary peristaltic waves,* which move it through the gastroesophageal junction and into the stomach. Effective stripping waves are necessary for timely movement of the bolus through the esophagus. Pressure changes at the cricopharyngeal sphincter and throughout the esophagus are also necessary for effective esophageal transit, but these pressures are generated over longer periods of time and do not reach pharyngeal pressure levels. As there are age-related changes in the oral-pharyngeal swallow, normal changes also occur in the function of the esophagus. These changes include decreased motility and increased age-related gastric reflux (Robbins, Ramig, & Shaker, 1996). Often, pharyngeal symptoms and complaints actually reflect esophageal phase dysfunction. The pharynx cannot be thought of as a separate entity from the esophagus. This is even more evident during a discussion of esophageal disease and dysfunction. Martin et al. (2001) noted that "abnormalities represent modulation of the swallow-related oropharyngeal motor sequence by factors associated with esophageal disease" (p. 29). One of these factors may be an alteration in cricopharyngeal function. Esophageal function is also important because the interaction between the gastrointestinal and upper airway tracts through various reflexes helps prevent retrograde aspiration of esophageal and stomach contents (Shaker, 1995, 2000). When tracheotomy and/or ventilator dependence is superimposed on esophageal dysfunction, whether related to changes secondary to aging or a disease process, the impact on oropharyngeal swallow function may be greatly heightened.

II. RELEVANT ANATOMY: STRUCTURES AND INNERVATION

Chapter 1 reviewed the functions and structures of the phonatory/respiratory system, including the muscular system and cranial nerve innervation. Anatomical components of the phonatory-respiratory tract are particularly relevant to the swallowing process. After a discussion of developmental issues, these structures are highlighted during this next section and in Figures 7-4 and 7-5.

A. Developmental Issues

1. Human anatomy has evolved to the point where the structures for speech, swallowing, and respiration are shared. This necessitated the development of a protective mechanism to ensure that these functions occur reciprocally and safely. Laitman and Reidenberg (1993) described the development of the specialized systems of deglutition and respiration in humans. They additionally compared human anatomy to more primitive systems, such as that of the reptile, where swallowing and respiration are separated, in an effort to understand the possible evolutionary process. In these less developed systems, including nonhuman primates and reptiles, the larynx is permanently positioned *high* in the neck, lifting it out of the path of a descending bolus. It was the descent of the larynx in human adults that demanded a mechanism for protecting the airway during swallowing (Laitman & Reidenberg, 1993).

2. Developmentally, the descent of the larynx in relation to other anatomy creates a space for the modulation of sound (i.e., a larger pharynx). However, this also places the larynx in direct path with a descending bolus, necessitating the closure pattern detailed in Figure 7-2. Infants (until age 2–3 years) still possess the elevated larynx which limits intricate speech production, but largely separates the channels used for deglutition and respiration. The channel for respiration leads essentially from the nose to the lungs, so that infants are primarily nose breathers. The capacity for mouth or oral breathing begins at approximately 4–6 months. Adults can use either the nasal or oral cavities for respiration (Laitman & Reidenberg, 1993). The differences in the adult versus the pediatric larynx are illustrated in Figure 7-3.

B. Oral and Nasal Cavities

Figure 7-4 illustrates the relevant anatomy of the adult oral and nasal cavities, pharynx, and larynx.

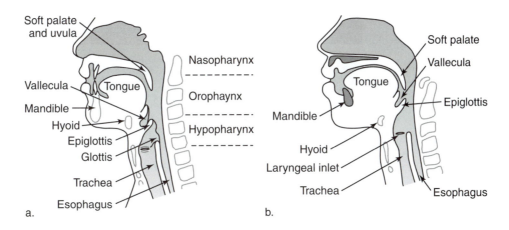

Figure 7-3. Views of **(a)** adult upper airways and **(b)** pediatric upper airways. Note the size differences and descent of the larynx in the adult. (From *Pediatric Swallowing and Feeding Assessment and Management,* by J. C. Arvedson and L. Brodsky, 1993, p. 6. Clifton Park, NY: Singular.)

1. Oral Cavity

   a. The lips, innervated by cranial nerve VII (facial), are responsible for sealing the oral cavity for oral preparation and propulsion of the actual swallow. The tongue is integral in oral preparation, oral transit, and in eliciting the pharyngeal swallow. The base of the tongue has a particularly important role. The base of the tongue is also partly responsible for the laryngeal elevation that is important in airway protection. The muscles responsible for the movements and sensation of the tongue are innervated by multiple cranial nerves including: V (trigeminal), VII (facial), IX (glossopharyngeal), X (vagus), XI (accessory), and XII (hypoglossal).

   b. Three pairs of *salivary glands,* the *parotid, sublingual,* and *submandibular,* are located on the cheek and the underside of the tongue and are responsible for secreting the lubrication necessary for management of the bolus in both the oral and pharyngeal phases. The parotid gland is innervated by fibers of cranial nerve IX (glossopharyngeal); the sublingual and submandibular glands by fibers of cranial nerve VII (facial) (Wilson-Pauwels, Akesson, & Stewart, 1988).

2. Nasal Cavity

The velum serves to close the nasal cavity from the rest of the hypopharynx and prevents nasal regurgitation. This action is accomplished via innervation from cranial nerve XI (accessory) and from the pharyngeal plexus.

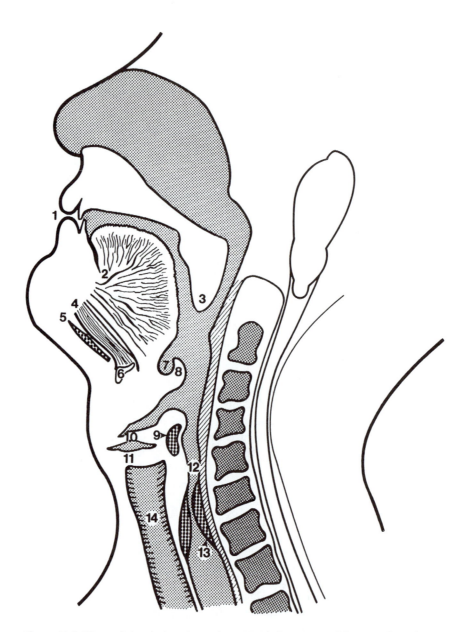

Figure 7-4. View of the oral and nasal cavities, pharynx, and larynx. The relevant structures for airway protection are pictured: **1.** lips; **2.** tongue; **3.** velum; **4.** geniohyoid muscle; **5.** mylohyoid muscle; **6.** hyoid bone; **7.** valleculae; **8.** epiglottis; **9.** arytenoid cartilage; **10.** false vocal folds; **11.** true vocal folds; **12.** pyriform sinuses; **13.** cricopharyngeus muscle; **14.** trachea. (From "Radiographic Contrast Examination of the Mouth, Pharynx, and Esophagus," by A. L. Perlman, C. Lu, and B. Jones, 1997, p. 157. In A. L. Perlman and K. Schulze-Delrieu [Eds.], *Deglutition and Its Disorders* [pp. 153–199]. Clifton Park, NY: Singular.)

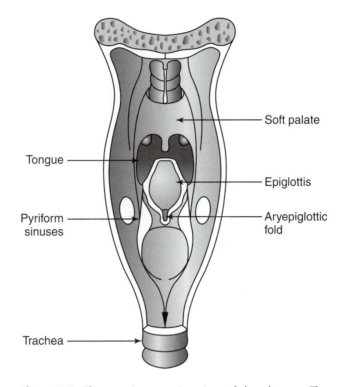

Figure 7-5. The anterior-posterior view of the pharynx. The pyriform sinuses, channels for food through the pharynx and around the larynx, lie between the pharyngeal constrictors and larynx. (From *Pediatric Swallowing and Feeding Assessment and Management,* by J. C. Arvedson and L. Brodsky, 1993, p. 10. Clifton Park, NY: Singular.)

C. Pharynx

Figure 7-5 illustrates the pharynx in an anterior-posterior view.

1. The pharynx, the muscular tube through which the bolus is propelled, contains the *valleculae,* recesses formed between the base of the tongue and the epiglottis. The *pharyngeal constrictors* (*superior, medial,* and *inferior*) add their muscular contractions to the forces propelling the bolus downward. Pharyngeal musculature is suspended in part from the *hyoid bone,* upon which the tongue rests. The hyoid bone is pulled superiorly and anteriorly from the action of the posterior tongue. When the mandible or tongue is fixed, the hyoid can also be elevated by actions of the suprahyoid muscles. The epiglottis, which serves to protect the airway by separating the respiratory and digestive tracts, is believed to have evolved into a secondary mechanism for airway protection.

Between the walls of the pharynx and the larynx are found the *pyriform sinuses,* another set of pharyngeal recesses through which a bolus passes during swallowing. These sinuses channel food away from the airway and into the esophagus.

The pyriform sinuses, like the valleculae, are important anatomical landmarks during the dysphagia assessment process, especially during objective dysphagia assessment procedures, such as fiberoptic assessment or videofluoroscopy.

D. Larynx

The bolus normally should not enter the *larynx* at any time during the swallowing process, although there is evidence that 45% of normal (not dysphagic) individuals do silently aspirate small quantities of saliva during sleep (Huxley, Viroslav, Gray, & Pierce, 1978). Also with age-related changes, the normal elderly may exhibit increased penetration and aspiration (Robbins, 2000). The larynx is protected from penetration by foreign substances at multiple levels. Mechanical elevation, via its attachments to the hyoid bone, pulls the larynx out of the pathway of the bolus. The intrinsic laryngeal muscles, innervated by cranial nerve X (vagus), close the larynx at the aryepiglottic folds, false vocal folds, and true vocal folds. This creates a seal that separates the airway and digestive tract.

E. Esophagus

Figure 7-6 depicts a radiographic image of a bolus passing through the PE segment and into the esophagus. At the top of the muscular esophagus lies the cricopharyngeal sphincter or upper esophageal sphincter (UES), the muscular band that must relax to allow passage of a bolus into the esophagus. The timing of this action is mediated by the brainstem. The UES opens via relaxation of the PE segment, the mechanical leverage provided by the elevation of the larynx, and the pressures generated by the pharyngeal stripping wave.

II. RELATIONSHIP BETWEEN SWALLOWING AND RESPIRATION

A. Shared Functions

Martin and Robbins (1995), Martin, Logemann, Shaker, and Dodds (1994), Martin (1991, 1994), and Shaker et al. (1992) have quantified and characterized the reciprocity between the respiratory-cardiac and digestive systems. This reciprocity is most evident at the larynx, the level of airway closure (Martin 1994). Disruption of the ability to coordinate airway closure at the appropriate time in the swallow can lead to airway compromise. Martin et al. (1994) and Martin (1994) stated that some of the factors that affect airway protection in the patient with pulmonary disease include:

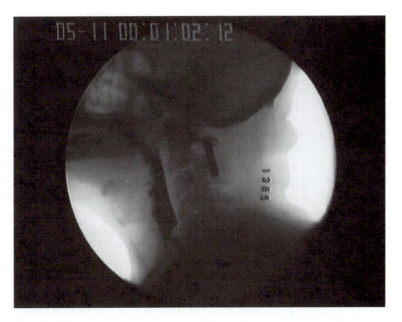

Figure 7-6. Lateral view of the esophagus illustrating cricopharyngeal prominence at the PE segment. (From "Radiographic Contrast Examination of the Mouth, Pharynx, and Esophagus," by A. L. Perlman, C. Lu, and B. Jones, 1997, p. 167. In A. L. Perlman and K. Schulze-Delrieu [Eds.], *Deglutition and Its Disorders* [pp. 153–199]. Clifton Park, NY: Singular.)

1. Alterations in the timing of airway closure during the swallow.

2. Interruption of the normally well timed pattern of swallowing and breathing.

3. Diminished respiratory defenses (e.g., diminished cough, reduced airway clearance).

A review of the literature, which follows, indicates that these are important aspects of normal swallowing. This literature supports the close relationship between respiration and swallowing function. For example, Shaker et al. (1992) demonstrated that when a respiratory system is stressed, as with a rapid respiratory rate (over 30 bpm), the duration of inspiratory phase diminishes and the time requirement for airway closure during swallowing is disrupted. Their findings suggested that:

> factors such as increased oxygen demand or an increase in arterial CO_2, etc., that result in tachypnea may influence the coupling of the swallowing with the phases of respiration. These findings provide further evidence for the presence of a sophisticated central communication between the deglutition and respiration centers. (p. 755)

Speech-language pathologists and other health care practitioners who work with dysphagic individuals must have an appreciation of the reciprocity of respiration and swallowing and should attempt to integrate this information into assessment and treatment.

B. Coordination of Swallowing and Respiration

The coordination of breathing and swallowing has been studied in normal adults. The results of this body of research begin to reveal how the aerodigestive tract has evolved to allow a shared passageway for food and air. In addition, these results reveal the potential for dysfunction in a compromised system (e.g., in the presence of respiratory insufficiency, diseased lungs, tracheostomy and/or ventilator dependence).

1. Smith, Wolkove, Colacone, and Kreisman (1989) used noninvasive monitoring tools to assess breathing in various conditions: normal breathing over a 5-minute interval, interspersed with eating a solid bolus and drinking water. In all conditions, the majority of swallows were expiratory events. That is, in young adult subjects, it was most typical for the swallow to interrupt expiration. Expiratory flow thus preceded and followed the swallow event. In this case, the swallowing sequence would occur as follows: inspiration, expiration, initiation of a pharyngeal swallow, onset of an *apneic interval* or cessation of respiration, passage of the bolus, and then resumption of the same expiratory breath. Expiration after the swallow may function as part of the body's airway clearance mechanism. Moreover, if the apneic interval is too short, safe swallowing may be impeded. Nilsson, Ekberg, Bulow and Hindflet (1996) used respirograms to detect misdirected swallows, that is, those that entered the larynx. They found that older subjects had shorter apneic intervals, with slightly longer pharyngeal passage time. A bolus was still traveling through the pharynx when airway closure ended and respiration commenced; therefore, the chance of aspiration increased.

2. In a separate study, Nishino, Yonezawa, and Honda (1985) reported that almost 80% of their normal, young adult male subjects initiated a swallow interrupting the expiratory phase of the respiratory cycle, with 20% initiating swallows during inspiration. Nishino et al. used terminology that differed slightly from Smith et al. (1989). When their definitions of "inspiration" and "expiration" are made consistent, the results of both studies are more similar. Therefore, both of these studies concluded that the majority of swallows in normal adults appear to interrupt expiration. If the swallow did not interrupt expiration, some normal adult male subjects initiated the swallow at the end of inspiration, so that they exhaled after the swallow (Smith et al., 1989). These studies further support the characteristic timing of respiratory events and swallowing in normal younger subjects.

3. Shaker et al. (1992) also demonstrated that most resting swallows (saliva swallows in this study) in young adults interrupted expiration. However, the authors also studied groups of healthy elderly and patients with diagnoses of COPD. The young subjects participated in physical exercise designed to increase their respiratory rates. Swallows were studied in these subjects at rest and during periods of increased breathing rates. Differences among all groups were evident. The results of this study indicated "that tachypnea, aging, bolus volume, and COPD modify the coordination between deglutition and phases of continuous respiration" (p. 753). The aged subjects swallowed significantly more often during *inspiration* than their young counterparts. Comparatively, patients with COPD swallowed even more often during the inspiratory phase than the normal age-matched subjects. Additionally, patients with COPD would resume breathing with an inspiration after the apneic interval. These results imply that normal elderly individuals and patients with compromised respiratory systems have alterations in the coordination of respiration and swallowing as compared with younger individuals. These alterations may place an individual with combined factors, such as age and respiratory disease, at a higher risk of disrupted airway protection due to difficulties with the timing of the swallow. The addition of variables such as tracheostomy and ventilator dependence may further compromise the ability of the respiratory and swallowing systems to function effectively.

C. Patterns of Respiration

1. Selley, Flack, Ellis, and Brooks (1989a) reported on respiratory patterns associated with swallowing for both normal adults and patients with neurological disease. They reported that 95% of all swallows in a normal adult subject were followed by an expiration. In a study of neurologically impaired adults with dysphagia, Selley, Flack, Ellis, and Brooks (1989b) found "identifiable differences from healthy subjects either in respiratory patterns, or in timings of some stages of the swallowing sequence" (pp. 174–175). For example, patients with cerebrovascular accident inhaled immediately after the swallow. A disruption in the respiratory control pattern was thus evidenced in individuals with neurological disease. Pickersgill, Dawson, and Wiles (1998) studied respiratory patterns related to anatomic lesions. They concluded that patients with brain, spinal cord, and peripheral neurological lesions can display abnormal patterns of deglutition apnea. For example, 18.9% of apneic intervals (periods of airway closure) in 20 patients were followed by inspiration, a pattern rare in the normal population. In other patients, apneic intervals were sometimes associated with more than one swallow, representing a discoordination or discrepancy between the apnea and the swallow.

2. Characteristic patterns have emerged during studies of breathing and swallowing. Nishino et al. (1985) reported the effect of the swallow on respiratory

patterns. The timing of the swallow affected the duration of the respiratory cycle, that is, the later a swallow occurred in expiration, the longer the expiratory phase. Smith et al. (1989) did not replicate these results in a later study. Martin et al. (1994) cited Nishino et al. (1985) in a discussion of the coordination of the swallow with the respiratory cycle and theorized that a pharyngeal swallow that occurred later in the expiratory phase would create a longer postswallow expiration. Martin et al. (1994) suggested that this pattern may be exaggerated in a dysphagic patient in order to provide additional airway clearance of a bolus retained in the pharynx. This would provide an additional protective mechanism for the airway.

3. Smith et al. (1989) examined patterns of respiration during eating and drinking, attempting to approximate a mealtime situation. Patterns of respiration during mealtime were less regular. Greater variations were seen in tidal volume, expiratory duration, and mean inspiratory flow rate. In addition, intraabdominal volume increased because of swallowed food and air, which limited diaphragmatic excursion, decreased the amount that the lungs could expand, and restricted lung volumes. Smith et al. (1989) hypothesized that such reductions in lung volume may be significant for individuals with compromised respiratory systems. They suggested that this decrease in lung volume might contribute to "breathlessness that occurs during eating in subjects with limited pulmonary function" (p. 582), such as individuals with severe COPD. Edgar (1994) also reported significant reductions in forced vital capacity for both normal subjects and individuals with COPD after a meal. These results correlate with our own observations of patients with COPD who complain of being "too full" and "out of breath" after eating only small portions of a meal, and who consequently take in restricted amounts of food.

4. The respiratory patterns may be somewhat different for successive swallows of large liquid boluses (Chi-Fishman & Sonies, 2000). During consecutive swallows, the airway remains closed for the duration of the swallows, with the larynx at least partly elevated. Expiration then begins after the completion of the last swallow, so that the breath must be held for a somewhat extended period. This pattern of prolonged airway closure may have implications for a compromised respiratory system. Successive swallows of large amounts of liquids might stress a patient with respiratory/pulmonary disease. Martin et al. (1994) demonstrated that large volume, successive liquid swallows did not result in respiratory discomfort in normal young adult subjects. However, they suggested that this pattern, multiple consecutive swallows with prolonged airway closure, may prove difficult for the patient with limited pulmonary endurance and reserves. Martin et al. (1994) stated

> Because this type of swallow requires prolonged apnea and airway closure to prevent aspiration of liquid, a patient may interrupt the sequence in an attempt to inhale or "catch his or her breath" and disrupt the tem-

poral respiration-swallowing pattern. It would appear that these individuals would be at greater risk for aspiration during these inspiratory attempts. (p. 721)

Bolus size in general affects aspects of the pharyngeal swallow (Martin & Robbins, 1995). Lazarus et al. (1993) noted that the duration of airway closure, laryngeal elevation, and UES opening appear at least partly related to bolus size. Longer durations of airway closure are required for pharyngeal passage of a large bolus. Alterations in apnea duration relating to bolus size may be responsible for changes in breathing patterns during mealtimes.

5. O'Connor (1994) demonstrated a relationship between deglutition and cardiopulmonary function reflected in increased pulse rate, respiratory rate, and systolic blood pressure during mealtime. For patients with compromised respiratory systems, this can lead to a degree of stress on the system while eating. Although this effort is negligible for an individual with a normal cardiac-respiratory system, it may increase a respiratory compromised patient's fatigue level during a meal. To maintain consistent minute ventilation during eating, the work of breathing may need to increase. In other words, patients may work harder to maintain consistent levels of O_2 and CO_2 in the blood during mealtime. Edgar (1994) reported that postmeal measures of maximum inspirations for individuals with COPD were significantly reduced when compared with premeal measures. Edgar (1994) suggested that this may reflect fatigue of the inspiratory musculature.

D. Role of Expiratory Airflow

The timing of the swallow within expiratory airflow reinforces the belief that expiratory airflow is important as an airway clearance mechanism in removing residual material pooled in the pharynx and larynx. Siebens, Tippett, Kirby, and French (1993) demonstrated that peak airflow velocities may reach 7 liters per second in normal subjects and that this is dramatically amplified in the small surface area of the larynx, resulting in a powerful expiratory force. The apneic pause that is part of the normal swallowing process ensures that the airway is closed during the swallow, while the resumption of expiratory airflow after the swallow serves to sweep the larynx/pharynx free of any residual material. The value of expiratory airflow has been described by Tippet and Siebens (1991) and Siebens et al. (1993). Muz, Mathog, Nelson, and Jones (1989) demonstrated that, when pulmonary air is not available for clearance, aspiration appears more likely to occur.

III. IMPACT OF TRACHEOTOMY ON SWALLOWING

Many individuals continue to eat with a tracheostomy tube. However, the potential for difficulty with deglutition is heightened in the presence of the tracheostomy tube, the

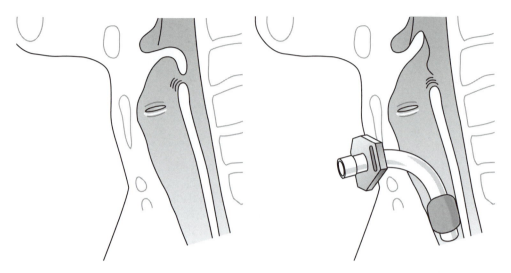

Figure 7-7. Laryngeal fixation.

surgical procedures, and neurological/respiratory impairments associated with tracheotomy. As described above, swallowing is a complex process and may be disrupted at a number of levels. Leder and Ross (2000) did not find a causal relationship between tracheostomy and aspiration and discussed the need for further study across multiple settings in patients requiring tracheostomy. Additionally, the patient with respiratory compromise is often at increased risk of pulmonary infections so that the consequences of aspiration are more serious. The potential impact of tracheotomy on swallowing can be loosely divided into mechanical and physiologic factors (Nash, 1988).

A. Mechanical Impact

1. Reduced Laryngeal Excursion

The tracheostomy tube itself may attach the larynx to the anterior portion of the neck, fixing it in position and limiting laryngeal elevation as illustrated in Figure 7-7. Laryngeal elevation is one of the major factors that ensures adequate airway protection and provides the leverage to create a cricopharyngeal opening. The degree of laryngeal fixation can be exacerbated by several factors, including incision type and surgical techniques, airway management procedures, equipment types, and cuff inflation.

a. A horizontal incision may increase the potential of laryngeal fixation by restricting the amount of movement in the vertical direction. The horizontal incision was traditionally considered more cosmetically acceptable than the vertical. However, because of the problems with laryngeal excursion reported in the surgical literature, the vertical incision is generally favored (Nash, 1988).

Anchoring of the tracheostomy tube to the surrounding musculature may limit laryngeal elevation. In a widely quoted article, Bonanno (1971) reported aspiration and dysphagia in 3 of 43 tracheostomized individuals. This aspiration appeared related to reduced laryngeal elevation secondary to laryngeal fixation. Logemann (1993) reported a single subject study utilizing videofluoroscopy with a tracheostomized individual in which laryngeal excursion was reduced but without significant impact on the functional aspects of the swallow. Laryngeal elevation should be assessed in any tracheostomized individual.

b.   Laryngeal excursion can also be adversely affected by decreased base of tongue movements. The movement of the hyoid bone and larynx is tied with base of the tongue movements. Patients who have been intubated for long periods of time may also present with decreased base of tongue movement. This reduced movement can decrease the piston-like driving action of the tongue base and the upward excursion of the larynx. The cause of this reduced function is most likely related to the continuous pressure and lever-like movement of the endotracheal tube on the base of the tongue. In some patients, upon extubation, the tongue has become a deconditioned muscle. Furthermore, de Larminat, Montravers, Durevil, and Desmonts (1995) stated that the negative impact on the pharyngeal swallow response begins on the first day of endotracheal intubation, leading to a delayed swallow. An improvement in the swallow response can occur 1 week post-extubation. Dikeman and Kazandjian, working in the acute care setting, routinely recommend that even for a premorbidly nondysphagic individual, oral feedings should not be initiated for at least 24 hours post-extubation. This recommendation is especially pertinent for the geriatric patient.

c.   The weight of equipment such as a T-piece or ventilator tubing may increase the sensation of dragging that the tracheostomized patient feels when trying to elevate the larynx. The physical restraints on the larynx may heighten the sensation of laryngeal fixation and impede upward movement, even if a swivel adapter is used to facilitate easier connection.

d.   Cuff inflation has been implicated in many of the dysphagic complications associated with tracheostomy. It has been a long-standing practice to permit oral eating in patients with inflated tracheostomy tube cuffs. Indeed, it was considered unsafe to let individuals with deflated cuffs take nutrition and hydration by mouth. In theory, the seal of the cuff to the tracheal walls was designed to reduce the risk of penetration from the larynx into the trachea. However, various researchers have documented difficulties with oral eating in the presence of cuffed tracheostomy tubes. Inflated cuffs do not stop aspiration from occurring. Cameron, Reynolds, and Zuidema (1973) demonstrated aspiration of blue dye placed in oral secretions in 42 of 61 tracheostomized patients with inflated cuffs. Bone, Davis, Zuidema, and Cameron (1974) demonstrated higher incidences of aspiration with low volume, high pressure cuffs than with low pressure cuffs or sponge cuffs. These older studies looked at the effect of high pressure cuffs, which were widely used at that time, and helped prompt the change to use lower pressure cuffs. Low pressure cuffs distribute the force of the seal more evenly and should not exceed a set level. However, their mechanical effects are still evident, and cuff overinflation may still occur if air volume is above recommended levels.

(1) Part of the disruption of normal airway protection relates to the mechanical anchoring of the larynx. A fully inflated cuff may drag along the tracheal walls during each attempt at elevation. This serves to further disrupt the smooth upward and forward movement of the larynx which is essential during the swallow. The friction created at the cuff site can be one of the predisposing factors for tracheal wall breakdown and the creation of a fistula. Even when caution is taken to keep the cuff inflated at an acceptable level, the cuff can still contact the tracheal walls, and the repeated efforts by the patient to elevate the larynx will result in the sensation of restriction. Many patients report a sensation of tightness when they swallow, which may be related to either the restricted movement or the cuff impinging into the esophagus.

(2) Partial obstruction of the esophagus by the inflated cuff may disturb the physical passage of the bolus and adversely affect the normal esophageal pressures generated during swallowing. The partial blockage of the esophagus can cause food and secretions to pool above the level of the cuff, eventually backing into the pharynx and perhaps entering the larynx as depicted in Figure 7-8. The presence of copious secretions or food being expelled at the stoma site, around the outer cannula, may be an indication that this has occurred and that the trachea above the cuff is actually filled with aspirated contents. This residue gradually builds up to the level of the stoma. The bacterial colonization of these contents poses a concern because an aspiration pneumonia may develop if they enter the lungs. A local irritation of the tracheal tissue can also be created, potentially leading to tracheomalacia.

(3) Manometry in animal subjects has demonstrated the disruption of esophageal pressures that appears related to the presence of the inflated cuff (Leverment, Pearson, & Rae, 1976). The complete esophageal stripping wave occurs in conjunction with timely cricopharyngeal relaxation and opening. This is partly dependent on the mechanical leverage provided by laryngeal elevation.

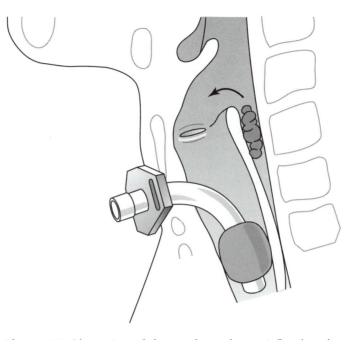

Figure 7-8. Obstruction of the esophagus by an inflated tracheostomy tube cuff.

2. Saliva and Secretion Management

Insufficient saliva can affect the ability to masticate and manage food in the mouth. Adequate lubrication is important for both speech *and* swallowing function. Excessive or thick saliva will detract from adequate swallowing function. Secretion production, if copious, may place a patient at heightened risk for aspiration and interfere with airway protection. Tracheostomized and ventilator-dependent patients may be at heightened risk for problems with saliva or secretions for several reasons.

a. Medication Side Effects

Medications that are associated with xerostomia, excessively dry mouth, include antihistamines, decongestants, sedatives, and antidepressants. These medications are frequently used in the tracheostomized and ventilator-dependent population (Eubanks & Bone, 1990).

(1) Antihistamines address the symptoms of colds and sinus conditions. Decongestants (**vasoconstrictors**) shrink mucosal tissue by constricting small arteries. If applied topically in spray form, the action is to reduce liquids in a particular area, decrease swelling, and open restricted passages (such as the nasal passage). Medication that is ingested can have similar results but will also produce a systemic effect.

(2) Anxiety is a common complaint of ventilator-dependent patients and may affect their ability to tolerate mechanical ventilation. To lessen anxiety, sedatives or hypnotics such as Buspar may be used (R. Fleming, personal communication, January 1995). Depression may certainly accompany anxiety and lessen the ability of an individual to participate in a rehabilitation program or weaning protocol. The tricyclics (e.g., Amitriptyline) are another group of drugs that are primarily used as antidepressants. Both types of medication also may be associated with decreased saliva production.

b. Secretions

An increase in secretion production is typically seen with tracheostomy placement. The defense systems of the upper airway, with its filtering and humidification function, are bypassed. **Nosocomial** infections, those acquired in a hospital or facility, are not unusual in the tracheostomized and ventilator-dependent individual (Levine & Neiderman, 1991). Chronic lung disease is also associated with increased bronchial secretions. Purulent secretions indicate infection and are treated by appropriate therapies. Another potential cause of viscous secretions is the inability to take in sufficient fluids with subsequent poor hydration of the entire body. Cuff deflation is often not an option for the patient with chronic aspiration of excessive secretions or the presence of copious secretions in the airway. Management of excessive secretions can be problematic. Pharmacological intervention, *percussion treatments* of the chest, and *postural (pulmonary) drainage* may be helpful. If these treatments are successful, cuff deflation may then be achieved, facilitating safe swallowing.

(1) Drugs helpful for excessive secretion production include *detergents* and *wetting agents, mucolytics,* and *bronchodilators.* Detergents and wetting agents (such as saline) serve to loosen mucus for easier removal during suctioning. Mucolytics work to reduce the viscosity of secretions. Similarly, antihistamines, as previously described, may be helpful in secretion reduction, because they promote removal and drying of material. Bronchodilators lessen secretions via drying action and promote opening of the airway. However, a medication with a drying effect would not be used in the presence of already viscous secretions. The drying function of the drug could increase secretion viscosity and potentially create a mucous plug. As with all pharmacological agents, these medications can have side effects and must be administered with caution. For example, many bronchodilators can predispose the patient to **tachycardia** (increased heart rate) or hypertension.

(2) Pulmonary drainage procedures may be helpful for the mobilization and removal of secretions and aspirated material (Eubanks & Bone,

1990). A pulmonary drainage program often follows the use of appropriate wetting agents which make the secretions thin enough to mobilize and, literally, drain during postural changes. The use of vibration or shaking and/or percussion or clapping of the chest wall follows. Suctioning is usually applied to fully remove the secretions from the airway. Pulmonary drainage programs may be carried out by specially trained nurses and physical therapists, and are commonly the responsibility of the respiratory care practitioner.

(3) There are multiple contraindications for both pharmalogical intervention and pulmonary drainage procedures. These procedures are initiated only on physician order and after careful selection of appropriate candidates. For example, the presence of excessive/thick secretions might impede the ability of a patient with a cardiac and respiratory condition to tolerate cuff deflation and eat orally. The patient's medical condition may preclude the use of certain drugs due to their side effects. A postural drainage program, with frequent changes in physical position, may also not be tolerated by an individual with **hypertension** (high blood pressure) or **hypotension** (low blood pressure).

B. Physiologic Impact

1. Disruption of Airway Pressures

A vital mechanism for the movement of the bolus through the pharynx and into the esophagus is the airway pressure generated by the base of the tongue. This pressure serves to propel the bolus downward in a stripping wave. Upon reaching the PE segment, the pressures shift into the esophagus after the UES relaxes. An open tracheostomy tube disrupts the maintenance of these pressures and will result in the accumulation of residue in the pharynx. Eibling and Diez-Gross (1996) discussed the contribution of subglottic air pressure to swallowing. They measured airflow and pressure peaks through the tracheostomy tube at the moment of the swallow. They noted that individuals with unoccluded tracheostomy tubes experienced expiratory air leakage through the tube that prevented the achievement of a pressure peak. The use of a specific one-way valve (Passy-Muir in this case) eliminated air leakage, restoring pressure accumulation. This pressure was theorized to relate to the ability to clear the pharynx, and these findings were confirmed during videofluoroscopic studies. Aspiration related to pharyngeal residue was eliminated in tracheostomized patients wearing Passy-Muir valves. In a related study, Stachler, Hamlet, Choi, and Fleming (1996) used scintigraphy to document aspiration reduction in tracheostomized individuals wearing Passy-Muir valves as compared with open tracheostomy tubes.

Leder, Tarro, and Burrell (1996) did not find that occlusion of the tracheostomy tube influenced aspiration prevalence. This study did not involve speaking valves. The authors theorized that, in their subjects, aspiration and overall dysphagic impairment might be related to factors other than occlusion of the tracheostomy tube, possibly other aspects of medical status.

These studies among others in the literature illustrate the difficulty in identifying the specific causal relationships between tracheotomy and swallowing. Kazandjian and Dikeman have seen, in their practice, dysphagic patients who derive benefits from tracheostomy tube occlusion and speaking valve placement and those who do not. Future research may support the theory that indeed multiple factors influence safe swallowing in tracheostomized patients. This should be assessed in the clinician's everyday practice by documenting any changes in swallowing function under varying conditions.

2. Reduction of Airflow Through the Glottis

a. Elimination of expiratory airflow

Tracheotomy causes a diversion of air from its normal flow pattern through the larynx. The presence of an inflated tracheostomy tube cuff will further reduce the potential for air to reach the vocal folds. The primary consequence is the loss of airflow. During the normal swallow, expiration is interrupted and then resumes following the swallow. Without airflow through the glottis, expiration cannot function to clear residual material from the airway.

b. Blunting of reflexive cough

Lack of airflow through the larynx will cause a gradual loss of laryngeal sensation. Laryngeal reflexes related to normal airflow, such as coughing, clearing the throat, and so on, will be eliminated (Feldman, Deal, & Urquhart, 1966; Tippett & Siebens, 1991). Eventually, this results in a decrease in the glottic closure response, the reaction of the larynx to aspirated material. The larynx is frequently exposed to aspirated material but does not have a normal response mechanism for clearance. Suctioning must be used to remove aspirated material from the area. Eventually, the cough will become ineffective.

c. Glottic closure response

Discoordination of the glottic closure response may also be a consequence of the long-term diversion of air due to placement of a tracheostomy tube. It is unclear how quickly this may occur following tracheostomy, but a significant effect has been noted by these authors within 3 months of the tracheotomy procedure. With a poorly coordinated laryngeal closure response, the bolus may enter the airway before the tiered laryngeal protection mechanism can respond.

IV. EFFECT OF MECHANICAL VENTILATION ON SWALLOWING

Many factors create an increased risk of dysphagia in the patient receiving invasive mechanical ventilation. Tolep, Getch, and Criner (1996) discussed swallowing dysfunction in patients receiving mechanical ventilation. They found that a large percentage (80%) of patients without concomitant neuromuscular disorders had abnormal videofluoroscopic findings.

A. Disruption of Normal Apneic Interval

In healthy subjects, respiration ceases during a swallow and usually continues with expiration following a swallow (Martin et al., 1994; Shaker et al., 1992; Smith et al., 1989). Ventilator dependence may serve to disrupt this pattern, especially if a patient is on a ventilatory mode that imposes a preset breath within a certain interval, regardless of the patient's response. In other words, the ventilator may push air in at a time the patient is trying to keep the airway closed. Although the air enters the system below the level of the vocal folds, the patient may find that this disparity disrupts the smooth sequence of swallowing. Systems that normally work in concert with each other are separated (Kazandjian, Dikeman, & Adams, 1991). If the cuff is inflated, the patient will not experience airflow through the upper airway and will be prone to many of the other complications that accompany eating in the presence of cuff inflation. However, if the cuff is deflated, air will divert upward through the airway during both inspiration and expiration. It has been demonstrated that patients can *learn* to use the expiratory airflow provided by the ventilator for airway clearance, mimicking the function of normal expiration (Siebens et al., 1993). Ventilator-dependent patients will thus benefit from cuff deflation when they eat.

B. Tube Feedings/Intubation

Langmore (1996) reported that endotracheal intubation, mechanical ventilation, and tracheostomy will impair swallowing more in the premorbidly dysphagic individual than in the nondysphagic patient. Dysphagic patients often have more difficulty tolerating extubation because of their decreased airway protection. Feeding tubes (nasogastric) are typically placed in this patient population and may increase aspiration risk. Langmore noted that the absence of oral intake in these patients decreased salivary flow and thus increased the potential for bacteria to colonize in the mouth. Both aspiration risk and the consequences of that aspiration are thus increased. Valles et al. (1995) demonstrated that the incidence of nosocomial pneumonia in mechanically ventilated (intubated) patients could be reduced by continuously

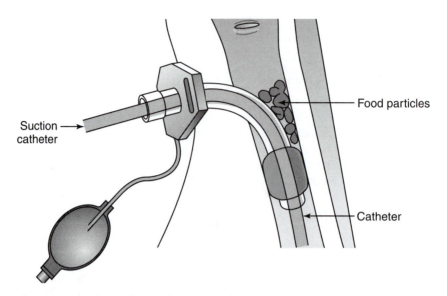

Figure 7-9. Food particles pooled on top of an inflated tracheostomy tube cuff.

suctioning subglottic secretions. The decreased risk was posited to result from reducing chronic microaspiration of gram-positive cocci and *Haemophilus influenzae* organisms, micro-organisms that more readily grow in the oral cavity.

C. Gastrointestinal Bleeding: Stress Ulcers

The tracheostomized and ventilator-dependent patient is at risk of gastrointestinal bleeding, which frequently accompanies stress ulcers (Bolton & Kline, 1994). This appears to be related to the increased physical and emotional stress of prolonged mechanical ventilation. For this reason ventilator-dependent patients are routinely placed on medications such as Zantac (ranitidine) and Carafate (sucralfate) (R. Fleming, personal communication, January 1995).

V. ORAL FEEDING IN THE PRESENCE OF CUFF INFLATION

A. Aspiration

1. There are several reasons that an inflated cuff does not prevent aspiration. The physical presence of the cuff in the trachea can *reduce* the potential that material will immediately contaminate the trachea if it enters the larynx and penetrates below the level of the vocal folds. Aspirated material pools on top of the cuff, as shown in Figure 7-9 and can be removed by tracheal suctioning when the cuff is eventually deflated. Difficulties arise when the amount of aspira-

tion is large, as potentially during a meal when both saliva and aspirated food boluses may enter the airway. Cuffs are not designed to prevent large volume aspiration.

a. Incomplete seal

To maintain the integrity of the tracheal tissue, cuff inflation should remain below capillary pressures. When the cuff pressure is controlled in this fashion, a minimal leak often exists. The cuff walls should not seal tightly against the tracheal walls. However, for the purpose of preventing aspiration, this means that material can fall between the trachea and the cuff, especially as the cuff slides with the movement of the larynx. Low pressure and sponge-type cuffs are more effective in producing a seal with the tracheal wall without causing tracheal abrasion. However, bacteria can easily move past the cuff into the airway, resulting in microaspirations. Over-inflation of the cuff can eventually lead to tracheal wall breakdown. This promotes a cycle of adding more air to compensate for the presence of a leak, leading to increased tracheal wall irritation, an incomplete seal, and a subsequent increase in cuff pressures (Feldman et al., 1966).

b. Accumulation of aspirated material

(1) If aspirated material, either saliva or food, collects on the cuff, bacterial colonization can occur. This places the patient at risk for aspiration pneumonia secondary to aspiration of oropharyngeal contents. The aspiration of **anaerobic** bacteria, which are found normally in the mouth, is increased in patients with airway protection problems. Patients with tracheostomy and mechanical ventilation also have been identified as being at higher risk for infection of the lower airways and lungs by **aerobic** bacteria. This may relate to the mechanical trauma of intubation and tracheostomy that damages cells, causes changes in the mucosa, and increases the ability of bacteria to attach to and colonize in tissue. Bacteria can then be more easily introduced into the airway. Sometimes patients who are treated for common anaerobic infections lose their ability to resist the aerobic infection (Kirsch & Sanders, 1988). Niederman, Ferranti, Ziegler, Merrill, and Reynolds (1984) discussed the increased incidence of bacterial colonization in patients with tracheostomy, especially long-term tracheostomy (persisting over several months). Clinically, this increased colonization resulted in various infectious complications. One of the most common pathogenic bacteria that colonized in the airway was *Pseudomonas aeruginosa.* Valles et al. (1995), although able to decrease colonized bacteria through continuous removal of secretions, found that the number of *Pseudomonas aeruginosa* organisms did not decrease. Niederman, Merrill et al. (1984) also noted that poor "nutritional status appeared to relate to both tracheal cell adherence

and colonization patterns in the lower airway" (p. 799). This may place tracheostomized patients with poor oral intake due to swallowing impairment at heightened risk of bacterial colonization and eventual infectious complications.

(2) At times, patients at risk for aspiration may be permitted to eat with the contingency that tracheal suctioning be completed before and after a meal. However, if a patient has aspirated, the material that has pooled on the cuff can fall into the airway when the cuff is deflated prior to suctioning. Although a percentage of the aspirated material will be removed by suctioning, some may enter the lower airways where it is more difficult to remove. Proper suctioning of pooled saliva or secretions can minimize this problem; however, even proper suctioning technique may not be sufficient to remove the aspirated material from above the cuff.

c. Destruction of cilia

A decrease in cilia has been identified at the cuff inflation site. Cilia are necessary for the removal of mucus and aspirated contents from the airway (Feldman et al., 1966). The reduction of cilia eliminates yet another level of protection from the tracheostomized and ventilator-dependent patient.

It is evident that multiple factors place tracheostomized and ventilator-dependent patients who present with dysphagia at special risk. The reciprocity of swallowing with the respiratory-cardiac systems and the shared functions of the aerodigestive tract must be considered during the assessment and treatment process discussed in Chapter 8.

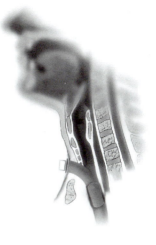

8

Assessment and Management of Dysphagia

Assessment of the dysphagic patient who is tracheostomized and ventilator dependent must acknowledge the potential effect of the disruption of airflow on the aerodigestive tract. Recall that airflow contributes to the propulsion of the bolus and to airway protection. Consequently, for the tracheostomized and ventilator-dependent patient, there is often a heightened potential for impairments in pharyngeal propulsion and airway protection. Determining the patient's candidacy for safe and adequate oral intake is primary. This intake may be contingent on diet modifications and special therapeutic techniques that are identified during the evaluation process. A treatment program will also directly relate to what is learned during each stage of the evaluation process. Periodic reassessment is necessary to modify the treatment program, as appropriate. The goal of assessment and management is to identify the nature and cause of the impairment, normalize airflow, treat underlying pathophysiology, and provide compensatory techniques for safe swallowing. However, the cause of the dysphagic impairment is not always obvious. Airflow return will not always be possible. Individual patients will differ in their ability to benefit from treatment techniques. The speech-language pathologist and the entire transdisciplinary team must assess the individual and the potential impact of tracheostomy, ventilator dependence, and an impaired respiratory system on deglutition.

I. CONTINUUM OF DISABILITY

The continuum of disability was described in Chapters 5 and 6 as a guide for the assessment of the tracheostomized and ventilator-dependent patient in multiple areas. The continuum can be used to identify the degree of dysphagia and describe the patient's status with regard to oral intake. The swallowing component of the continuum of disability is detailed in Table 8-1. The scope of impairment moves from full oral feeding, to supplemented or modified oral intake, to therapeutic or recreational feedings, to

Table 8-1. Continuum of disability: Swallowing subsystem. (Adapted from "Continuum of Disability" by C. Salciccia, 1986. In C. Salciccia, L. Adams, & G. Kapassakis, *Communication Management of Respiratorily-Involved Quadriplegic Adults.* Paper presented at Goldwater Memorial Hospital, New York, NY)

Swallowing					
Normal swallowing	Mild oral-pharyngeal weakness. Difficulty with solids and/or liquids.	Moderate oral-pharyngeal dysphagia. Management of altered diet.	Moderate-severe oral-pharyngeal dysphagia. Oral intake supplemented with alternative feeding or pleasurable/recreational feeding.	Severe oral-pharyngeal dysphagia. Pleasurable feeding.	NPO

Note: NPO = non per os; nonoral feeding only.

nonoral status. It also may be considered a range of either deterioration or improvement, depending on the direction of change. It is common for patients to receive nutrition and hydration simultaneously via oral and alternative methods, especially as they are participating in therapeutic swallowing and feeding programs.

The speech-language pathologist is most commonly and appropriately the team member who carries out dysphagia assessment and intervention. As in any aspect of care for the tracheostomized and ventilator-dependent patient, however, a team approach is optimal, and the physician(s), nurse, respiratory care practitioner, registered dietitian, occupational therapist, and physical therapist all function as essential members. Team leaders and roles also vary across facilities.

II. ASSESSMENT

A. Clinical Examination

1. Purpose/Description

The dysphagia evaluation process typically begins with the clinical or bedside evaluation, so named as the clinician is often initially called to the patient's bedside to determine candidacy for oral intake (Groher, 1992, 2000). Valuable but limited information is gathered during this assessment. Depending on the patient's medical status, the clinical evaluation typically leads to requests for other objective evaluation procedures, such as fiberoptic assessment or video-fluoroscopy. The clinical assessment rarely is the final step in the dysphagia evaluation process. Only if the clinician is *completely* confident of a patient's ability to manage oral intake will a recommendation for oral feeding be made based solely on the bedside assessment. More commonly, bedside evaluations stand alone when the patient is already eating and there are questions regarding management of a particular diet, or an upgrade to a different level diet. The bedside evaluation can take place over several sessions, especially if other objective assessment techniques are not yet available or if the patient is medically fragile. For example, a patient with a history of aspiration pneumonia who is currently NPO and presents with a wet vocal quality, may be initially assessed with a dye mixed with saliva *prior* to providing any food bolus. Contingent on the results of this evaluation, the clinician may later proceed with an actual dyed food bolus, perhaps 24 hours later.

2. Indications

A comprehensive clinical evaluation of swallowing should be part of the total swallowing evaluation of the tracheostomized and ventilator-dependent individual with dysphagia. This assessment is ordered by a physician when a patient is admitted to a facility with a diagnosis of dysphagia or begins demonstrating dysphagic symptoms in a particular setting, such as a long-term care facility. It is most effectively conducted with patients who have some degree of cooperation, especially for assessment of airway protection abilities. The clinical examination is described succinctly by Groher (2000) who stresses that typically dysphagic etiologies are multifactorial. The most significant etiologies are neurogenic in origin: obstructive respiratory disease, other respiratory impairments, and metabolic insufficiency.

3. Procedure

a. History taking

During the bedside examination, the clinician begins with a careful review of the medical history taken not only from the medical record, but from the physician, respiratory care practitioner, nursing staff, family and, if possible, the patient. A careful review is essential. Hendrix (1993, p. 69) writes that "history taking is the first step in the translation of the patient's symptoms and concerns into a diagnosis which in turn should lead to a rational treatment plan." In addition to inquiry into the medical diagnosis, the clinician should consider such factors as the current medical condition, the relevant medical history, patient medications, and other concomitant symptoms, such as repeated aspiration pneumonia or weight loss. Questions that will further guide the history-taking process include (Hendrix, 1993; Kazandjian et al., 1991):

(1) What are the dysphagic complaints/symptoms, including a general localization of difficulty? What consistencies create the dysphagic symptoms? When was the onset of the dysphagia? Did it follow intubation and/or tracheotomy?

(2) How is the patient currently receiving nutrition and hydration? Is a feeding tube present (nasogastric or gastrostomy tube)? How long has it been in place?

(3) Are there incidents of choking/coughing and when do they occur? Have any food consistencies been expelled from or around the tracheostomy tube? If the patient is eating orally, is the cuff deflated or inflated? Can the cuff be deflated? How long can the patient tolerate cuff deflation during the day? Is the cuff partly or fully inflated?

(4) What is the type and size of the tracheostomy tube? Are both the inner and outer cannulae fenestrated? What is in place during the evaluation?

(5) How frequently must the patient be suctioned? Are secretions copious? Viscous? Does the patient receive respiratory treatments and how frequently? Does the patient appear to become breathless or fatigued during a meal? Are respiratory treatments frequently needed after a meal?

(6) Is the patient on or off the ventilator during the day? What about during mealtime? How much time off the ventilator is available?

(7) Are there complaints of **odynophagia,** or pain on swallowing? regurgitation? heartburn? (indicating possible esophageal difficulties).

(8) Is there a history of anatomic abnormalities (e.g., fistulas, granuloma, stenosis) related to intubation and/or tracheotomy?

The case example presented at the end of this chapter illustrates the problem-solving process that is initiated with history taking. The history should give the clinician a good sense of how to proceed with the actual clinical evaluation and if, for example, test swallows will be performed during the assessment process. The decision to give food or liquids during the assessment is based on medical and clinical judgment. A conservative approach takes the patient from trial dry swallows to controlled amounts of other food boluses, as appropriate. The administration of food and/or liquids must be done with the understanding that this test is blind and that the clinician's information is quite subjective. The presence of a tracheostomy tube does provide access to the airway that is not available with nontracheostomized individuals. Despite this access to the airway, a tremendous amount of inference is still necessary during the clinical examination. A sample clinical evaluation form is found in Appendix C.

b. Oral-peripheral examination

The clinical evaluation continues with a visualization of the oral cavity, including oral health, reflexes, sensation, and saliva management. This information will directly impact on aspects of the oral preparatory and oral phases of swallowing. Tracheostomized and ventilator-dependent patients often have special concerns related to long-term nonoral feeding status, the presence of a tracheostomy tube, and loss of oral/nasal airflow.

(1) Dentition and mucosa should be inspected for general health and any postintubation damage. Bacterial colonization of inflamed gingiva is common. Gingivitis may therefore increase the chance of a bacteria-associated pneumonia in patients who aspirate oropharyngeal contents (Kirsch & Sanders, 1988). Individuals who have inflated cuffs require stringent oral care because the normal mechanisms for evaporation of secretions and saliva flow have been disrupted. The patient's overall saliva management, quantity and type of secretions, or other conditions such as xerostomia should be noted. A dry mouth may interfere with test swallows, especially if an individual has not taken oral intake for some time. Xerostomia over a long period of time may also lead to oral infections, tooth decay, and a burning sensation in the mouth and on the tongue (Hudson & Mills, 2000). Moistening the mouth with water or glycerine swabs may facilitate oral movements and the triggering of an effective swallow.

(2) The presence of any primitive oral reflexes should be documented. The presence or absence of a gag reflex, when noted during the assessment, does not preclude oral alimentation but will provide information about the integrity of cranial nerves IX (glossopharyngeal) and X (vagus) in the upper airway. Although the dysphagia clinician will frequently encounter the statement, "NPO secondary to absent gag," research with normal subjects has indicated that a significant part of the normal population may not possess a gag (Logemann, 1993). In addition, although the status of the gag reflex *will* provide information regarding neurological (cranial nerve) status, no link between the presence or absence of a gag and the presence or absence of a swallow has been demonstrated (Leder, 1996a, 1997).

(3) Movements of the lips, tongue, mandible, and palate are evaluated for range and strength. During intubation, the pressure exerted against the base of the tongue by the endotracheal tube may have impeded function, and lingual strength should be carefully assessed by resistance techniques. The base of tongue movement contributes to the driving force so important for moving the bolus through the pharynx.

(4) Cuff inflation and the cessation of airflow through the nasal/oral cavities will interfere with taste and smell; therefore, reliable testing of these sensations may be difficult.

c. Cuff deflation/test swallows

To continue the evaluation of the pharyngeal stage of the swallow, partial cuff deflation *must* be achieved. ***As always, this is done only after clearance*** *by the physician.* This will allow the clinician to briefly occlude the tracheostomy tube to normalize airflow and assess airway competence and airway protection abilities, perhaps identifying strategies that will be used in later treatment programs. Partial cuff deflation means that the cuff must be deflated enough to allow the patient access to the airway for coughing, clearing the throat, expectorating secretions, and vocalizing. Although a patient may be able to trigger a swallow with the cuff fully inflated, the clinician will not be able to detect suspected aspiration. Symptoms such as vocal changes or leakage of material from the stoma may go unrecognized. An aspirated bolus may gradually work its way around the sides of the cuff, and be removed via tracheal suctioning, but the clinician will be uncertain about the timing and amount of aspiration. Without cuff deflation, a clinician can assess only the oral stage and the ability to trigger a pharyngeal swallow. Furthermore, because oral intake in the presence of a fully inflated cuff should not be encouraged, cuff deflation should be an eventual goal if total oral alimentation is to be considered. Patients who eat in the presence of a fully inflated cuff are at risk for numerous complications. These complications were discussed in detail in Chapter 7. A cuff that cannot be deflated due to copious secretions or an unstable pulmonary status will alert the clinician to existing airway issues prior to the bedside assessment.

(1) If the reality of the situation is that the speech pathologist cannot obtain an order for cuff deflation from a physician who is concerned about aspiration risk or ventilation issues, it is the clinician's responsibility to explain the limitations of an assessment of swallowing conducted in the presence of an inflated cuff and to begin the process of inservicing the medical team. Ideally, oral intake should be deferred until at least partial cuff deflation is achieved. The goal should be to move toward full cuff deflation as quickly as possible. An individual who is so medically fragile as to preclude cuff deflation is usually not a candidate for significant oral intake. The speech pathologist should remind the medical team that, if a patient will be eating in the presence of a fully inflated cuff, the recommendations made during the dysphagia assessment will be useless! Any benefits derived from reestablishing airflow will be lost, and mechanical limitations may be imposed upon the patient. Again, *partial* cuff deflation may be one option that the clinician can explore.

(2) After medical clearance and proper suctioning, the cuff is deflated. For ventilator-dependent patients, ventilatory modifications, with the assistance of a respiratory care practitioner, may be needed before the patient can tolerate a period of cuff deflation. If cuff deflation has been established in the restoration of oral communication, those ventilator settings will usually be appropriate during the dysphagia assessment. See Chapter 5 for a more in-depth discussion of suggested ventilator modifications. The patient should be given time to become

adjusted to the change in settings as well as the airflow through the upper airway. Suctioning should be performed as needed. If the patient has been tolerating speaking valve placement, it may be used during the evaluation in an effort to normalize pharyngeal pressures. However, if a patient uses only a one-way valve for brief intervals due to symptoms of increased work of breathing, the clinician may choose to minimize the number of variables present and defer use of a valve until a baseline estimate of the patient's abilities is achieved.

(3) During speaking valve use or tracheal occlusion, the clinician should determine gross vocal fold status by assessing the patient's ability to phonate, cough, or clear the throat. A patient who is not accustomed to tracheal occlusion can be occluded briefly, 5 to 10 seconds at a time, to grossly assess airway management. Vocal quality during these tasks may indicate ability to manage secretions. Laryngeal elevation can be examined during dry swallows or pitch variation tasks, especially during attempts to reach falsetto. During this assessment of laryngeal function, if the patient is aphonic, the clinician will be uncertain whether tracheostomy tube size or impaired vocal fold movement is interfering with phonation. An otolaryngology (ENT) report of vocal fold status may be necessary to resolve this issue. Although the patient with decreased pulmonary support may demonstrate decreased intensity or duration of voice production, the patient should be able to achieve at least some phonation. Poor breath support can significantly affect the ability to perform an effective cough. If the patient can phonate, clear the throat, and expectorate secretions, however, the evaluation can progress to include trial swallows.

(4) Trial swallows are attempted with the tracheostomy tube briefly occluded. With the ingestion of a controlled bolus, oral transit/control and the speed of initiation of the pharyngeal swallow can be noted. The presence and timing of a cough (immediate or delayed) should be recorded. A change in vocal quality, with a wet sound detected, is an important indicator of potential penetration of material. The patient's awareness of that sound, and his ability to cough or clear material, whether volitionally or cued, is also of importance. The patient's ability to clear the airway will factor into the eventual transition to safe oral feeding, perhaps by utilizing alternate swallow and throat clearance as therapeutic techniques. This may be an important strategy during dysphagia treatment or oral feeding.

d. The incorporation of a procedure known as the blue dye test into the clinical evaluation can be helpful in determining at least gross airway competence (Gilardeau, Kazandjian, Dikeman, Bach, & Tucker, 1995).

The blue dye procedure has been debated in the literature. In a widely reviewed article, Thompson-Henry and Braddock (1995) described false negative results in five out of five tracheostomized patients. The blue dye failed to detect aspiration that was later documented on instrumental assessment. Elapsed time between the blue dye and instrumental procedures was variable. The authors suggested caution in using this approach in tracheostomized patients, especially those with a compromised pulmonary status. Methodological issues in this study were addressed by Tippett and Siebens (1996) and Leder (1996b). However, despite these concerns, the experience of Thompson-Henry and Braddock supports the clinical experience of Kazandjian and Dikeman who have found the blue dye procedure unreliable in consistently detecting aspiration. However, it can be a helpful screening tool as part of the clinical assessment.

(1) The blue dye test consists of the placement of a few drops of sterile water mixed with blue or green food coloring placed on the tongue or in a small amount (1 cc) of sterile water. A syringe can be used to accurately measure the bolus amount. Sterile water, although perhaps more easily aspirated in some individuals, is a relatively benign substance and also can be removed via tracheal suctioning compared with more viscous consistencies. Ice chips can also be used. The patient is suctioned immediately and at 15-minute intervals over a 1-hour period. The presence of any dye in the tracheal secretions is recorded. A positive test results from the presence of dye on tracheal suctioning. A negative test result is the absence of dye. This test has obvious and numerous limitations. For example, if dye is found, it will be unclear *why* the aspiration occurred, *when* it occurred, or *what* quantity of material has been aspirated, as the 1-cc bolus mixes with saliva and secretions. Therefore, the provision of oral feeding after a negative blue dye test has been obtained with dye applied to the tongue may overlook many contexts in which the patient *will* aspirate. Essentially, a positive blue dye test will alert the clinician to a connection between the mouth and trachea that should not be present. This may certainly have implications for speech and swallowing.

(2) Blue dye can also be useful mixed with various food consistencies. This should be done one consistency at a time (e.g., with liquid at one time in the day and semisolids at another). An individual may demonstrate a negative test for one consistency or amount, such as liquids, and a positive test for another, such as a semisolid. When more viscous foods such as pudding or applesauce are used, the potential for pharyngeal retention increases. Since this retention cannot be documented visually, the patient should be suctioned at least several times, at intervals, after the administration of a single bolus. Aspiration occurring well after the swallow may be detected in this fashion. The later suctioning intervals are especially important for documentation of tolerance of the semisolid boluses secondary to this potential for pharyngeal retention. A notation should be made

Table 8-2. Protocol for test swallows, utilizing blue dye during the clinical evaluation.

For *tracheostomized* patients who normally maintain inflated cuffs, the optimal procedure for test swallows is:

1. Deflate cuff fully or partially (follow suctioning protocol)
2. Occlude tracheostomy tube
3. Dry test swallow
4. Check vocal quality; encourage cough/throat clear
5. Bolus test swallow
6. Check vocal quality; encourage cough/throat clear
7. Suction (cuff deflated)
8. Rest interval (+5 minutes; reinflate cuff partially if risk of aspiration is high)
9. Resuction
10. *Negative:* continue with larger amounts of different consistencies; *positive:* terminate test; try different bolus types.

For *ventilator-dependent* patients with inflated cuffs, the test swallow procedure is:

1. Deflate cuff fully or partially (follow suctioning protocol)
2. Institute ventilator modifications as tolerated; allow patient time to adjust to settings
3. Dry test swallow
4. Check vocal quality; encourage cough/throat clear utilizing ventilator flow if possible
5. Bolus test swallow
6. Check vocal quality; encourage cough/throat clear
7. Suction (cuff deflated)
8. Rest interval (+5 minutes; partially reinflate cuff if needed between suctioning intervals)
9. Resuction
10. *Negative:* continue with different consistencies; larger amounts; *positive:* terminate test.

regarding cuff status during the suctioning, because retained material from the pharynx may pool on top of a partly inflated cuff and may be detected only when the cuff is fully deflated or after leaking into the airway around the sides of the cuff. A protocol suggested for test swallows utilizing blue dye is presented in Table 8-2.

(3) Although helpful, a blue dye test should be interpreted conservatively and never used exclusively to determine candidacy for oral feeding. *The clinician must interpret the results of a blue dye test in the context of the total clinical evaluation.* A negative blue dye test will allow the clinician to proceed with further test swallows and collect more information regarding the patient's swallow. A positive blue

dye test will the alert the clinician to the presence of aspiration and dictate a conservative approach to any further assessment. Blue dye tests are optimally performed over several sessions during a 48- to 72-hour period. Nursing and respiratory care staff, and any individuals involved in the suctioning protocol, should be aware that the test is in progress. A tracking sheet can assist staff in documenting the presence of blue dye at any time. Refer to Appendix D for an example of a tracking sheet. Difficulties will arise for less experienced personnel who must grade the results regarding degree of dye present (e.g., trace or tinged to more significant amounts of dye). The subjectivity of the assessment becomes very evident at this time.

(4) Blue dye can also be mixed with **enteral** feedings, or those provided via nasogastric or gastrostomy tubes to document the presence of gastrointestinal contents in tracheal secretions. This technique is often utilized if aspiration is suspected despite a nonoral feeding status and presence of an inflated cuff. This aspiration may be secondary to the reflux of formula. Reflux refers to the retrograde flow of material from the stomach into the esophagus. At times, it may even extend into the pharynx where it then may be aspirated. Chapter 10 describes a sample transdisciplinary protocol for the use of blue dye in enteral feedings.

Kazandjian and Dikeman have found the blue dye procedure helpful in identifying gross aspiration of secretions, not as the sole factor in making decisions regarding oral feeding. Tippett (2000) developed an algorithm for use of the blue dye procedure and has reported good success with the use of this conservative approach. Recently, there has been concern with potential systemic effects of food coloring. To date, scattered adverse reactions have been documented when patients have been given large bolus amounts, for example, in enteral feedings (Ideno et al., 1991; Metheny & Clouse, 1997). Further research is needed to quantify what amounts of blue or green food coloring, if any, are truly unsafe.

e.   Glucose oxidase testing

Detection of aspirated contents in tracheal secretions can be accomplished via use of glucose oxidase test strips, which measure the amount of glucose in a substance. This method has been used to document the presence of aspirated enteral feedings (i.e., those from the gastrointestinal tract) in tracheal secretions. The test strip is dipped into either contents obtained from suctioning or material expelled from the tracheostomy tube or around the stoma. Glucose oxidase testing was found to be more sensitive than blue dye visualization in detecting pulmonary aspiration of enteral feedings in intubated individuals (Potts, Zaroukian, Guerrero, & Baker, 1993).

f. Fenestrated tracheostomy tubes

The clinician should note the presence of a fenestrated tracheostomy tube during the assessment. If the inner cannula is nonfenestrated, the fenestration is nullified, but if the inner cannula is fenestrated, there is another potential source of entry of secretions or food through that area. For example, aspirated material pooled on top of the tracheostomy tube can fall through the fenestration. This would occur despite cuff inflation as the fenestration site is above the cuff. (For this reason, most individuals at risk for aspiration are not maintained with fenestrated tracheostomy tubes.) Eventually, the use of a fenestration and cuff deflation can assist in optimizing airflow for airway clearance. To reduce the number of variables the clinician must evaluate simultaneously, the nonfenestrated inner cannula should be in place during the initial dysphagia assessment. Trials utilizing the fenestrated cannula can be deferred.

g. Compensatory strategies/postural changes

Postural changes and compensatory strategies can be introduced during the bedside assessment, although their value will not be as clearly demonstrated as during a radiographic evaluation. For example, if a patient clearly presents with lingual weakness, the risk of premature leakage of the bolus into the pharynx may be heightened and neck flexion may be of value. Unfortunately, the clinician will be able to see only the end result of the swallow, that is, aspiration or perhaps a wet vocal quality, to suggest what strategies were and were not helpful.

h. Ventilator issues

If a patient is ventilator dependent, it is prudent to wait until objective measures can be utilized before giving significant amounts of food by mouth. A blue dye test can provide helpful information for both pulmonary medicine, respiratory therapy, and speech pathology regarding gross airway competence. An individual who is tolerating cuff deflation, possibly with a Passy-Muir speaking valve in-line with the ventilator, will have a more stable pulmonary status. They may tolerate a blue dye test, trial swallows, and the use of food and liquid during the clinical assessment. Some patients actually benefit from the assistance of the positive pressure from the ventilator to assist in airway clearance. This will be discussed more extensively during treatment options. However, it is generally more difficult to have a patient cough or clear the throat against the ventilator, and it can be stressful for the patient to be repeatedly suctioned during the evaluation process.

4. Contraindications: Clinical Evaluation

a. Patients who are not alert, extremely anxious or agitated, or severely cognitively/linguistically impaired will not be candidates for the comprehensive clinical evaluation, which demands a degree of cooperation from the patient.

b. Patients who are medically unstable and extremely fragile may be poor candidates not only for cuff deflation but also for the repeated suctioning, swallows, and coughing that accompany the administration of the different boluses. Fluctuating blood pressures and oxygen saturations, tenuous cardiac status, and purulent secretions are also potential contraindications to cuff deflation and ventilator modifications. The clinician must look at these factors when assessing whether a patient can participate in the assessment or is a viable candidate for oral intake.

The clinician must integrate a tremendous amount of information while determining an individual's candidacy for oral alimentation or the need for objective assessment techniques. Other assessment procedures will be helpful during the clinical evaluation. One of these techniques is **cervical auscultation.**

B. Cervical Auscultation

Cervical auscultation is a technique used to detect sounds of a swallow via a stethoscope placed on the larynx (Bosma, 1992). The clinician can learn to detect not only the presence or absence of a pharyngeal swallow, but, via respiratory sounds, the possibility of a compromised airway (Hamlet, Penney, & Formolo, 1994; Zenner, 2000; Zenner, Losinski, & Mills, 1995). This technique can be effectively incorporated into the clinical evaluation and may add to the information provided by the blue dye test. It is easily tolerated by patients because it involves only the placement of a stethoscope or microphone on the larynx. The microphone is connected to a tape recorder. Placement may be more difficult with tracheostomized and ventilator-dependent patients because of interfering apparatus or positioning. Research is being conducted to quantify the sounds of the swallow and to increase the objectivity of this technique (Selley et al., 1994; Takahashi, Groher, & Michi, 1994; Zenner et al., 1995). Zenner (2000) provides a helpful review of breath sounds associated with respiration in her discussion of the role of cervical auscultation in the clinical evaluation. Huckabee and Pelletier (1999) also discuss the possible use of auscultation as a biofeedback tool to facilitate correct use of treatment techniques, such as a supraglottic swallow with a breath hold.

With the information obtained during these procedures, the clinician will move to more objective (and invasive) assessment techniques. Fiberoptic assessment, integrated into many dysphagia evaluation protocols, has been especially helpful with tracheostomized and ventilator-dependent patients who present with decreased mobility and possibly limited access to other techniques.

C. Pulse Oximetry

Pulse oximetry has previously been described as a noninvasive monitoring tool measuring levels of arterial blood oxygenation. Its use in the dysphagia assessment process has been described by various researchers who explored changes in pulse oximetry readings correlated with aspiration. Zaidi et al. (1995) documented decreases in pulse oximetry readings when aspiration occurred. Sellars, Dunnet, and Carter (1998) did not find a clear-cut relationship between aspiration and changes in oxygen saturation readings. These researchers did find that changes in respiratory status can occur during feedings. Tamura, Shishikura, Mukai, and Kaneko (1999) described alterations in pulse rate (increased) and oxygen saturation levels (decreased) during meals in disabled subjects. They theorized that oral feeding can stress the circulatory system. Similar changes in respiratory status are often noted in patients with severe COPD, who at times cannot tolerate a full meal. Pulse oximetry can be helpful in monitoring a patient's tolerance of oral feeding over a specific time period. Colodny (2001) documented that patients with COPD had lower levels of oxygen saturation than dysphagia patients with other disorders. Colodny theorized that normal aging changes in swallowing and pulmonary status, combined with a disease such as COPD, can contribute to dysphagia as well as compromise pulmonary functioning. Again, monitoring of oxygen saturation levels during meals may be helpful in these cases.

D. Fiberoptic Assessment of Swallowing

1. Description and Purpose

    a.   The fiberoptic assessment of swallowing is an assessment procedure that utilizes a fiberoptic nasopharyngoscope to directly visualize the pharynx and larynx before, during, and after the swallow. Langmore, Schatz, and Olsen (1988) and Langmore (1993) defined the term *FEES* for her fiberoptic examination of swallowing safety. Langmore's FEES protocol is carefully defined and incorporates administration of graduated bolus sizes and types. This protocol is the most comprehensive method of assessing swallowing abilities during a fiberoptic examination. A fiberoptic assessment of swallowing, however, may need to be modified according to the tolerance of the patient. Some patients may not be able to tolerate passage of the scope for lengthy periods in order to complete the full assessment. When possible, completion of the FEES protocol would be

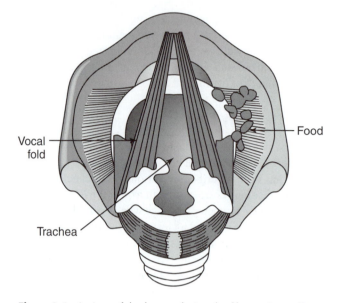

Figure 8-1. A view of the larynx during the fiberoptic swallowing assessment.

optimal. During the procedure, the fiberoptic scope is inserted into the nares and passed over the velum into a position to view the pharynx and larynx. Swallows are performed using dyed boluses with the scope in place. Although the actual swallow cannot be visualized secondary to airway closure, the passage of the bolus can be monitored. The study assists in the observation of:

(1) gross pharyngeal and laryngeal anatomy, especially airway closure abilities.

(2) premature leakage of a bolus from the oral cavity into the pharynx.

(3) speed of the triggering of the pharyngeal swallow.

(4) velopharyngeal closure.

(5) retention in the pharyngeal recesses.

(6) preferential passage of the bolus as indicated by location of residual material to the right or left.

(7) aspiration *before* the swallow, as material spills into the larynx.

(8) aspiration *after* the swallow, from retained material.

(9) estimated amount of aspiration.

A view of the larynx during the fiberoptic swallowing study, with a depiction of aspirated food particles near the vocal folds, is shown in Figure 8-1.

b. Compensatory strategies and postural changes can be utilized during this study, as visual imaging continues throughout the swallows and the impact of these techniques can be monitored.

c. If this is the first fiberoptic evaluation for the patient, the presence of any anatomical or structural problems should be noted. A general assessment of vocal fold function should also be performed.

d. The fiberoptic examination should ideally be conducted with the tracheostomy tube cuff at least partially deflated to allow access to the upper airway for clearance of penetrated or aspirated material. Occlusion of the tube by a speaking valve or cap should maximize this benefit. Digital occlusion may also be attempted; however, its benefits and the effects on other biomechanical aspects of the swallow appear less consistent (Leder, Joe, Hill, & Traube, 2001).

2. Indications

The fiberoptic assessment is used for any individual who requires a comprehensive swallowing evaluation. It typically follows the clinical examination. The procedure is especially helpful for individuals, including tracheostomized and ventilator-dependent individuals, who have limited mobility or decreased ability to follow directions required for procedures such as videofluoroscopy.

3. Procedure

The fiberoptic study is performed by a health care professional trained not only in the technique of scope placement but also in the observation of actual swallows. This procedure is usually performed by an otolaryngologist and a speech-language pathologist. In some facilities the study may be performed by a speech-language pathologist who has received special, extensive training in the technique. Individuals who perform invasive procedures obviously must be properly trained and must present documentation that attests to this training. Protocols differ from facility to facility. Some facilities will not allow the procedure to be performed unless a physician is in attendance. Others mandate that a physician be present in the facility. Contingency plans for medical emergencies should be in place prior to performing fiberoptic studies. Concerns and considerations for use of this instrumental technique were also outlined by the American Speech-Language-Hearing Association's Ad Hoc committee in their position statements (ASHA, 1992a, 1992b). ASHA also regularly updates training guidelines for nasal endoscopy.

a. Videotaping of the fiberoptic assessment is accomplished for later review by the clinician and physician, especially if the physician was not involved in the actual study. This recorded study is often referred to as a video-fiberoptic or videoendoscopic swallowing study and usually follows a more formalized protocol (Bastian, 1993; Langmore, 2000).

b.   The patient is screened to determine that there are no particular con-traindications to the procedure, such as a history of laryngospasm during, for example, suctioning procedures. The completion of the clinical assess-ment should guide the clinician through the fiberoptic swallowing proto-col, especially in terms of which consistencies (if any) and amounts to give the patient. The use of pulse oximetry will be a helpful addition to more objectively documented tolerance of this procedure. Changes from baseline can be monitored.

c.   A decongestant (e.g., Neosynephrine or Afrin) is often used to shrink the nasal passages for better insertion of the scope tip. A local anesthetic (e.g., xylocaine, lidocaine) may then be applied to the nares to ease pas-sage of the scope into the nasal cavity. The solutions may be either sprayed or applied to a cotton tip applicator which is then placed into the nares. Spraying must be limited to the nasal passages to avoid numb-ing the pharynx. Because this is difficult to accomplish, most practitioners favor either packing the area with treated cotton or avoiding the use of anesthetics.

d.   The scope is introduced transnasally and first moved into position to view the velum. Velar function generally is observed before advancing into the hypopharynx, to image the tip of the epiglottis, valleculae, aryepiglottic folds, arytenoid cartilage, pyriform sinuses, and glottis. Again, if this is the first visualization of the pharyngeal and laryngeal areas, the otolaryn-gologist (whether during the actual evaluation or when reviewing the tape) should examine the area for anatomical abnormalities, functional impairments (vocal cord paralysis), and mucosal irritation/infections. The presence, amount, and quality of secretions should be noted and related to the clinical impression of secretion management. To reduce the risk of laryngospasm, the scope should not touch the false vocal folds, arytenoids, or true vocal folds (Langmore, 1993).

e.   Pooling of secretions in the pharynx and penetration into the laryngeal vestibule can be viewed during the procedure. This can be more easily and effectively documented with the introduction of either blue or green food coloring, which mixes with oral secretions, onto the patient's tongue or with test substances. The dye will allow the tracking of material from the oral cavity through the pharynx and larynx. This will allow the clini-cian to visualize the overall ability of the patient to manage secretions. If the patient had a "positive" blue dye test during a prior clinical assessment with a fully deflated cuff, the cuff may be left partially inflated during the initial dyed saliva swallow. However, the inflated cuff will decrease any use of the airway for clearance of secretions. Murray, Langmore, Ginsberg, and Dostie (1996) reported that accumulation of visible oropharyngeal secretions in the laryngeal vestibule during FEES was highly predictive of aspiration of boluses presented during the study.

f. For trial swallows, several options exist. As with blue dye testing, administration of a benign substance, in measured quantities, is preferred in the event that aspiration occurs. Bolus amounts may proceed from liquids to soft solids. Langmore (2000) describes the FEES ice-chip protocol for medically fragile patients who would be less able to tolerate aspiration. The ice-chip protocol is recommended for many tracheostomized and ventilator-dependent patients for this reason.

g. Fiberoptic assessment can document impairments in both the oral and pharyngeal stages of the swallow. As the scope is positioned in the pharynx, assessment will assist in demonstrating the following specific impairments:
   (1) a delay in the pharyngeal swallow, or impairments in oral phase function seen as premature spilling of a bolus from the oral cavity (premature leakage).
   (2) lack of laryngeal elevation.
   (3) vallecular residue.
   (4) pyriform sinus residue (unilateral or bilateral).
   (5) penetration/aspiration of material into the laryngeal vestibule before the swallow, or penetration/aspiration of material *after* the swallow from vallecular or pyriform residue. All events *during* the swallow are obliterated from view due to the movement of the epiglottis and sphincteric action of the larynx. Residue may be demonstrated in the laryngeal vestibule or on the vocal folds *after* the swallow when the larynx reopens and the airway is visible.
   (6) airway protection abilities as a patient reacts to the aspirated material by coughing or trying to eliminate material from the airway.

h. Fiberoptic assessment will not directly document oral stage dysfunction, although it can be implied from other symptoms, such as vallecular residue, often associated with decreased base of tongue movement. Aspiration during the swallow cannot be identified at the moment of the swallow but is inferred from the presence of material on the vocal folds after the swallow. Therefore, the fiberoptic assessment is most effectively utilized in conjunction with a comprehensive clinical evaluation, and with videofluoroscopy, particularly if aspiration during the swallow is suspected.

i. The esophageal phase of the swallow cannot be assessed via FEES; however, esophageal-pharyngeal backflow can be observed during the study.

The clinician will, however, have little insight into the cause, for example, anatomic obstruction versus actual reflux.

4. Contraindications: Fiberoptic Study

a.   Most individuals can tolerate a brief fiberoptic assessment of swallowing. Patients should be alert and not experiencing acute medical difficulties. Special care should be taken if the patient has a history of laryngospasm or bronchospasm during suctioning, which might predispose them to problems during the fiberoptic assessment (Langmore, 1993). Monitoring tools such as pulse oximetry used during the procedure can indicate subtle changes in status, especially for communicatively impaired patients who cannot report the sensations that accompany the increased work of breathing.

b.   The information regarding airway protection status provided by the fiberoptic study is especially relevant for the tracheostomized and ventilator-dependent patient. For example, evaluation of a patient's ability to use breath-hold maneuvers during oral intake can be used to identify useful strategies for safe oral intake. Fiberoptic assessment also provides a more comprehensive and objective picture of the pharyngeal phase of swallowing than that obtained during a clinical examination. The fiberoptic assessment does not replace the most comprehensive assessment tool for dysphagic patients, videofluoroscopy, a radiographic evaluation that provides a real time image of the entire swallowing process and documents deficits in each stage. The efficacy of therapeutic maneuvers and postural changes, such as speaking valve use during the swallow, can also be documented.

c.   FEESST (fiberoptic endoscopic evaluation of swallowing with sensory testing) is a modification of FEES that incorporates endoscopic sensory testing of the pharynx and larynx into the procedure (Keen, Debell, & Blitzer, 1993; Aviv, Kim, Thomson, Sunshine, Kaplan & Close, 1998). This technique would appear to have applicability with the tracheostomized and ventilator-dependent population, as sensory deficits are typically suspected with this population. During FEESST, measured air pulses are delivered to the larynx. Quantification of the amount and placement of the air pulses has been difficult. However, because sensory loss and increased risk of aspiration pneumonia do appear related, FEESST can be another useful tool for the dysphagia clinician.

E. Videofluoroscopy

1. Description and Purpose

a.   Videofluoroscopic assessment of swallowing is a comprehensive radiographic evaluation of the swallowing process, defining transit and motility problems and identifying the timing and degree of aspiration (Logemann,

1998). Tracheostomized and ventilator-dependent patients with dysphagia who can participate in the procedure are assessed with a range of bolus consistencies and amounts. These boluses document management during the oral, pharyngeal, and esophageal stages of the swallow and, most importantly, identify therapeutic maneuvers that are useful in facilitating safe and adequate oral intake. Therefore, videofluoroscopy is a dynamic study which integrates both evaluation of function and efficacy of treatment approaches.

(1) During the videofluoroscopic procedure, patients are often positioned with special seating devices to facilitate the use of postural changes and allow imaging of lateral, anterior-posterior, and possibly oblique views. Figure 8-2 illustrates the anterior-posterior and lateral views during a videofluoroscopy. Graduated bolus amounts and varying consistencies are presented in a hierarchial manner (e.g., thin liquids, thick liquids, semisolids, soft solids, solids in 1-cc, 3-cc, 5-cc, 10-cc, and 20-cc amounts, and gulps or successive swallows). To limit radiation exposure time, each consistency need not be given in each amount; rather, problematic consistencies can be more carefully evaluated. Management of each consistency is recorded and, where deficits exist, therapeutic options attempted. Frame by frame analysis of the swallows assists in this process. Treatment options include those unique to tracheostomized and ventilator-dependent patients such as cuff deflation and use of the expiratory flow of the ventilator for airway clearance and speaking valve use during the swallow. Based on patient tolerance, videofluoroscopy can document improvement in swallowing status if used serially.

(2) When indicated, the imaging of the oral-pharyngeal phase of the swallow can be paired with a study of the motility and structure of the thoracic esophagus. This type of study may be requested when the swallowing complaint cannot be localized and may involve esophageal structure and function (Robbins & Fagerholm, 1992).

b. The purpose of a videofluoroscopic study is to:
(1) Evaluate oral/pharyngeal transit times and motility problems.
(2) Identify anatomical abnormalities in the oral cavity and pharynx.
(3) Identify presence and etiology of aspiration.
(4) Implement therapeutic maneuvers and strategies to address above deficits.
(5) During a complete study, document function of upper esophageal sphincter and image cervical/thoracic esophageal structure and motility.
(6) Integrate findings into the total clinical picture to determine candidacy for either oral or nonoral feeding.
(7) Generate referrals for related tests (fiberoptic evaluation of swallowing, endoscopy, manometry, scintigraphy) and to other specialties as indicated.

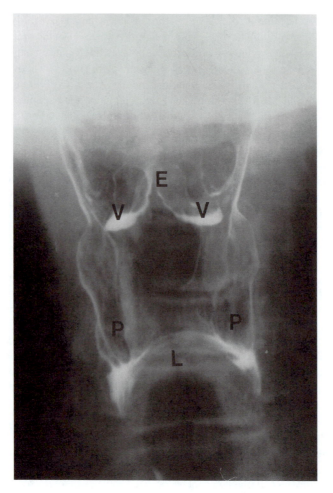

Figure 8-2a. Anterior-posterior view of the swallow during videofluoroscopy. The relevant structures are depicted as follows: E, epiglottis; V, valleculae; P, pyriform sinuses; L, larynx.

2. Indications

a. Most individuals who can maintain alertness for at least an hour, are medically stable enough to tolerate transport to the procedure, and are able to participate sufficiently in the test protocol can receive a videofluoroscopy. Since the goal is to determine therapeutic techniques, individuals who can follow directions and learn new information can benefit

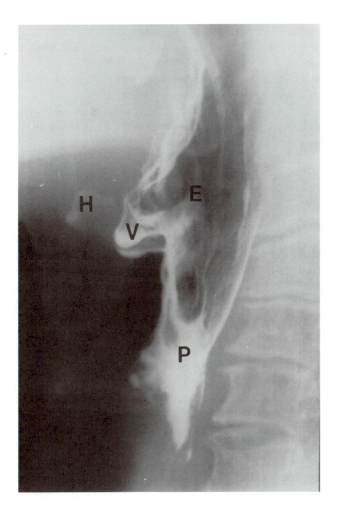

Figure 8-2b. Lateral view of the swallow demonstrating coating of the pharyngeal structures with barium.

the most. Many tracheostomized **and** ventilator-dependent patients can participate in this assessment. The presence of the ventilator, while posing challenges to positioning, should not inhibit successful completion of a videofluoroscopy. A portable ventilator obviously will facilitate transport to the radiology suite, and specialized devices for positioning can assist in physically arranging the equipment. The general indications for a video-fluoroscopic study for the tracheostomized and ventilator-dependent patient, as well as any dysphagic individual, are listed below.

b. General indications for requesting a videofluoroscopic swallowing study include (Fienberg, 1993):

(1) A suspected pharyngeal stage swallowing deficit.

(2) Swallowing deficit of unknown origin not explained by a clinical evaluation.

(3) Clinical sequela suggestive of dysphagia such as unexplained weight loss or suspected respiratory related infections.

(4) Suspicion of aspiration without a clearly defined source.

(5) Abnormalities of the pharyngoesophageal segment impacting on oral intake.

3. Procedure

a. Transportation to and positioning in the videofluoroscopy suite often pose the initial challenge, especially for the ventilator-dependent patient. If the patient can be placed on a special seating unit that both provides transportation and can be utilized in the radiology suite, manipulation of the patient can be minimized. An example of one type of device is pictured in Figure 8-3. This is less taxing for all involved in the study. It is vital that the clinician know the dimensions and limitations of the fluoroscopy equipment and be prepared to compensate for them. This may involve requesting the assistance and presence of the respiratory care practitioner who can monitor the patient's ventilatory needs, while the clinician concentrates on physically arranging the examination.

b. Once the patient is positioned for the study, the hierarchial administration of graduated boluses can begin. Imaging in the lateral view generally is preferred in order to detect aspiration as well as to obtain the most complete picture of the oral-pharyngeal swallowing sequence. The clinician must now decide when and if the tracheostomy tube cuff will be deflated during the study. As during the clinical evaluation, to obtain a true picture of the patient's abilities, the cuff must be deflated. This will minimize the mechanical and physiologic interference of the cuff and allow introduction of therapeutic techniques. To ensure patient safety, several principles must be considered:

(1) For either a tracheostomized or ventilator-dependent patient, this should not be the first time the cuff is deflated. As was discussed in detail in Chapter 5, a patient will experience physiologic changes and, frequently, concomitant anxiety when the ventilatory settings change. Because the videofluoroscopic evaluation can be an intimidating experience, other new variables, such as first time cuff deflation, should be minimized.

(2) Second, it is the clinician's responsibility to be familiar with the patient's abilities in order to minimize any risk of aspiration of barium during the evaluation. A patient who demonstrated a positive blue dye test and is a suspected aspirator will benefit from a videofluoroscopic examination that can identify the etiology of aspiration. However, the

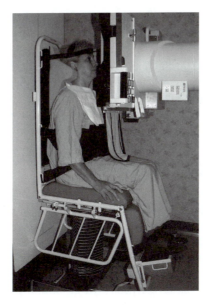

Figure 8-3. A specially designed chair for videofluoroscopic evaluation. (Photo courtesy of Stevis Corporation)

clinician must use special care when presenting the first bolus. This means administration of minimal material, and ensuring that suctioning is immediately available. The presentation of a 1-cc liquid bolus is often suggested during videofluoroscopic protocols (Logemann, 1998). If aspirated, this amount of material should not create airway obstruction, but it should be sufficient to image the swallow adequately and identify contributing causes of the aspiration.

(3) The tracheostomy tube cuff also can be left partially inflated during the initial swallows. This is a clinical judgment that is based partly on the patient's tolerance of cuff deflation and partially on the patient's status as documented during the clinical evaluation. If fully inflated, however, the cuff will interfere with the usefulness of many of the therapeutic techniques that should be attempted during the study. It appears most advantageous to bring a patient into the radiology suite when he is ready to tolerate at least a period of cuff deflation.

c. The protocol for the tracheostomized and ventilator-dependent patient should continue with the administration of graduated size boluses and different consistencies in a hierarchial fashion. Prior to the provision of any consistencies, the clinician can also observe the patient's management of secretions in the airway. Modifications that facilitate safe oral intake should be attempted as soon as indicated. Therapeutic maneuvers can include postural changes (neck flexion, head rotation) and compensatory strategies (effortful swallow, alternate liquid/solid swallows, supraglottic swallow) that are incorporated into any videofluoroscopic evaluation as appropriate to the patient's specific dysphagic impairment (Logemann, 1998). Although determining useful therapeutic techniques is a major component of the assessment, the clinician should remember that this is an invasive procedure which involves exposure to radiation. Swallows should be performed when they add diagnostic or therapeutic information to the study. Specific procedures can also be used for the tracheostomized and ventilator-dependent patient that will utilize available airway clearance and protection techniques. These include:

(1) Occlusion of the tracheostomy tube can be used to restore expiratory airflow, permitting the patient to use an effective cough, throat clear, or other technique that necessitates the accumulation of subglottic air pressure, such as a supraglottic swallow (Siebens et al., 1993). (If the patient cannot self-occlude the tracheostomy tube, the speech-language pathologist or radiologist should use a lead-lined glove because his or her hand will be in the field of exposure during this time.) For those individuals who tolerate speaking valves, an initial baseline swallow can be obtained, then contrasted with swallows with the valve in place.

(2) The leak obtained from the ventilator when the cuff is deflated can be used to provide airflow for airway clearance. Tippett and Siebens (1991) and Siebens et al. (1993) describe techniques for using the tidal volume from the ventilator, which is often increased when the cuff is deflated, to clear retained material from the pharynx and laryngeal vestibule. In one case study (Siebens et al., 1993), a patient was able to eat safely when receiving mechanical ventilation, but not during free time from the ventilator. The air provided by the ventilator aided in clearing retained material from the upper airway. The usefulness of this technique can be documented during the videofluoroscopy. If necessary, in order to minimize radiation exposure, the clinician can briefly stop the procedure and practice utilizing expiratory airflow with the patient, then document the usefulness of the strategy under videofluoroscopy.

(3) Placement of a speaking valve in the ventilator circuitry can increase the patient's ability to obtain subglottic pressure and increase the potential for clearance of any material retained in the pharynx. While wearing a speaking valve the patient does not have to wait for the push of air during the inspiratory phase of the ventilator. Air pressure accumulates in the upper airway and tracheostomy tube, and so may be available for clearing material from the pharynx or larynx.

d. At the completion of the study, the clinician should have identified what consistencies, if any, are acceptable for oral intake and, most importantly, under what conditions oral intake can be tolerated. This may include, for example, a recommendation that a patient eat a puree diet utilizing a neck flexion posture and a speaking valve. Of course, the clinician may also decide to recommend that oral intake be deferred until a period of indirect or direct dysphagia treatment is completed. Treatment options will be discussed in the next section.

4. Contraindications: Videofluoroscopy

a. Videofluoroscopy is an invasive procedure in that it exposes a patient to radiation. Precautions to limit radiation exposure to both patients and health care practitioners should be maintained. Actual limitations on radiation exposure time often vary between facilities but generally do not exceed 5 minutes. Radiation precautions also include judicious use of reevaluations and use of protective equipment (i.e., lead-lined vests, gloves, and thyroid shields).

b. Videofluoroscopy is also a somewhat strenuous procedure that cannot be tolerated by all tracheostomized and ventilator-dependent individuals. The transdisciplinary team, familiar with the protocol in their particular facility, must decide together if a patient can physically participate in the procedure. As mentioned previously, unstable medical status can certainly be a limiting factor, as can severe language and/or cognitive impairment, fluctuating alertness level, and agitation. The clinician who is aware of the rigors of this particular procedure and fellow team members should weigh the risks and benefits of videofluoroscopy for each patient.

F. Additional Dysphagia Assessment Procedures

Depending on a patient's particular dysphagic impairment, team members may recommend other diagnostic procedures as part of the total assessment of swallowing. These recommendations will be contingent on the tracheostomized and ventilator-dependent patient's ability to tolerate the procedure. Techniques that the dysphagia clinician may utilize include:

1. Ultrasound

Ultrasound utilizes sound waves to image muscle and soft tissue. In the assessment and treatment of dysphagia, this technique has been used most extensively for the oral cavity. It has also demonstrated applicability to imaging the pharynx and obtaining information regarding the pharyngeal phase of the swallow by tracking movements of the hyoid bone (Sonies & Baum, 1988). Ultrasound has been used to image movements of the tongue during swallowing of liquid boluses and has provided normative data regarding lingual movement during bolus propulsion (Sonies & Baum, 1988). Ultrasound may also be used as a biofeedback modality. Treatment paradigms have been created to address impaired lingual mobility and laryngeal excursion. Although it does image via sound waves which move through soft tissue, ultrasound is considered less invasive than a radiographic procedure and therefore may be repeated more frequently. The procedure may be applicable to tracheostomized and ventilator-dependent patients as a biofeedback treatment tool due to its noninvasive nature and relatively low cost.

2. Manometry

Manometry is a technique that quantifies pressure changes within a particular structure. Traditionally, it is used in the esophagus in the assessment of motility disorders, and often contributes to the total dysphagia evaluation for patients who come to swallowing centers complaining of dysphagic symptoms. Esophageal manometry is an invasive procedure that involves the insertion of a probe or probes into the stomach and esophagus (Feussner, Kauer, & Siewert, 1993). Pressure readings are obtained at various portions of the esophagus. When paired with the results of videofluoroscopy and visual assessment of the esophagus, such as fiberoptic endoscopy, it is useful in the diagnosis of disorders such as achalasia (a failure of a sphincter to relax) or esophageal spasm.

    a.   Oropharyngeal manometry has been used to study the propulsive forces of the oral cavity and pharynx which contribute to the opening of the upper esophageal sphincter. A lack of propulsion can be inferred from videofluoroscopy, as when pharyngeal residue is seen, but probes placed in the pharynx can identify this pattern. Pharyngeal manometry is most useful in the treatment of the dysphagic patient when paired with videofluoroscopy, because the pressure readings can be coordinated with the events of the swallow. Figure 8-4 pictures simultaneous manometry and videofluoroscopy. A more medically fragile individual may find this procedure difficult to tolerate.

3. Scintigraphy

Scintigraphy studies assess bolus movement by tracking a radionuclide within a bolus via special equipment including a camera and computer. The bolus can be followed as it moves through the stages of the swallow. Material retained in the pharynx can be quantified by recording the level of radionuclide in that area (Hamlet, Muz, Farris, Kumpuris, & Jones, 1992). In addition, scintigraphy can follow the movement of an aspirated bolus and aid in documenting the amount of material that penetrates the airway (Muz, Mathog, Miller, Rosen, & Borrero, 1987; Silver & Nostrand, 1992). The technique is being paired with videofluoroscopy to assist in increasing the objectivity of the evaluation of pharyngeal dysphagia and documenting the lung's ability to clear unwanted

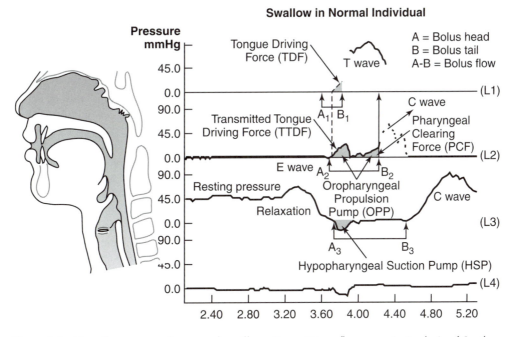

Figure 8-4. Manofluorogram of a normal swallow. (From "Manofluoroscopic Analysis of Swallowing," by F. M. S. McConnel, D. Cerenko, and M. S. Mendelsohn, 1988, p. 626. In Y. P. Krespi and A. Blitzer [Eds.], *Otolaryngologic Clinics of North America: Aspiration and Swallowing Disorders.* Philadelphia: W. B. Saunders. Copyright 1988 by W. B. Saunders Company. Reprinted with permission)

material over a period of time. This test may provide information regarding the risk of pulmonary infection following aspiration of saliva or oral intake.

4. Electromyography (EMG)

Electromyography (EEMG) utilizes needle electrodes placed within muscle bodies to record myoelectric signals during swallowing. Although used more extensively in the assessment of oral movements, EMG can be utilized to record contractions in the pharynx and larynx as well (Perlman, 1993). This technique may have implications for assessing the ability of the muscles of the mouth, pharynx, and larynx to function in a coordinated fashion, and therefore could have application with the tracheostomized and ventilator-dependent population. Due to its invasive nature, this technique is not commonly used with a patient population. Martin, Logemann, Shaker, and Dodds (1994), as well as others (Cook et al.,1989; Shaker, Dodds, Dantas, Hogan, & Arndorfer, 1990), described the use of noninvasive, submental electromyography, using surface electrodes placed under the chin, in the assessment of breathing and swallowing. This procedure may be tolerated more easily by patients and has applicability in clinical as well as research settings. Clinical surface electromyography (SEMG) is used diagnostically to assess the function of swallowing muscles pre- and postintervention. SEMG has been used more extensively as a biofeedback tool in many areas of physical medicine and rehabilitation. In their review of the literature in this area, Huckabee and Pellitier (1999) discuss the growing clinical applications and success of this technique as a biofeedback treatment tool. It is a noninvasive technique that does require considerable patient effort, especially in learning techniques such as the supraglottic swallow. Clinicians should use the same judgment in applying SEMG to tracheostomized and ventilator-dependent patients as they would in using any effortful treatment technique with this population.

The results of all of the evaluation tools outlined above can add to the clinician's treatment planning abilities. Treatment of swallowing disorders must incorporate not only the results of the total dysphagia evaluation but a sensitivity to the special needs of the tracheostomized and ventilator-dependent patient. Groher (1994) discussed the decision-making process in determining oral versus nonoral feeding with an extensive review of the many variables that must be considered by the clinician and the team. One issue discussed by Groher is the difficulty in predicting the effects of aspiration in a dysphagic patient. Aspiration during instrumental examinations is often documented in narrative terms. Robbins, Coyle, Rosenbek, Roecker, and Wood (1999) described the use of an eight-point scale to quantify aspects of penetration and aspiration, for example, whether material is expelled from the airway spontaneously or upon cueing. It can be very helpful for the clinician to quantify aspiration in the tracheostomized and ventilator-dependent population, especially since aspiration tolerance is difficult to predict. Groher (1994) also stated, "the upper limit of how much aspiration, and what type of material can be tolerated safely in the lungs is not known, although a volume of 25 ml of highly acidic contents carries more risk than clear fluids" (p. 232). The risk of pneumonia after aspiration is also not clear. The multiple risk factors of dysphagia, respiratory compromise, or long-term tracheostomy and ventilator dependence are still not understood. The need for a careful assessment leading to treatment planning and feed/no feed decisions is underscored in such cases.

III. TREATMENT APPROACHES

A. Swallowing and Respiration: Interrelationships

The first consideration in treatment should be to evaluate the interrelationships between swallowing and respiration as discussed in Chapter 7.

1. Recent research with individuals with tracheostomy and dysphagia has demonstrated that normalization of subglottal air pressures and resumption of airflow

through the upper airway can reduce the potential for aspiration in high-risk individuals (Gross, Dettlebach, Zajac, & Eibling, 1994; Snyderman, Johnson, & Eibling, 1994; Stachler, Hamlet, Choi, & Fleming, 1994). Gross et al. (1994) demonstrated that an individual who aspirated thin liquids with an unoccluded tracheostomy tube did not aspirate while wearing a Passy-Muir speaking valve. Pressure measurements indicated a tenfold increase in subglottic pressure with the speaking valve in place. Snyderman et al. (1994) also demonstrated that placement of a Passy-Muir speaking valve was effective in preventing aspiration in tracheostomized patients. The authors prescribed a trial of valve use prior to evaluating individuals for surgical management of aspiration. Objective documentation on the benefit of normalized pharyngeal air pressures was demonstrated by Stachler et al. (1994). Using scintigraphy, they demonstrated significantly reduced amounts of aspiration in patients known to aspirate when the patients wore a Passy-Muir speaking valve. Leder et al. (2001) did not demonstrate consistent benefit (aspiration reduction) from light digital occlusion of a tracheostomy tube during FEES. Studies such as those cited will assist in quantifying the efficacy of the use of speaking valves or other intervention techniques in the assessment and treatment of dysphagic individuals.

2. It has been demonstrated that pulmonary and cardiac status interrelate with swallowing function and that, in patients with pulmonary disease, dysphagic symptoms may be exacerbated (Martin, 1994; O'Connor, 1994). Martin (1994) states that "decompensations in airway protection, particularly at the level of the larynx, and decreased swallowing efficiency may lead to exacerbations of pre-existing respiratory problems and significantly interfere with acquisition of safe and adequate oral nutrition" (p. 4). Furthermore, Martin (1991) reported that the strategies that may be employed to facilitate safe oral intake in dysphagic patients can stress a patient with cardiac, pulmonary, and swallowing impairment. Martin (1991) suggested that these strategies can even be counterproductive. Tracheostomized and ventilator-dependent patients often have multiple comorbidities such as diabetes and smoking history, conditions which also impact safe swallowing status (Borgstrom, Olsson, Sundkuist, & Ekberg, 1988). The clinician must constantly monitor the tracheostomized and ventilator-dependent patient's health status as it pertains to dysphagia treatment. Prescribed treatments may have an adverse effect on an already decompensated system. Based on this information, the clinician should monitor the patient during dysphagia therapy or oral intake with measures such as pulse oximetry, which can detect the effects of fatigue or stress on a cardiopulmonary system.

B. Treatment Decisions: Indirect Versus Direct Therapy

1. Treatment Planning

a. Recommendations regarding the safety of beginning oral feedings, continuing oral feedings, or remaining on nonoral status are made by the speech-language pathologist and the entire treatment team. These recommendations are based on the results of the dysphagia evaluation and the patient's complete clinical picture. Recommendations serve as points on the continuum of disability previously discussed in this chapter. A range of options exists in between. For example, tracheostomized and ventilator-dependent patients may eat orally only under specific conditions or with modified diets. They may receive nutrition and hydration partly by mouth and partly by alternate means. They may receive oral intake only during direct dysphagia treatment with a speech-language pathologist, or they may maintain a nonoral status but commence an indirect dysphagia treatment program. These recommendations are made in the interest of maintaining *safe* and *adequate* nutrition and hydration for a particular individual. Naturally, this type of treatment planning is not unique to the tracheostomized and ventilator-dependent patient, but is used for all patients with oropharyngeal dysphagia regardless of their diagnosis.

2. Indirect Therapy

    a. Indirect therapy methods involve the prescription of techniques to remediate deficits contributing to the dysphagia *without* the use of food or liquid by mouth. This type of intervention is usually recommended for the patient who cannot achieve safe and adequate intake even with the use of modified diets, postural changes, or compensatory strategies. Intake restrictions usually are imposed because of the patient's fragile medical status and potential for aspiration as well as the severity of the dysphagia. During therapeutic intervention, the cuff should be deflated as maximally as possible while repeated swallows and maneuvers are being conducted. For airway protection exercises, the tracheostomy tube should be momentarily occluded with the finger, so that the patient can attempt to utilize the upper airway. If tolerated by the patient, one-way speaking valves should be used when possible. When respiratory monitoring indicates that the work of breathing increases during the swallowing therapy, and puts the patient at medical risk, valve use may be deferred for another period during the day (i.e., not during mealtime). Depending on patient tolerance, treatment sessions may last from 15–30 minutes. Patients also may be able to tolerate airway protection exercises more easily when they are interspersed with other therapy tasks such as less strenuous oromotor exercises or when rest periods are provided.

    b. Indirect therapy methods can include:
      (1) Oromotor exercises such as resistance techniques (with or without bite blocks that increase the level of difficulty of an exercise) to increase the strength of the lips, tongue, or mandible. Base of tongue weakness has been identified as a frequent concern with this population. If diagnosed, it can be addressed with the use of target words

(e.g., Ka-La, Coke, Huk, and Toega) and direct pressure on a gauze pad placed in the back of the mouth. There are also commercially available devices designed for various types of oral weakness which may be considered by the clinician. Although there is limited evidence that oral exercises are efficacious, specific isometric strengthening exercises for the tongue have been noted to increase lingual strength and endurance (J. Robbins, 2001, personal communication). Clinicians should evaluate the effectiveness of these exercises with their individual patients. Perhaps the benefits that patients derive from these types of exercises are related more to the increased attention to an area of decreased function.

(2) Laryngeal excursion exercises, such as pitch variation and the use of falsetto, are used to address poor laryngeal elevation. Patients also may be instructed in the use of an effortful swallow, Mendelsohn maneuver, supraglottic swallow, or super-supraglottic swallow. These techniques facilitate a degree of laryngeal elevation and laryngeal closure (Logemann, 1998). Martin et al. (1993) discussed the effect of breath-hold maneuvers on laryngeal valving patterns in normal adults, and documented complete airway closure when patients were asked to perform a hard or effortful breath hold. These authors also discussed the application of fiberoptic studies in the assessment of a patient's ability to effectively perform these therapeutic maneuvers. For the tracheostomized and ventilator-dependent patient, these techniques may provide optimal airway closure. However, the effort and coordination required in performing these tasks could easily stress a weakened system, and some patients may not be able to sustain them throughout an entire treatment session (or meal).

(3) Vocal fold adduction exercises to address incomplete glottic closure can be performed during the airway protection exercises described above. Other specific techniques for vocal fold adduction were described in Chapter 5 and include forceful phonation (e.g., /ha-ha/), coughing, clearing the throat, and applying pressure against a resisting force (e.g., pushing on the sides of a wheelchair, pressing the hands together firmly). Quadriplegic patients can perform resistance exercises with their foreheads or shoulders. *It is strongly recommended that medical clearance be obtained before attempting any effortful maneuvers or exercises.* These techniques could stress a patient with concomitant swallowing, cardiac, and respiratory problems.

(4) Thermal stimulation is a technique used to address a delayed or absent swallow (Logemann, 1998). Reports in the swallowing literature regarding its efficacy vary (Lazzara, Lazarus, & Logemann, 1986; Neumann, Bartolome, Buchholtz, & Prosiegel, 1995; Rosenbek, Robbins, Fishback, & Levine, 1991). However, it is one technique that can be attempted while the patient's pharyngeal swallow is reassessed periodically. Thermal stimulation can be used while encouraging repeat dry/saliva swallows. Repeat swallows are a help-ful technique in addressing weakened pharyngeal musculature.

3. **Direct Therapy**

   a. Direct therapy methods incorporate all of those discussed above with the addition of controlled amounts of food and/or liquid. Direct therapy is recommended for patients who can tolerate limited amounts of oral intake only under specific, therapeutic conditions, and who cannot maintain safe swallowing for the duration of a meal. Direct therapy can be used to instruct patients in the effective use of compensatory strategies which will be incorporated into mealtimes. For tracheostomized and ventilator-dependent patients, the bolus may be tinged with food coloring to document its presence or absence during tracheal suctioning.

   b. Patients who are able to tolerate placement of a speaking valve during dysphagia treatment may benefit from the increasing normalization of sub-glottic air pressure then available for passage through the upper airway (Gross et al., 1994; Stachler et al., 1994). Clinicians may utilize speaking valves during objective assessment procedures, such as videofluoroscopy, to determine the effectiveness of these devices during direct dysphagia treatment. For example, some individuals may receive oral intake only when a one-way speaking valve is in place.

   c. When reassessment documents that a patient can utilize postural changes and compensatory strategies effectively enough to tolerate increased in-take, a therapeutic diet is usually prescribed. At this time the speech-language pathologist may wish to instruct the team members involved with feeding in the appropriate techniques to ensure carryover. The patient may continue to be monitored periodically at mealtime by the speech-language pathologist. The clinician will assess the need for ongoing use of compensatory strategies and postural modifications originally described during the treatment program.

4. **Alternate Feeding Methods**

   Patients who cannot complete the transition to full oral feeding will need a continued alternate feeding method. Nasogastric tubes, with their concomitant patient discomfort and associated medical difficulties, usually are not retained for more than a month, especially when the dysphagia is severe. For patients with a severe swallowing disability, placement of a **percutaneous gastros-tomy tube (PEG)** may be appropriate. This is placed after consultation with a gastroenterologist who determines if the patient is a candidate for this method of nutrition and hydration. A surgical procedure such as insertion of a gastros-tomy or jejunostomy tube is indicated for some individuals. The registered dietitian or nutritionist will then determine the caloric needs of the patient and recommend a particular formula for feeding.

Management of dysphagia in the tracheostomized and ventilator-dependent patient is a complex process that requires integration of many of the components of the respiratory, cardiac, and digestive systems. Maintenance of safe and adequate nutrition and hydration will play a major role in the patient's successful rehabilitation.

IV. CASE EXAMPLE: KENNY

This case example illustrates the management of dysphagic impairments that result from the interactions of disordered respiratory, cardiac, and digestive systems. Kenny illustrates many of the components of the assessment and treatment process previously discussed.

A. Introduction

Kenny was introduced through the case vignettes in nonoral communication, Chapter 6, section IV.C.2. Kenny was a 26-year-old man who sustained a C1–C2 fracture and right subdural hematoma. His communication diagnosis was aphonia secondary to tracheostomy tube cuff inflation and 24-hour ventilator dependence, dysarthria, and dysphagia. He was admitted to a long-term care/rehabilitation facility receiving alternative feedings via gastrostomy tube. At the time of his admission, Kenny had been receiving nonoral feedings for approximately 4 months secondary to moderate-severe dysphagia and repeated aspiration pneumonias.

On Kenny's admission to the long-term rehabilitation unit, his physician consulted the speech-language pathologist for a dysphagia evaluation (in addition to the communication evaluation discussed earlier) to assess his candidacy for oral intake. This young patient was highly motivated to eat again. Swallowing (and communication) issues had not been addressed in the acute care facility due to numerous medical concerns.

B. History Taking

1. The process of Kenny's clinical evaluation began with a careful review of his medical history, with an emphasis on questions relevant to this tracheostomized and ventilator-dependent individual. The onset of Kenny's presenting dysphagic symptoms began immediately following the motor vehicle accident. There was documented impairment of cranial nerves IX (glossopharyngeal), X (vagus), and XI (accessory) due to the subdural hematoma. The patient was intubated on an emergency basis at the accident scene. He had incidents of repeated aspiration pneumonia in the acute care facility. There

were also incidences of fluctuating blood pressures and unstable O_2 saturation levels. At the time of his admission, Kenny was maintained with full mechanical ventilatory support: assist control mode with a rate of 12, a FIO_2 of 45%, and TV 750 ml. He had a size 8 cuffed, nonfenestrated tracheostomy tube in place. He maintained full cuff inflation at all times. There was no free time from the ventilator, and there were no attempts at weaning secondary to his fragile medical status (repeated pulmonary infections) and copious secretions. He required suctioning by nursing and respiratory staff on at least an hourly basis to prevent mucous plugs.

2. Kenny's medical history contained information relevant to the dysphagia assessment process. This patient's pulmonary status had been severely affected not only by his presenting physical injury, but by a compromised airway protection mechanism. This was evident from his history of repeated respiratory-related infections and ineffective secretion management. The long-term cuff inflation and large size tracheostomy tube were considered additional potential risk factors in this patient's ability to protect his own airway. They were also limiting factors for the clinician beginning the clinical evaluation. Additionally, this patient clearly presented with a tenuous medical status that demanded a conservative approach and careful monitoring.

C. Clinical Evaluation

1. Oral Peripheral Examination

Kenny's oromotor evaluation revealed significant weakness of the oral mechanism, including the base of the tongue as assessed via resistance techniques and indirectly via target articulatory tasks. The patient presented with a significantly reduced gag reflex that accompanied the known cranial nerve impairment.

2. Cuff Deflation/Blue Dye Test

a. At the time of this initial evaluation, the patient was maintained with only a minimal leak in the cuff pressure. Although it was necessary to achieve at least partial cuff deflation to continue with an accurate clinical assessment, the speech-language pathologist and respiratory care practitioner decided not to initiate significant changes in ventilatory settings. This decision was based on the history of fluctuations in blood pressure and oxygen saturation and suspected potential for aspiration. First, baseline measures of oxygen saturation and pulse rate were obtained as the patient was monitored via pulse oximetry. Oxygen saturation was 95% during this initial monitoring. The respiratory care practitioner then slowly removed air from the cuff, 1 cc at a time, while the patient was suctioned by the nurse. The speech-language pathologist encouraged the patient to attempt vocalization and throat clearance. When the patient could produce a weak vocalization on /a/, the respiratory care practitioner stopped removing air from the cuff. The patient's ventilatory status was monitored carefully for several moments. When O_2 saturation began to trend downward slightly, to 91%, the respiratory care practitioner increased the tidal volume slightly. This stabilized the patient's O_2 saturation at 95%. The speech-language pathologist then proceeded with the clinical assessment of the pharyngeal phase of the swallow. The patient initiated a pharyngeal swallow after 4 seconds. Laryngeal elevation was judged to be moderately decreased. On dry test swallows, the patient demonstrated an intermittent wet vocal quality which he was able to clear on the clinician's cues. Cervical auscultation assisted the clinician in identifying changes in inspiratory sounds after the swallow. The clinician detected breath sound wetness intermittently during the dry swallows. At this time, two drops of blue vegetable dye were placed on Kenny's tongue. He initiated a swallow after approximately 3 seconds. Again, a wet vocal quality was noted. Tracheal suctioning was then performed. The blue dye test was immediately positive with significant amounts of blue secretions removed from the trachea.

b. With these results, the blue dye study was terminated. The cuff was reinflated to a minimal leak and a consult generated to the physician requesting a fiberoptic swallowing study. The positive blue dye test, and the other clinical signs of pharyngeal and laryngeal impairment prompted this request for a more objective assessment of airway protection. Further test swallows with any type bolus were thus deferred.

D. Fiberoptic Swallowing Study

1. Before beginning the swallowing study, the patient's vocal fold status was first assessed with nasopharyngolaryngoscopy. The patient's cuff was partially deflated during the procedure. Pulse oximetry was used to monitor any changes in O_2 saturation and pulse rate. The direct fiberoptic examination revealed incomplete adduction of the vocal folds during phonation attempts, with a large posterior vocal chink demonstrated. Vocal quality was hoarse. Intermittent changes in vocal quality accompanied inadequate secretion management documented by visualization of secretions pooling in the larynx and falling between the vocal folds. The patient did not demonstrate a reflexive response to this laryngeal penetration and aspiration. Given these results, no food or liquid boluses were administered. Instead, food coloring was again placed on the tongue and the patient was instructed to dry swallow. There was premature leakage of dyed saliva into the valleculae. Pooling of saliva was noted in the valleculae and left pyriform sinus after the swallow. Approximately 4 seconds after the dye dropped into the valleculae, the swallow triggered. After the swallow, blue-tinged material was detected upon the vocal

folds. The patient was able to clear the material using throat clearing with the clinician's prompting.

2. The results of the clinical evaluation and the fiberoptic study were integrated into treatment planning for Kenny. Videofluoroscopy was deferred because it was felt it would not provide additional information at this time. Kenny's airway protection status was clearly compromised, at least partly due to impaired vocal fold closure. The combined clinical and fiberoptic studies identified oral and pharyngeal stage deficits that placed the patient at risk for aspiration, and that could be addressed via indirect therapy techniques. Given the patient's history of repeated pulmonary infections and compromised airway protection, an indirect treatment program was initiated, and the patient continued to receive nutrition and hydration via the gastrostomy tube only.

E. Indirect Treatment Program

1. Treatment

a. Lingual strengthening exercises with an emphasis on base of tongue movement against resistance, selected articulatory tasks, lingual elevation and lateralization, and anterior to posterior transit (using a gauze pad dipped in nectar and thoroughly dried).

b. Thermal stimulation to address the pharyngeal swallow delay.

c. Vocal fold adduction exercises included coughing, clearing the throat, repeated swallows, and applying limited head movements against the resistance of the clinician's hand. Due to the history of fluctuating blood pressures and oxygen saturation, the patient was monitored via pulse oximetry during these potentially taxing exercises. Oxygen saturation and pulse rate were observed continuously.

2. Cuff Deflation

a. To assist in normalizing airflow for airway clearance, periods of cuff deflation were increased. This was incorporated into therapy sessions with the assistance of a respiratory care practitioner who specialized in pulmonary rehabilitation. The cuff was maintained with partial deflation while tidal volume and FIO_2 were increased slightly. The pulmonary rehabilitation specialist also added pressure support to the respiratory settings during these time periods. With these changes, the patient was able to tolerate up to 40 minutes of cuff deflation without changes in PaO_2 and $PaCO_2$, as measured by dual oximetry and capnography. Kenny also was able to achieve fair voice production and clear secretions from the airway during the indirect dysphagia treatment described above. The patient appeared to effectively coordinate his throat clearing with the inspiratory phase of the ventilator, upon which he received additional airflow. Kenny was directed to "wait for the air, then try to get a little cough." Airway clearance was monitored with the use of vocal changes and cervical auscultation during treatment sessions. In addition, the exsufflator was used to promote clearance of secretions from the airway. The nurse used the exsufflator before and after the patient's dysphagia treatment session.

b. Kenny eventually was able to tolerate partial cuff deflation for two 30- to 40-minute periods during the day. Full cuff deflation was gradually introduced and was tolerated well for these periods. Kenny was assessed with a Passy-Muir speaking valve in-line with the ventilator circuitry. He achieved improved voice production and more forceful throat clearance, but reported a sensation of increased breathing effort and tightness after about 20 minutes of valve use. Kenny was encouraged to consistently blow out air during valve usage, especially when he was not speaking. He was felt to be an eventual candidate for longer periods of speaking valve use.

F. Fiberoptic Study 2 and Videofluoroscopy

1. Repeat Fiberoptics

Due to Kenny's improving clinical status and his enhanced airway protection abilities, he was scheduled for a repeat fiberoptic study. Vocal fold adduction had improved. The administration of dye on the patient's tongue demonstrated some mild premature leakage prior to the swallow, an improved pharyngeal swallow (4 second delay), and pooling in the valleculae and pyriform sinuses after the swallow. However, no material was detected in the larynx after the swallow. Graduated size boluses (1 cc, 3 cc) of dyed applesauce and water (1 cc) were thus administered. For the semisolids, the above noted improvements in function were also seen. For the liquid bolus, a tinge of dye was noted on the vocal folds after the swallow. However, the patient reflexively cleared the residue by using throat clearing, an action not seen prior to treatment.

2. Videofluoroscopy

Based on these improvements in airway protection status and his overall increased medical status, Kenny was seen for videofluoroscopy. He was transported to the radiology suite with the help of the respiratory care practitioner. Secondary to positioning restraints, the test was conducted in the lateral and oblique views. Full cuff deflation was maintained, and the patient was reminded to use the airway clearance strategies introduced in indirect therapy techniques during the assessment. The evaluation revealed oral stage weakness, premature leakage of liquid boluses into the valleculae prior to the swallow, decreased laryngeal elevation during the swallow, pooling in the valleculae and pyriform sinuses after the swallow, and penetration of 5-cc amounts of liquids and semisolids after the swallow. Kenny tolerated smaller bolus amounts (1 cc, 3 cc) but could not clear the larger amounts through the pharynx quickly enough to avoid laryngeal penetration. When the clinician cued Kenny to use his treatment strategies, he cleared the material from the airway prior to any aspiration occurring. Kenny required clinician cues to achieve clearance because he stated he "did not know" when material was entering the larynx. Based on these results, his nonoral status was maintained, but direct dysphagia therapy was implemented.

G. Direct Dysphagia Therapy

Administration of 1- to 2-cc bolus amounts of dyed thickened liquids were incorporated into the direct treatment paradigm. Repeated effortful swallows and airway clearance methods were emphasized. Due to the decrease noted in laryngeal elevation, pitch variation tasks were added to the therapy sessions. Although a Mendelsohn maneuver might have addressed the decreased elevation and retention of material in the pharynx, Kenny was unable to coordinate this movement with the phases of the ventilator. Oromotor exercises continued. Kenny began taking larger amounts of food on a recreational basis, under supervision, and tolerated increasing periods of cuff deflation. He was discharged from the long-term care facility to a facility closer to his home, where the professional staff then aided him in the transition to a more complete oral diet.

Kenny's case illustrates the impact of tracheostomy and ventilator-dependence on the complex interrelationship between swallowing and respiration.

9

Case Examples

Comprehensive management of the tracheostomized and/or ventilator-dependent patient is best illustrated via detailed case examples. Specific cases can demonstrate the roles of team members and present the concept of coordinated care. It is with team effort that effective management of the tracheostomized and ventilator-dependent patient takes place. This transdisciplinary team concept requires participation of a variety of specialized professionals. This chapter will present five case examples and discuss the input of individual team members.

I. ROLE OF THE TRANSDISCIPLINARY TEAM

A. Coordinated Care

The transdisciplinary team concept is more than multiple disciplines working in isolation; it is a coordinated effort of care. Each discipline appreciates the roles of the others. Table 9-1 details the members of the team who work to successfully manage the tracheostomized and/or ventilator-dependent patient. The role of each team member is often defined by the specific treatment setting. As previously discussed, settings may include:

1. **Acute Care/ICU**

2. **Rehabilitation**

3. **Subacute**

4. **Extended Care**

5. **Home Care**

Table 9-1. Members of the Transdisciplinary Team. (From "Transdisciplinary Team Concept," by M. S. Kazandjian and K. J. Dikeman, 1993, p. 258. In M. F. Mason (Ed.), *Speech Pathology for Tracheostomized and Ventilator Patients.* Newport Beach, CA: Voicing! Inc. Copyright 1993 by Voicing! Inc. Reprinted with permission.)

Medical

Primary care physician and consulting physicians may include any of the following:

Pulmonologist	Physiatrist
Internist	Trauma Surgeon
Otolaryngologist	Thoracic Surgeon
Pediatrician	Neuro Physician/Surgeon
Neurologist	Intensive Care/Critical Care M.D.
Cardiologist	Geriatrician
Orthopedist	

Medical Professionals

Respiratory/Pulmonary Therapist

Nurse Specialists (Otolaryngology, Pulmonary, Rehabilitation)

Nurse/Nurse Technician/Nurse's Aide

Dietician/Nutritionist

Feeding/Swallowing Team

Pharmacist

Physical

Physical Therapist

Licensed Physical Therapist Assistant

Physical Therapy Technician

Occupational Therapist

Certified Occupational Therapist Assistant

Rehabilitation Engineer

Vocational/Recreational

Vocational Therapist

Recreation Therapist

Special Educator/Teacher

Psychosocial

Social Worker/Case Manager

Psychologist/Psychiatrist

Chaplain

Patient/Family

Communication

Audiologist

Speech-Language Pathologist

The focus of care will vary depending on the setting in which the patient is placed. For example, in the acute care/ICU setting, care is directed at stabilization and survival. Communication and swallowing intervention often must take a "back seat" to more life-threatening issues. However, at times communication and swallowing are intertwined with immediate medical decisions and require the assistance of the speech-language pathologist to facilitate total care. In the rehabilitation and extended care settings, treatment can be directed toward more long-term communication/swallowing strategies which may involve more aggressive intervention (e.g., gradual cuff deflation). Similar intervention may occur in the home setting; however, availability of team members may be limited in this environment.

II. CONTINUUM OF DISABILITY: CASE EXAMPLES

Transdisciplinary team members join together in addressing the areas highlighted on the Continuum of Disability as illustrated in Table 9-2. The Continuum of Disability is used to provide a complete composite of each tracheostomized and/or ventilator-dependent patient and identify his or her particular needs. As patients begin treatment, movement through the continuum may be evident and can occur in either direction.

The following case examples illustrate the clinical courses of several tracheostomized and ventilator-dependent patients. Some details have been altered and clinical pictures combined to protect confidentiality and facilitate the descriptive process.

III. PATIENT AC

A. Background History

1. Setting: Ventilator Unit of an Extended Care Facility

AC was a 76-year-old female with a diagnosis of COPD. She demonstrated the typical pink puffer pattern with heightened anxiety, a thin barrel-chested frame and use of her accessory muscles during respiration. On admission she was tracheostomized and ventilator-dependent. Her mode of ventilation was assist control (A/C) with a rate of 12. Ventilatory settings included an FIO_2 of 40% and a tidal volume (TV) of 750 ml. She maintained a $PaCO_2$ of 63 until the respiratory therapist increased TV, increasing minute ventilation and consequently alveolar ventilation. $PaCO_2$ decreased to 50 at this time, very typical for a patient with this medical diagnosis. She had a cuffed, nonfenestrated #6 tracheostomy tube and required frequent suctioning. AC had a long history of cigarette smoking. She had difficulty maintaining her weight in recent years. She was initially admitted from home to an acute care hospital due to exacerbation of the COPD. Once placed on the ventilator and stabilized, she was transferred to the extended care setting for long-term management with a plan

Table 9-2. Components of the Full Continuum of Disability. (Adapted from "Continuum of Disability" by C. Salciccia, 1986. In C. Salciccia, L. Adams, & G. Kapassakis, *Communication Management of Respiratorily-Involved Quadriplegic Adults.* Paper presented at Goldwater Memorial Hospital, New York, NY.)

Physical Motor

Normal UE ROM and fine motor. Good endurance.	Adequate UE ROM and fine motor. Fair endurance.	UE weakness. Gross movement adequate. Limited ROM. Poor endurance.	Significant weakness. Limitations in ROM. Poorly coordinated UE function. Severely limited endurance.	Quadriplegia. No upper/ lower extremity function.	Pentaplegia. No movement including head.

Speech/Voice

Phonation with good vocal intensity. Articulation WNL.	Phonation with decreased intensity. Good articulation.	Phonation poorly coordinated with ventilation.	Aphonic with good mouthing.	Aphonia with mild dysarthria.	Aphonia with moderate dysarthria.	Aphonia with severe dysarthria.

Cognitive-Linguistic

No deficits, intact status.	Mild deficits (memory, orientation, reasoning, anomia).	Moderate deficits (impairments in language expression/ reception).	Severe deficits.	Profound deficits.

Behavior

Patient indicates concerns, highly motivated for treatment.	Mild anxiety, but can be reassured.	Moderate anxiety, difficulty in transitioning through intervention stages. Treatment is interfered with.	Severe anxiety. No intervention possible.

Swallowing

Normal swallowing.	Mild oral-pharyngeal weakness. Difficulty with solids and/or liquids.	Moderate oral-pharyngeal dysphagia. Management of altered diet.	Moderate-severe oral-pharyngeal dysphagia. Oral intake supple-mented with alternative feeding or pleasurable/ recreational feeding.	Severe oral-pharyngeal dysphagia. Pleasurable feeding.	NPO

Note: UE = upper extremity; ROM = range of motion; WNL = within normal limits; NPO = non per os, nonoral feeding only.

for eventual weaning and discharge to home. She was a widow with three children. According to AC's family, she enjoyed watching television, reading, and visits from her grandchildren.

B. Presenting Initial Status on Evaluation

1. AC's Continuum of Disability

Table 9-3 illustrates AC's status at the beginning of the assessment process. AC presented with essentially normal physical-motor abilities. However, her endurance was considered only fair because of the increased work of breathing caused by daily activities. Even getting out of bed was difficult for AC. She often felt short of breath and occasionally required the additional ventilatory assistance of manual bagging. In terms of speech and voice, AC was aphonic with good mouthing. She presented with a fully inflated tracheostomy tube cuff. AC's cognitive-linguistic function was characterized by mild deficits primarily in short-term memory, orientation to place, and concentration/attention to task. Periods of confusion were evident at different times of the day particularly when she was unable to obtain a full night's sleep. Behaviorally, AC had moderate-severe anxiety. She became visibly nervous when anyone attempted to make modifications to the ventilator settings and complained of "trouble breathing" even when monitoring equipment revealed adequate O_2 and CO_2 exchange and uncompromised cardiac status. Due to her continued complaints of being "hot" and feeling like "there is no air in this room," she often would fully undress in her bed with no regard for visitors or open doorways. AC tolerated a regular diet and exhibited no oral-pharyngeal swallowing deficits.

2. Needs Assessment

AC's communication needs related primarily to her anxiety and current medical condition. Communicative locations included her bed, the chair in her room, and the activity room of the ventilator unit. Occasionally, she would visit the main dining area and porch in the main lobby of the facility. AC's initial method of message transfer was through writing with pen and paper. However, during periods of heightened anxiety, she rapidly mouthed her messages and became increasingly frustrated when her communication partners could not understand. Communication partners ranged from her family, regular nurses, therapists, and doctors to unfamiliar visitors and staff such as temporary nurses or new volunteers.

C. Diagnostic Intervention

1. Stages of Communication Intervention

All transdisciplinary team members were inserviced and aware of AC's communication goals. Each member made attempts to facilitate communication

Table 9-3. Continuum of Disability: "AC." (Adapted from "Continuum of Disability" by C. Salciccia, 1986. In C. Salciccia, L. Adams, & G. Kapassakis, *Communication Management of Respiratorily-Involved Quadriplegic Adults.* Paper presented at Goldwater Memorial Hospital, New York, NY.)

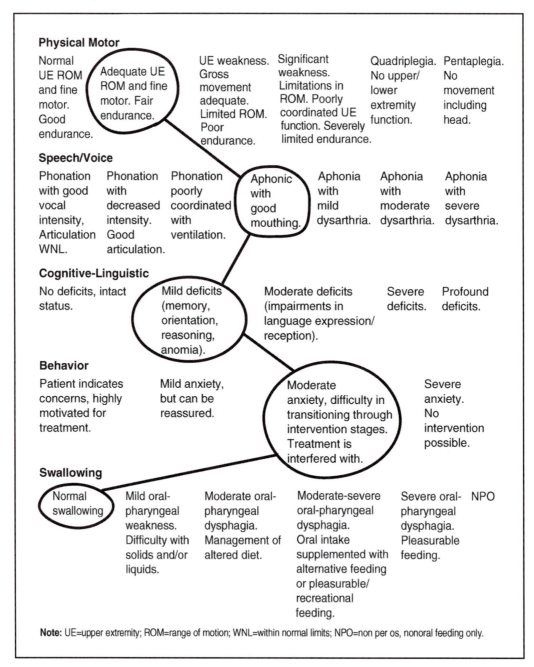

Physical Motor

| Normal UE ROM and fine motor. Good endurance. | Adequate UE ROM and fine motor. Fair endurance. | UE weakness. Gross movement adequate. Limited ROM. Poor endurance. | Significant weakness. Limitations in ROM. Poorly coordinated UE function. Severely limited endurance. | Quadriplegia. No upper/ lower extremity function. | Pentaplegia. No movement including head. |

Speech/Voice

| Phonation with good vocal intensity, Articulation WNL. | Phonation with decreased intensity. Good articulation. | Phonation poorly coordinated with ventilation. | Aphonic with good mouthing. | Aphonia with mild dysarthria. | Aphonia with moderate dysarthria. | Aphonia with severe dysarthria. |

Cognitive-Linguistic

| No deficits, intact status. | Mild deficits (memory, orientation, reasoning, anomia). | Moderate deficits (impairments in language expression/ reception). | Severe deficits. | Profound deficits. |

Behavior

| Patient indicates concerns, highly motivated for treatment. | Mild anxiety, but can be reassured. | Moderate anxiety, difficulty in transitioning through intervention stages. Treatment is interfered with. | Severe anxiety. No intervention possible. |

Swallowing

| Normal swallowing | Mild oral-pharyngeal weakness. Difficulty with solids and/or liquids. | Moderate oral-pharyngeal dysphagia. Management of altered diet. | Moderate-severe oral-pharyngeal dysphagia. Oral intake supplemented with alternative feeding or pleasurable/ recreational feeding. | Severe oral-pharyngeal dysphagia. Pleasurable feeding. | NPO |

Note: UE=upper extremity; ROM=range of motion; WNL=within normal limits; NPO=non per os, nonoral feeding only.

by encouraging the use of new systems introduced by the speech-language pathologist. Weekly progress updates were given to the transdisciplinary team during ventilator rounds so that continuity of care was maintained.

a. Leak speech

A transdisciplinary team approach was especially necessary in managing AC's case. She required the coordination of several services to optimize her communication and socialization. Initial intervention was directed at restoring oral communication. Treatment sessions were conducted by respiratory therapy and speech-language pathology. The protocol to deflate the tracheostomy tube cuff and create leak speech was initiated. During this process, AC was monitored by both oximetry and capnography. Baseline measurements were SaO_2 of 96%, PCO_2 of 45, and a pulse rate of 97. As the cuff was deflated, the respiratory care practitioner made modifications to the tidal volume of the ventilator to compensate for the minimal loss of volume created by the leak of air. Tidal volume was increased by 100 ml during periods of cuff deflation. Initially, AC began to cough and expressed the feeling of "having air tickle my throat." After the coughing subsided, she was instructed to begin voicing. The speech-language pathologist presented AC with various automatic speech tasks, such as counting, in an attempt to assist her in using the airflow for voicing. AC initiated many comments and coordinated the airflow to say one or two words per breath cycle. These initial sessions focused on providing a partial leak and allowing AC to become accustomed to the sensation of airflow moving through the upper airway. Full cuff deflation was then attempted. Tidal volume was increased by 200 ml. This number was obtained by having AC exhale into a spirometer after cuff deflation. AC was closely monitored for CO_2 retention and possible increased back pressures resulting from the increase in tidal volume. SaO_2 and PCO_2 levels remained close to baseline. AC required continual reassurance that she was okay. She was returned to full cuff inflation in 5 to 10 minutes. Attempts were made to coordinate short visits from a family member, another resident, or staff member with periods of cuff deflation and oral communication to motivate AC and provide her with positive feedback.

b. Speaking valve use

Once AC adjusted to full tracheostomy tube cuff deflation for short periods of time, placement of a one-way speaking valve in-line with the ventilator tubing was attempted. AC was first introduced to the Passy-Muir speaking valve by meeting other ventilator-dependent residents who successfully used the device. She was given the opportunity to ask questions, share experiences with these residents, and hear concerns similar to her own. The staff psychologist often joined these treatment sessions to facilitate questions and probe feelings of anxiety. The first attempt to place the speaking valve in-line was marginally successful. The resident complained of "not getting enough air" despite the measures obtained by the objective monitoring devices. The clinicians maintained the valve in-line for approximately 3 minutes. Later treatment sessions focused on gradually increasing the length of valve wear time. It was demonstrated to AC that she could speak in extended sentences without coordinating each word with the breath cycle. AC eventually tolerated a wear time of 30 minutes before clinical and objective assessment documented increased work of breathing. This was evident via increased pulse rate and PCO_2 compared to initial measures. Given AC's baseline pulmonary status, 30 minutes of valve use was considered quite successful.

c. **Nonoral communication methods**

AC communicated with her family during periods of valve use and oral communication. The team also made attempts to coordinate her valve use with recreational activities that she enjoyed, such as bingo. She was greatly reinforced by her ability to call out, "Bingo!" when she had the number-letter combinations to win the game. However, because AC could tolerate the speaking valve for a maximum of 30 minutes, nonoral communication methods were necessary to meet her needs for the other hours of the day and night. AC was most comfortable with writing and was given a small dry erase board for communicating her daily needs. The speech-language pathologist also created a phrase board which AC used to quickly communicate messages to the staff when her anxiety or condition interfered with writing. The phrase board included messages such as "I need to go back to bed," "Please get the respiratory therapist," "I am not getting enough air," "I am feeling scared," "I need a respiratory treatment now." Other oral methods of communication (i.e., mouthing, use of an electro-larynx) were presented; however, AC's anxiety and inability to coordinate her rapid mouthing with the activation of the devices limited their success.

2. **Stages of Swallowing Intervention**

a. **Clinical evaluation of swallowing**

As discussed previously, AC initially presented with adequate swallowing function. Due to her edentulous status, she did require a mechanical soft diet. Approximately 3 months following her admission, two changes in AC's status were noted. She had increased difficulty tolerating full cuff deflation and using a Passy-Muir speaking valve in-line with the ventilator. Additionally, the nurses on the day shift noted what appeared to be food escaping around the sides of the tracheostomy tube after meals. The attending physician was alerted and a consult was generated to speech pathology for a swallowing evaluation. The speech-language pathologist scheduled the evaluation during lunch time. AC was first observed at baseline status, eating with a partially deflated tracheostomy tube cuff. No changes were made initially; however, blue food coloring was added to solid food for easy visualization of aspiration. Because a blue dye test can only rule in aspiration (not rule out), and cannot differentiate between consistencies, liquids were not tested at this time. The clinical swallowing evaluation documented adequate oral stage functioning. After AC ate approximately one-quarter of her tray, small amounts of blue dyed food were noted first in the tracheostomy tube and then expelled around the sides of the tracheostomy tube following a cough. There were intermittent changes in vocal quality. The clinician theorized that the expulsion of food around the sides of the tracheostomy tube was secondary to pooling of food above the partially inflated cuff which was then forced out on the reflexive cough. Oximetry monitoring during the evaluation revealed increased heart rate and slightly decreased O_2 saturation levels.

The second stage of the swallowing evaluation was performed the next day. Clearance for full cuff deflation and placement of the Passy-Muir speaking valve was obtained. The patient was once again given blue-dyed food from her tray. Following several swallows, AC was suctioned and large amounts of blue dyed material was removed. A recommendation for a fiberoptic evaluation of swallowing with otolaryngology (ENT) and a temporary nonoral feeding status was made by the speech-language pathologist.

b. Fiberoptic evaluation of swallowing

A swallowing evaluation via direct fiberoptics was performed with speech pathology and ENT. The tracheostomy tube cuff was maintained partially deflated for the period of the study. Direct visualization of the airway revealed adequate vocal fold closure on phonation. One teaspoon of blue-dyed semisolid consistency was presented. The patient triggered a timely swallow. Retention of some of the material was evident in the pyriform sinuses bilaterally. AC was prompted to trigger dry swallows in an effort to clear the material from the pharynx. An additional teaspoon of semisolid consistency was provided. Pharyngeal retention and a reflexive cough were evidenced. Aspiration after the swallow was noted, with aspiration during the swallow suspected. Optimally, a speaking valve would have been placed in-line to address the suspected reduction in pharyngeal pressures, evidenced by pharyngeal retention. However, AC was not tolerating the speaking valve at this time and could not maintain adequate ventilation with a fully deflated cuff. This occurred as she reached the final stages of COPD.

c. Tracheostomy tube size change

In an attempt to continue cuff deflation and maintain adequate ventilation, the size of AC's tracheostomy tube cuff was increased from a size #6 to a size #8. The patient was observed again with small amounts of dyed food. Evidence of poor airway protection was again noted by dyed food observed during suctioning. However, AC was able to maintain adequate ventilation with a partial leak. Although her secretions had been increasing, frequent suctioning allowed her to maintain this partial leak. Even with this small amount of airflow, AC was able to expectorate secretions orally. This partial leak allowed for voicing of short utterances to make at least basic needs and concerns known. Under these conditions, oral feedings were continued for several weeks.

d.   Long-term management of nutrition and hydration

Eventually, recommendations were made to maintain a nonoral feeding status and provide long-term alternative feeding. AC was unable to tolerate even small amounts of food or liquid without evidence of aspiration. The transdisciplinary team theorized that, as AC's pulmonary status deteriorated, the work of breathing during cuff deflation was increasing. AC's ability to tolerate the back pressures generated by the one-way speaking valve was also decreasing. AC's condition deteriorated, allowing only maintenance of a minimal leak in cuff pressures. This drastically reduced the amount of airflow through the upper airway. Because she was able to tolerate only a minimal leak and unable to wear the valve, AC lost the mechanisms available for airway clearance. She was unable to utilize ventilator flow during coughing or generate sufficient pressures to clear retained material from the pharynx. AC was transferred to the acute care hospital for placement of a PEG. She lived for several more months, maximizing her quality of life through nonoral communication methods and therapeutic recreation activities. AC suffered a cardiac arrest approximately 5 months following admission. As she did not have a do-not-resuscitate (DNR) order, cardiopulmonary resuscitation was attempted, but efforts were unsuccessful and AC died enroute to the emergency room. Although weaning from mechanical ventilation had not been achieved, AC's quality of life had been a focus of care throughout her stay in the extended care setting.

IV. PATIENT BT

A. Background History

1. Setting: Respiratory Unit of a Rehabilitation Hospital

BT was a 27-year-old man with a diagnosis of amyotrophic lateral sclerosis (ALS), a progressive neurological disease. Prior to his admission to the hospital, BT had been living at home and was an artist and photographer. He made the decision to enter the respiratory unit of the hospital as the progression of his ALS required ventilatory assistance at night (BiPAP™) and made it difficult for him to remain at home.

B. Presenting Status on Evaluation

1. BT's Continuum of Disability

Table 9-4 illustrates BT's status during the initial assessment process. BT presented with severe physical-motor deficits, limiting his movements to slight ranging of the hands and head. Head control was fair at the time of admission. When fatigued the patient had tremendous difficulty maintaining his head in an erect position. He could not lift it if it fell forward. Speech and voice function was judged to be aphonic with moderate-severe dysarthria. Speech was characterized by severe hypernasality, imprecise articulatory contacts, reduced breath support, and low vocal volume. Speech intelligibility was poor and understood only by familiar communication partners such as family members. BT's cognitive-linguistic ability was within normal limits. He was highly motivated to continue with his art work and design and was eager to participate in treatment directed toward maximizing communication. At the time of admission, BT presented with a moderate oral/pharyngeal stage dysphagia. He tolerated a mechanical soft diet. However, he was unable to maintain adequate nutrition and hydration by mouth, primarily due to fatigue during meals, and therefore received supplemental intake via a PEG.

2. Needs Assessment

BT's message needs were extensive. Rapid and accurate requests/comments to hospital staff were a daily necessity. He was highly motivated to continue his work in art and photography and therefore expressed a specific desire to assist him in making this possible. BT also required a nonoral communication system to supplement his oral attempts at message transfer. It was necessary for this communication system to be portable, allowing him to use it in multiple positions in bed, in the chair, and in the various areas in and outside of the hospital. Communication partners ranged from unfamiliar medical staff and outside consultants to familiar friends and family. He additionally required a sophisticated method of written communication so that he could not only detail questions and comments to the medical staff, but also instruct assistants. He would direct his assistants in the mechanical aspects of his art and photography. In other words, BT had to give specific instructions to people regarding the settings of the camera, the lighting, and the setting and position of each subject. This sophisticated communication system had to be computer-based to allow for the integration of specialized software in graphic design. BT also needed to communicate any difficulty that he was experiencing with daily medical care and his current diet. BT needed to direct the nurse aide in the

Table 9-4. Continuum of Disability: "BT." (Adapted from "Continuum of Disability" by C. Salciccia, 1986. In C. Salciccia, L. Adams, & G. Kapassakis, *Communication Management of Respiratorily-Involved Quadriplegic Adults*. Paper presented at Goldwater Memorial Hospital, New York, NY.)

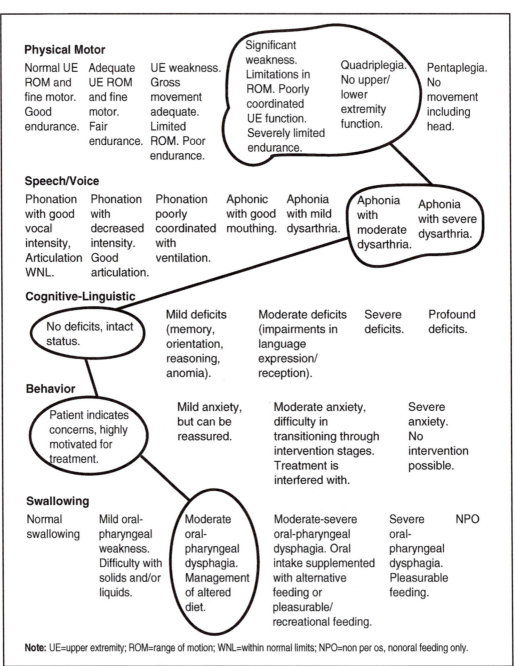

Physical Motor

Normal UE ROM and fine motor. Good endurance.

Adequate UE ROM and fine motor. Fair endurance.

UE weakness. Gross movement adequate. Limited ROM. Poor endurance.

Significant weakness. Limitations in ROM. Poorly coordinated UE function. Severely limited endurance.

Quadriplegia. No upper/lower extremity function.

Pentaplegia. No movement including head.

Speech/Voice

Phonation with good vocal intensity, Articulation WNL.

Phonation with decreased intensity. Good articulation.

Phonation poorly coordinated with ventilation.

Aphonic with good mouthing.

Aphonia with mild dysarthria.

Aphonia with moderate dysarthria.

Aphonia with severe dysarthria.

Cognitive-Linguistic

No deficits, intact status.

Mild deficits (memory, orientation, reasoning, anomia).

Moderate deficits (impairments in language expression/reception).

Severe deficits.

Profound deficits.

Behavior

Patient indicates concerns, highly motivated for treatment.

Mild anxiety, but can be reassured.

Moderate anxiety, difficulty in transitioning through intervention stages. Treatment is interfered with.

Severe anxiety. No intervention possible.

Swallowing

Normal swallowing

Mild oral-pharyngeal weakness. Difficulty with solids and/or liquids.

Moderate oral-pharyngeal dysphagia. Management of altered diet.

Moderate-severe oral-pharyngeal dysphagia. Oral intake supplemented with alternative feeding or pleasurable/recreational feeding.

Severe oral-pharyngeal dysphagia. Pleasurable feeding.

NPO

Note: UE=upper extremity; ROM=range of motion; WNL=within normal limits; NPO=non per os, nonoral feeding only.

quantity of each spoonful of food and indicate, during meals, when the food was too difficult to manage. Message needs therefore also encompassed quick, personally related communication to direct his daily care.

C. Diagnostic Intervention

1. Stages of Communication Intervention

The tracheostomized and ventilator-dependent patient with a degenerative disease will require intervention techniques to address the changing needs of an individual whose physical-motor function and speech will deteriorate. BT illustrates this degenerative course.

a. Call buzzer/alerting signal

During the initial stages of treatment the speech-language pathologist and occupational therapist worked closely to adapt the nursing call buzzer. This allowed BT to alert the staff when he required attention. The standard cylindrical call buzzer, present in most hospitals, was modified to fit a specially adapted glove, which allowed him to hold and manipulate the buzzer. BT could activate the buzzer in his many positions whether in the bed or in a wheelchair.

b. Nonelectronic communication system (eye gaze)

Daily message needs were addressed first via nonelectronic communication. Message transfer in all positions and locations was accomplished by oral communication supplemented with the use of an Eye-Link. BT could utilize this method of communication while in bed, in the chair, and on BiPAP™ at night. BT would verbally produce the letter as he eye-pointed to the target letter on the Eye-Link. All communication partners were instructed in the use of this nonelectronic eye-gaze system. Most people immediately became proficient in its use. The speech-language pathologist did periodic inservices with the medical staff to ensure that all new personnel were comfortable in this method of nonoral communication.

c. Switch access

Next, BT was evaluated by the speech-language pathologist and occupational therapist for switch access that would allow him to operate his integrated communication system. The occupational therapist fabricated foam wedges and splints to position BT's arms and hands. Two small round switches were attached to the wedges allowing for finger activation with each hand. Once BT could activate each switch with rapid, accurate movements, dual switch Morse code was introduced. Morse code was introduced to provide BT with a quicker access mode than allowed by single switch scanning. BT began daily treatment sessions to learn the various codes that represented letters, numbers, and punctuation.

d. Computer access

An IBM computer was donated to BT. This nonportable device allowed him to continue with his art and design work. Because physical-motor impairment interfered with his ability to direct select, an alternative access method was evaluated. As described above, BT was able to utilize dual switches for Morse code. A keyboard emulator was obtained which allowed BT to access his software packages via Morse code. With Morse code, BT also was able to do word processing and therefore write detailed messages to his communication partners. Consultants, including a computer programmer who specialized in adapting computers for the disabled, were called on to develop and modify programs to meet BT's special needs. For example, specific architectural design programs were modified and became accessible via switch access.

e. Dedicated communication system

The Eye-Link and the nonportable writing system were effective in meeting most of BT's communication needs while in the hospital; however, the systems did not meet his communication needs when communicating with unfamiliar partners outside the facility. This became evident during the planning stage of an art show in which BT was being honored. Special plans were made to transport BT from the hospital to a local gallery where his art was being displayed. During this time, BT would have to communicate with large numbers of people who would not be able to understand his verbal output or use an Eye-Link. A portable dedicated electronic communication system was provided to allow for Morse code access, speech synthesis, and hard copy print. This provided BT with the flexibility to communicate with a variety of communication partners through speech or print. Comments and short paragraphs that could be easily retrieved to increase the rate of communicative exchanges were preprogrammed into the device. Abbreviation-expansion was also utilized to increase the speed of message transfer. This portable alternative communication system allowed BT the independence to communicate in a novel environment.

f. Nonelectronic communication board

As BT's physical-motor function deteriorated, he was unable to maintain an upright head position, especially when he was seated in the wheelchair. Head posture was often forward and could not be changed without the assistance of his communication partner. As a result, the eye gaze system which BT had utilized became nonfunctional while he was in the chair. The occupational therapist made several attempts to fabricate assistive devices, such as a head strap and neck brace, to assist in head control, but BT refused these adaptive devices. BT was then introduced to a row-column letter/word/phrase board which the clinician presented via visual and auditory modalities, pointing to and repeating items. BT produced a verbal "yeh" when the communication partner indicated the intended target. This scanning system was successful in obtaining daily needs from the patient and was thus integrated into his multi-modality communication approach, replacing the Eye-Link. The Eye-Link continued to be his primary method of message transfer while in bed. This was due to the interference of the oral/nasal BiPAP™ mask, which prevented his production of the verbal "yeh" for confirmation.

2. Stages of Dysphagia Intervention

a. Inservicing

BT had a percutaneous endoscopic gastrostomy tube (PEG) on admission, but did continue to tolerate a mechanical soft diet. Initial intervention techniques centered primarily on inservicing the nursing staff and family in techniques to facilitate safe swallowing and feeding. The speech-language pathologist instructed staff in postural modifications and optimal presentation of food. This included ensuring an upright position, providing small bolus sizes, and being aware of any vocal changes during solid or liquid intake. The dietitian monitored BT's oral intake closely.

b. Postural modification

As BT's disease progressed his ability to tolerate oral intake decreased. Nursing reported occasional wet vocal quality on solid as well as liquid intake. Secondary to a delayed pharyngeal swallow, the patient found it advantageous to maintain a fully flexed head posture to reduce the possibility of losing control of the bolus. The usefulness of this technique was confirmed by a videofluoroscopic evaluation that documented elimination of aspiration of liquid consistencies when a chin tuck was utilized.

c. Use of a mechanical CoughAssist

Secretion management became increasingly difficult as pulmonary reserve decreased and BT was unable to produce a productive cough. Three to five times daily, a mechanical CoughAssist was utilized by nursing and respiratory therapy to clear secretions from the distal airways. The CoughAssist was the treatment of choice because the patient was not tracheostomized. Had suctioning been performed, it could have been performed transnasally, but would have been uncomfortable for the patient as well as less effective in clearing retained secretions.

3. Bioethical Concerns

The rehabilitation hospital had instituted a Bioethical Committee to address issues relating to right-to-die and advance directives. The team consisted of the director of rehabilitation medicine (an MD), the attending physiatrist and internist, psychologist, patient advocate, lawyer, clergyman, social worker, and speech-language pathologist.

a.   As one member of the team, the speech-language pathologist evaluates the nonspeaking patient who is unable to make needs known verbally and determines communicative competency (Kazandjian & Dikeman, 1990). Communicative competency requires that the patient demonstrate consistent and reliable responses to questions posed by the communicative partner. The goal of determining communicative competency and mental competency for the bioethical team is to assess the patient's capacity to make decisions regarding his medical care, including the issues of right-to-die (determination) and advance directives. For example, the patient in the ICU who is ventilator-dependent and aphonic may require only the provision of an alternative communication system such as a letter/alphabet board to indicate wishes concerning his medical care. Communicative competency is easily established in such a case. However, a patient with physical, cognitive, and linguistic deficits may be limited to only a yes/no communication system. Even in this case, the speech-language pathologist can assist in determining reliability of the patient's communication. At this point, the psychiatrist can proceed with an assessment of the patient's competency and decisional capacity. Often the speech-language pathologist remains present throughout the actual evaluation to assist in modifying language to a level that a linguistically impaired patient can understand. Although it may be common for the bioethical team to deal with issues typical to the tracheotomized and ventilator-dependent individual, such as removing mechanical ventilatory support, each case is individual and reflects the needs of the patient and the patient's designated representative (Maynard & Muth, 1987).

b.   BT's case was reviewed frequently by this group. BT had numerous concerns that were relevant to the Bioethical Committee. He had established a DNR and living will. BT not only did not want a tracheostomy and invasive mechanical ventilation, but refused all other life-prolonging procedures. He was aware that noninvasive ventilation was slowly becoming ineffective as his bulbar signs increased. The Bioethical Committee met several times to clarify BT's wishes and document any current modifications of the living will. Eventually, BT's respiratory capacity did deteriorate. He died according to his wishes, without any of the life sustaining methods he had declined.

V. PATIENT EB

A. Background History

1. Setting: Intensive Care Unit

EB was a 61-year-old man with a medical diagnosis of AIDS and previous history of left CVA. His communication diagnosis was severe nonfluent aphasia and mild dysarthria. EB had been receiving speech and language treatment; however, due to severe depression, he had begun refusing all therapy. This refusal persisted despite antidepressant medication. He also presented with pain on swallowing and consequent avoidance of oral intake. This was due to significant candidiasis. Approximately 2 months after admission to an extended care facility EB's medical status deteriorated significantly. He was diagnosed with pneumocystis carinii pneumonia (PCP) and subsequent respiratory failure. He was admitted to an ICU and was intubated and placed on mechanical ventilation. This procedure was performed as there were no advance directives to the contrary.

Three weeks later, after stabilizing his immediate condition, the physician and patient advocate called the speech-language pathologist, psychiatrist, and family for a consultation to assess the patient's communicative competency. The physician required consent from the patient in order to proceed with a tracheostomy for pulmonary toilet as well as connection to mechanical ventilation. The patient had been intubated for several weeks and maintenance of pulmonary toilet had become difficult. He was alert and visibly anxious. When the patient's significant other arrived at the hospital from out of town, he informed the physicians that EB would not have wanted invasive mechanical support, specifically a tracheotomy. Although he was not the designated representative, the significant other requested that the patient not be maintained on mechanical ventilation and that the endotracheal tube be removed. The patient had no advanced directives or living will. He had previously signed only a DNR order.

B. Presenting Status on Evaluation

1. EB's Continuum of Disability

Table 9-5 illustrates EB's status during the initial assessment. In terms of physical-motor status, he presented with a right hemiplegia and immobilized

Table 9-5. Continuum of Disability: "EB." (Adapted from "Continuum of Disability" by C. Salciccia, 1986. In C. Salciccia, L. Adams, & G. Kapassakis, *Communication Management of Respiratorily-Involved Quadriplegic Adults*. Paper presented at Goldwater Memorial Hospital, New York, NY.)

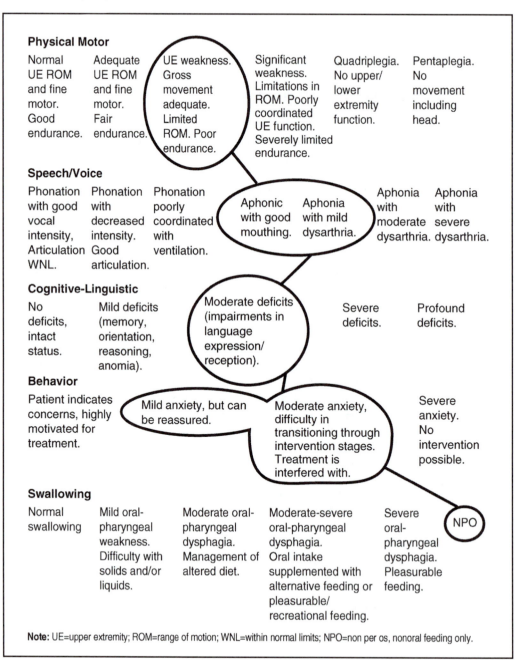

Physical Motor

| Normal UE ROM and fine motor. Good endurance. | Adequate UE ROM and fine motor. Fair endurance. | UE weakness. Gross movement adequate. Limited ROM. Poor endurance. | Significant weakness. Limitations in ROM. Poorly coordinated UE function. Severely limited endurance. | Quadriplegia. No upper/ lower extremity function. | Pentaplegia. No movement including head. |

Speech/Voice

| Phonation with good vocal intensity, Articulation WNL. | Phonation with decreased intensity. Good articulation. | Phonation poorly coordinated with ventilation. | Aphonic with good mouthing. | Aphonia with mild dysarthria. | Aphonia with moderate dysarthria. | Aphonia with severe dysarthria. |

Cognitive-Linguistic

| No deficits, intact status. | Mild deficits (memory, orientation, reasoning, anomia). | Moderate deficits (impairments in language expression/ reception). | | Severe deficits. | Profound deficits. |

Behavior

| Patient indicates concerns, highly motivated for treatment. | Mild anxiety, but can be reassured. | | Moderate anxiety, difficulty in transitioning through intervention stages. Treatment is interfered with. | | Severe anxiety. No intervention possible. |

Swallowing

| Normal swallowing | Mild oral-pharyngeal weakness. Difficulty with solids and/or liquids. | Moderate oral-pharyngeal dysphagia. Management of altered diet. | Moderate-severe oral-pharyngeal dysphagia. Oral intake supplemented with alternative feeding or pleasurable/ recreational feeding. | Severe oral-pharyngeal dysphagia. Pleasurable feeding. | NPO |

Note: UE=upper extremity; ROM=range of motion; WNL=within normal limits; NPO=non per os, nonoral feeding only.

left arm and hand due to IV lines. He was aphonic secondary to the endotracheal tube. In terms of cognitive-linguistic status, he was known to have at least a moderate nonfluent aphasia with fair comprehension. Behavioral assessment revealed EB to be alert with heightened anxiety secondary to being in the ICU setting, aphonic, and aphasic. Swallowing status was nonoral. The patient was intubated and was receiving IV fluids.

2. Needs Assessment

EB required a quick and reliable method of immediate message transfer so that his attending physicians, nursing, and respiratory staff could understand his needs and respect his wishes regarding his medical care. He was positioned with his head slightly elevated in bed. The ICU environment was noisy and busy. Communication partners ranged from his family and familiar physicians and nurses to the several specialists called for consultation who were meeting this individual for the first time.

3. Diagnostic Communication Intervention

Restoring oral communication was not considered an option due to his aphasia, poor medical status, and urgency of the physician's request. A simple augmentative communication system was therefore attempted. The speech-language pathologist looked for a reliable motor movement to use, in addition to his head nods and shakes, with which the patient could indicate "yes" or "no." EB was presented with the words printed in large letters on a clipboard. This graphic response was used to clarify any nonverbal head nods/shakes that he demonstrated. In establishing communicative competence, the clinician progressed from simple, concrete questions to more abstract material. For example, the speech-language pathologist asked: "Are you a man? woman?" "Are you sick?" "Are you in the hospital?" "Are you having trouble breathing?" "Do you know that the doctor can help you breathe with a tube in your throat?" "Do you want a machine to help you breathe?"

The psychiatrist was present and participated in the evaluation. However, these questions were phrased for the comprehension level of an aphasic. Additionally, these questions were presented several times to ensure EB's response reliability. The role of the speech-language pathologist was to establish communicative competency for a reliable yes/no response. The psychiatrist was then able to determine competency and obtain consent for the tracheotomy procedure which was performed. The patient indicated that, despite his previous expressions of refusal of mechanical ventilation, he was not yet ready to die. His case demonstrates the interdependence of the transdisciplinary team and the importance of establishing communication in even the most acute settings.

VI. PATIENT AG

A. Background History

1. Setting: Respiratory Unit of a Rehabilitation Hospital/Home Care

AG is a 30-year-old man with a medical diagnosis of C4–C6 spinal cord injury, quadriplegia, tracheostomy, and respiratory insufficiency secondary to a motor vehicle accident. The patient, unresponsive at the scene of the accident, was intubated and placed on full mechanical support. He was weaned from the ventilator in an acute care facility approximately 14 days after the accident and tracheostomized for long-term management of his respiratory insufficiency. A size #6 cuffed Shiley tracheostomy tube was placed. AG was placed on trach collar with an FIO_2 of 35%. Two weeks later, AG was able to tolerate room air. He was considered stable and ready for transfer to a specialized tracheostomy and ventilator unit for rehabilitation services. He had an involved family who visited him daily. Prior to his accident, AG was employed as a private detective. He was a college graduate and was living in a second-floor apartment with his girlfriend. Regarding his leisure interests, AG enjoyed sports, not only as a spectator, but as a player.

B. Presenting Status on Evaluation

1. AG's Continuum of Disability

Table 9-6 illustrates AG's presenting status during the assessment at bedside. AG presented with quadriplegia. Head and slight shoulder movement was available. His speech and voice function was characterized by aphonia with good mouthing. With deflation of the tracheostomy tube cuff and occlusion of the tracheostomy tube, his voice was judged to be hoarse with moderately reduced vocal volume and monopitch. Breath support for speech was poor. His average maximum sustained phonation time was 2 seconds. AG's cognitive-linguistic ability was within normal limits. Behaviorally, he reported mild anxiety but could be easily reassured. AG was fed via nonoral methods on admission. He had several episodes of aspiration pneumonia in the acute care facility and was fed via NG tube. A dysphagia workup was pending. Oral secretion management was adequate. On admission, the patient did not require frequent suctioning of secretions.

2. Needs Assessment

AG was highly motivated to participate in therapy to improve his voice quality and initiate oral feedings. His goal was to resume the greatest degree of independence possible. Communicative locations included all areas within and outside of the hospital accessible to AG in his chair and in all positions in

Table 9-6. Continuum of Disability: "AG." (Adapted from "Continuum of Disability" by C. Salciccia, 1986. In C. Salciccia, L. Adams, & G. Kapassakis, *Communication Management of Respiratorily-Involved Quadriplegic Adults*. Paper presented at Goldwater Memorial Hospital, New York, NY.)

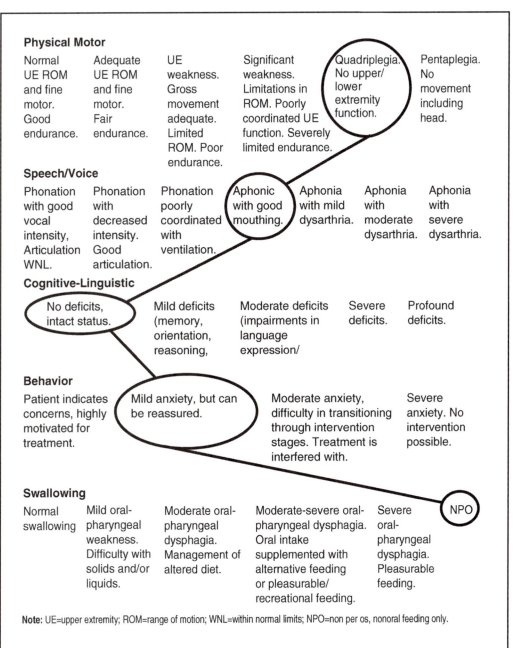

Physical Motor

Normal UE ROM and fine motor. Good endurance.	Adequate UE ROM and fine motor. Fair endurance.	UE weakness. Gross movement adequate. Limited ROM. Poor endurance.	Significant weakness. Limitations in ROM. Poorly coordinated UE function. Severely limited endurance.	Quadriplegia. No upper/ lower extremity function.	Pentaplegia. No movement including head.

Speech/Voice

Phonation with good vocal intensity, Articulation WNL.	Phonation with decreased intensity. Good articulation.	Phonation poorly coordinated with ventilation.	Aphonic with good mouthing.	Aphonia with mild dysarthria.	Aphonia with moderate dysarthria.	Aphonia with severe dysarthria.

Cognitive-Linguistic

No deficits, intact status.	Mild deficits (memory, orientation, reasoning,	Moderate deficits (impairments in language expression/	Severe deficits.	Profound deficits.

Behavior

Patient indicates concerns, highly motivated for treatment.	Mild anxiety, but can be reassured.	Moderate anxiety, difficulty in transitioning through intervention stages. Treatment is interfered with.	Severe anxiety. No intervention possible.

Swallowing

Normal swallowing	Mild oral-pharyngeal weakness. Difficulty with solids and/or liquids.	Moderate oral-pharyngeal dysphagia. Management of altered diet.	Moderate-severe oral-pharyngeal dysphagia. Oral intake supplemented with alternative feeding or pleasurable/ recreational feeding.	Severe oral-pharyngeal dysphagia. Pleasurable feeding.	NPO

Note: UE=upper extremity; ROM=range of motion; WNL=within normal limits; NPO=non per os, nonoral feeding only.

bed. With tracheal occlusion AG could make his needs known orally; however, independent tracheal occlusion was not possible secondary to his physical motor status. Therefore, he was aphonic and could not call for help. The standard call system was inaccessible to him. He could not use his upper extremities for writing. Communication partners consisted of his family and friends, staff, and other patients throughout the hospital. Many other patients in the hospital were also quadriplegic and could not assist AG in accessing a method of message transfer such as a manual communication board. AG's method of message transfer had to be as independent as possible.

C. Diagnostic Intervention

1. Stages of Communication Intervention

a. Call buzzer

AG could not access the standard nursing call buzzer. The occupational therapist and the speech-language pathologist assessed AG with several switches that could be utilized to call for help when in bed. A sip and puff or pneumatic switch was selected, given AG's intact oral control and good secretion management. The switch was connected to a flexible gooseneck arm and clamped onto the side rail of the bed. This was easily removed and repositioned as AG was turned in the bed.

b. ENT evaluation

Given AG's presenting vocal symptoms of hoarseness and reduced volume, an assessment by otolaryngology was indicated to obtain objective information regarding the status of the airway, as well as for clearance for voice therapy. Direct fiberoptic evaluation of the laryngeal mechanism revealed a 2-mm anterior chink or opening of the vocal folds on phonation. The arytenoid cartilages were edematous. This appeared to be secondary to intubation trauma. No evidence of pooled secretions was noted. The otolaryngologist gave clearance for voice treatment, cuff deflation, trial speaking valve use, and hyperfunctional voice techniques to facilitate vocal fold approximation.

c. Tracheostomy tube change

Voice therapy focused on occlusion of the tracheostomy tube for utilization of the upper airway. Prior to initiating treatment, AG's tracheostomy tube was changed to a cuffless size #6. The tube type was changed to allow more airflow through the system and reduce drag during laryngeal elevation. Although AG received nonoral feedings due to a history of aspiration-related pneumonia, secretion management was good and was not a deterrent in removing the cuff.

d. Speaking valve

A speaking valve was attempted almost immediately. AG required his communicative partner to occlude the tracheostomy tube to allow for voice production. In an effort to reduce the need for manual occlusion and provide AG with an immediate means of communicating orally and independently, a Passy-Muir speaking valve was utilized. To monitor SaO_2 levels, oximetry was used during placement attempts. Clinically, he was considered at low risk for CO_2 retention due to his intact cognitive status and lack of any intrinsic lung disease. AG tolerated his initial valve placement for 25 to 30 minutes before his work of breathing increased and O_2 saturation decreased from baseline. He adjusted easily to a more normalized exhalation pattern. The patient did report fatigue after the initial valve placement. Daily treatment sessions continued to focus on gradually increasing wear time until AG was able to tolerate valve use during all waking hours. AG was able to reach this goal within 3 months.

e. Voice therapy

AG wore the speaking valve during voice therapy. Voice therapy involved techniques to facilitate increased vocal fold closure. Common hyperfunctional methods, described by Froeschels, Kastein, and Weiss (1955), involving interlocking the fingers and pulling in opposite directions or pushing against a stable surface such as a table or wall, could not be utilized secondary to AG's physical-motor disability. Instead, AG was cued to phonate an /i/, and push his head against the clinician's hand placed on his forehead. In another technique, downward pressure was placed on his shoulders as AG pushed upward while phonating. Modeled production of a hard glottal attack was used to demonstrate better voice production (Aronson, 1985). Singing scales and producing falsetto were used to achieve vocal fold approximation and laryngeal elevation. Speech instrumentation was especially useful in working with pitch and loudness parameters. This provided AG with visual feedback to assist him in discriminating between inadequate and improved voicing. The Visipitch™ interfaced with the computer provided the clinician with data to compare treatment sessions and monitor AG's progress in pitch (frequency) and loudness (amplitude).

Breath support for speech was reduced. Phrenic nerve dysfunction was confirmed with EMG studies performed by the physiatrist. Exercises to improve speech intelligibility and vocal loudness were initiated. AG was instructed in using phrasing techniques to maximize breath support during an extended utterance. He was cued to "take a breath between every three words and then continue with the sentence." An oral manometer (U-tube manometer) was also utilized for estimating the subglottal air flow and providing visual feedback during the treatment task (Netsell & Hixon, 1978). Incentive spirometry was utilized to improve breath support and facilitate better subglottic air pressure and diaphragmatic support. AG's maximum sustained phonation was 2 seconds on admission, but increased to 20 seconds over 10 months of treatment. The physiatrist prescribed a diaphragmatic binder to further assist breath support during the day.

f. Electronic communication system for written communication

AG was exposed to several methods of computer access for written communication. He was initially instructed in dual switch Morse code via a sip and puff switch. A dedicated portable communication device was used during the instruction phases of treatment. AG used Morse code with fair effectiveness; however, his motivation for a written communication method was limited. He reported that writing was not a priority for him while in the hospital and he decided not to pursue further training in computer access at that time.

2. Stages of Swallowing Intervention

a. Fiberoptic evaluation of swallowing 1

AG was very anxious to remove the NG tube and resume oral feedings. On admission, a fiberoptic evaluation of swallowing was performed to observe AG's ability to manage small (1 teaspoon) size boluses of blue-colored water and applesauce. Oral management was within normal limits. Adequate elevation of the velopharynx was observed. The patient triggered a timely pharyngeal swallow. AG presented with reduced laryngeal elevation that, in the absence of any other significant neurological symptomatology (i.e., brainstem involvement), may have been related to laryngeal fixation secondary to the tracheostomy tube. Bilateral retention of the bolus in the pyriform sinuses was noted. Aspiration of the blue material was evident after the swallow. Aspiration was also suspected during the swallow secondary to blue-tinged material noted on the vocal folds. Intermittent wet vocal quality was also noted while the aspiration was observed. AG was cued to cough and clear the airway; however, his cough was weak and not effective as a clearance mechanism. Placement of the speaking valve assisted the patient to generate a more productive cough. However, use of the speaking valve did not significantly change the results of the fiberoptic study. The patient could not safely manage even small amounts of food orally. AG was instructed to utilize a supraglottic swallow and Mendelsohn maneuver during the evaluation to assess their effectiveness for protecting the airway. Initially, AG could not use these strategies well. It appeared difficult for him to coordinate airway closure with a swallow. The patient continued to practice these strategies in therapy sessions.

b. **Videofluoroscopic evaluation 1**

The initial videofluoroscopic evaluation was performed to confirm and elaborate on the information obtained via the fiberoptic evaluation. Testing was performed with and without tracheal occlusion to determine if any improvement in pharyngeal transit and airway clearance was evidenced. Regardless of occlusion, AG presented with severe pharyngeal dysphagia characterized by retention of the contrast material in the pyriform sinuses, decreased laryngeal elevation, aspiration during and after the swallow, and poor airway clearance. Indirect dysphagia treatment was recommended given the poor management of even a 1-cc size bolus. Focusing on postural techniques and compensatory strategies was suggested. With the neurological history of unconsciousness at the time of the injury the patient's dysphagia was considered related to anoxic encephalopathy, the intubation trauma, interference from the tracheostomy tube and nasogastric tube, and general deconditioning. AG refused a PEG and continued to receive his nutrition and hydration through the NG tube.

c. **Fiberoptic evaluation of swallowing 2**

Six weeks of intensive dysphagia treatment incorporated techniques to facilitate vocal fold closure, eliminate the laryngeal chink, and improve laryngeal excursion and airway clearance. A repeat fiberoptic swallowing examination was then performed. Results of this examination indicated not only closure of the anterior chink, but no aspiration of the dyed semisolid bolus before and after the swallow. There was no evidence of aspiration during the swallow. A repeat videofluoroscopic evaluation was then recommended to obtain detailed information regarding the pharyngeal stage of the swallow and determine if oral feedings could be initiated.

d. **Videofluoroscopic evaluation 2**

The results of the second videofluoroscopic evaluation revealed a significant improvement from the previous evaluation. The study was performed with a speaking valve, which AG wore during most waking hours, in place. AG continued to present with a moderate dysphagia characterized by decreased pharyngeal transit and continued risk of aspiration. There was no actual aspiration during the study, although the patient was at significant risk of aspiration after the swallow due to retained pharyngeal material. With minimal bolus sizes of 3–5 cc there was laryngeal penetration, which AG cleared upon clinician cuing. The concern was that AG would aspirate quantities larger than a 5-cc bolus. In light of his history of aspiration and weakened pulmonary defenses, it was recommended that AG continue nonoral feedings. However, he began direct dysphagia treatment using small (1- to 2-cc boluses) of thickened liquids under the supervision of the speech-language pathologist. A repeat study was suggested in 3 weeks.

e. Patient and family education

The techniques used in indirect dysphagia treatment were incorporated into a direct therapy program. Over the course of a 45-minute treatment session the patient was initially given 2 to 3 teaspoons of semisolid boluses. This gradually increased to one quarter/one half cup of semisolids and thick liquids. Clinical techniques were used to monitor aspiration, including the use of dyed consistencies, cervical auscultation, and intermittent monitoring of vocal quality. In addition, strategies were introduced to begin the process of transitioning AG toward oral feeding. The manual cough technique was demonstrated to assist AG in secretion or bolus clearance. The patient was instructed in self-discriminating between wet and clear voice in order to appropriately utilize laryngeal clearing techniques. Physical therapy instructed the patient's family in percussion techniques to assist in clearing any food or secretions from the airway, as well as to maintain satisfactory pulmonary health. As AG began to take increased amounts of oral intake, compensatory swallowing techniques were taught to family members and unit staff for reinforcement.

f. Videofluoroscopic evaluation 3

After approximately 3 weeks of additional treatment addressing the above clinical signs, a follow-up videofluoroscopic evaluation was performed to document swallowing function. Since this was the third assessment for this patient, this evaluation was kept to minimum amount of radiation exposure. It was important to document adequate airway protection before removing the nasogastric tube. This brief reevaluation documented improved pharyngeal clearance of the bolus and no aspiration or laryngeal penetration. Therefore, AG began an oral diet of soft solids and nectar-thickened liquids. His nasogastric tube was removed. Over the next 6 months, AG was advanced from semisolids and thickened liquids to a regular diet.

One year after admission, AG was discharged to his mother's home with 24-hour nursing assistance. The apartment had been fully renovated to allow for wheelchair accessibility and independent living.

D. Intervention: Home Care

1. Environmental Control/Computer Access

Following discharge home, AG was seen by therapists representing all of the rehabilitative disciplines to ensure that his needs were met in his new environment. The occupational therapist and speech-language pathologist worked closely with the rehabilitation engineer to install an environmental control unit. This allowed AG to control his immediate surroundings including the lights, the door, the radio, the bed position, and emergency calling system. The rehabilitation team worked to assist AG in computer and on-line bulletin board access and written communication. The team selected voice-activated software, which allowed this quadriplegic patient full computer access.

2. Decannulation

AG exhibited no signs of aspiration over the latter part of his hospital stay and while at home. He wore a speaking valve all waking hours, demonstrated adequate airway protection and no longer needed the tracheostomy tube for pulmonary toilet. Approximately 1 month after returning home, AG's tracheostomy tube was capped. He was decannulated 2 weeks later.

AG lived at home and maintained his independence with a motorized wheelchair, computer system, and adaptive devices. Over the years he had multiple hospital admissions related to bowel obstruction and urinary retention. He died at age 41, secondary to complications from these problems.

VII. PATIENT JW

A. Background History

1. Setting: Subacute Ventilator Unit

JW was a 74-year-old male admitted to Silvercrest Extended Care Facility, Subacute Ventilator Unit, following coronary artery bypass graft (CABGx2) with subsequent respiratory failure and inability to wean secondary to multiple medical complications. Contributory history included COPD. The patient was tracheostomized in the acute care setting. A PEG was also placed about 2 weeks after the CABGx2. The patient was fed totally by nonoral methods. He was admitted to Silvercrest with a ventilation mode of AC 12. He had a #8 (Shiley) tracheostomy tube in place, cuffed and nonfenestrated. He was tolerating some trials off the ventilator during the day, although his CO_2 did trend upwards after several hours. This appeared at least partly related to increasing anxiety, verbalized by the patient. JW had a long history of cigarette smoking and noncompliance with cardiac lifestyle modifications. He was unmarried and retired from the construction business. He had a nephew who was involved in his care.

B. Presenting Initial Status on Evaluation

1. JW's Continuum of Disability

Table 9-7 illustrates JW's status at the beginning of the initial assessment process. JW presented with functional physical-motor abilities. Endurance was limited. Daily activities, including dressing, created increased work of breathing. JW was aphonic when receiving mechanical ventilation and dysphonic when receiving oxygen via T-piece ventilation. Cognitive-linguistic status was intact. In terms of behavior, the patient exhibited mild anxiety but could be reassured. As noted, he was NPO, receiving all nutrition via PEG. There was no premorbid history of dysphagia.

2. Needs Assessment

JW's communication needs related primarily to the limitations of his physical endurance. Until he was strong enough to attend physical therapy, his communication locations included his room (in and out of bed) and the activity room of the subacute unit. Occasionally, he would visit the main dining room of the facility, which doubled as an activity center for movies and musical events. When receiving mechanical ventilation, he was able to write legibly but preferred to mouth words. As he entered the weaning process, he was off the ventilator for longer periods of time and was able to communicate via vocal methods. He was moderately dysphonic.

C. Diagnostic Intervention

1. Stages of Communication Intervention

JW's communication goals were discussed weekly during team rounds. As the speech-language pathologist explored communication options, these were presented to the team for carryover by all disciplines.

a. Speaking valve use

JW did well in the weaning process and advanced rapidly to T-piece ventilation for most waking hours, about 8:00 A.M. to 8:00 P.M. He received 5 liters of oxygen. He tolerated cuff deflation without difficulty. A speaking valve (Passy-Muir speaking valve 2001) was placed by the speech-language pathologist after receipt of a physician's order and discussion with the respiratory care practitioner. The patient did not have difficulty

Table 9-7. Continuum of Disability "JW." (Adapted from "Continuum of Disability" by C. Salciccia, 1986. In C. Salciccia, L. Adams, & G. Kapassakis, *Communication Management of Respiratorily-Involved Quadriplegic Adults*. Paper presented at Goldwater Memorial Hospital, New York, NY.)

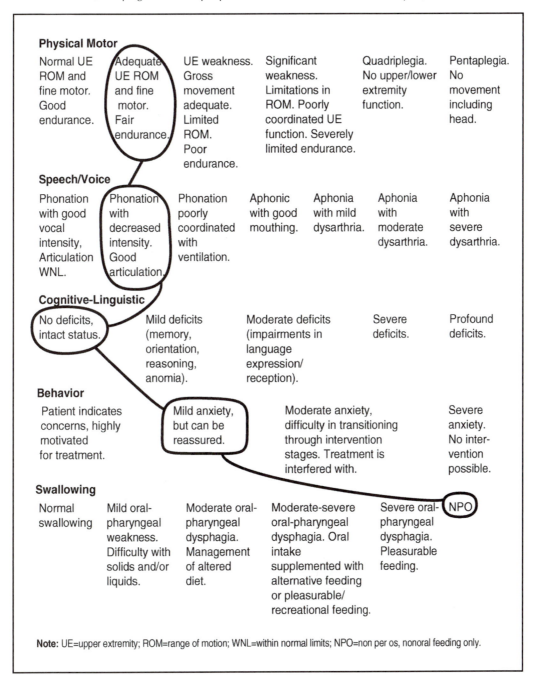

Physical Motor

Normal UE ROM and fine motor. Good endurance.	Adequate UE ROM and fine motor. Fair endurance.	UE weakness. Gross movement adequate. Limited ROM. Poor endurance.	Significant weakness. Limitations in ROM. Poorly coordinated UE function. Severely limited endurance.	Quadriplegia. No upper/lower extremity function.	Pentaplegia. No movement including head.

Speech/Voice

Phonation with good vocal intensity, Articulation WNL.	Phonation with decreased intensity. Good articulation.	Phonation poorly coordinated with ventilation.	Aphonic with good mouthing.	Aphonia with mild dysarthria.	Aphonia with moderate dysarthria.	Aphonia with severe dysarthria.

Cognitive-Linguistic

No deficits, intact status.	Mild deficits (memory, orientation, reasoning, anomia).	Moderate deficits (impairments in language expression/reception).	Severe deficits.	Profound deficits.

Behavior

Patient indicates concerns, highly motivated for treatment.	Mild anxiety, but can be reassured.	Moderate anxiety, difficulty in transitioning through intervention stages. Treatment is interfered with.	Severe anxiety. No intervention possible.

Swallowing

Normal swallowing	Mild oral-pharyngeal weakness. Difficulty with solids and/or liquids.	Moderate oral-pharyngeal dysphagia. Management of altered diet.	Moderate-severe oral-pharyngeal dysphagia. Oral intake supplemented with alternative feeding or pleasurable/recreational feeding.	Severe oral-pharyngeal dysphagia. Pleasurable feeding.	NPO

Note: UE=upper extremity; ROM=range of motion; WNL=within normal limits; NPO=non per os, nonoral feeding only.

with valve placement during this time. Baseline oximetry and capnography measures remained stable at SaO_2 of 97%, PCO_2 of 42, and a pulse rate of 92. Voice quality was slightly improved with valve use, and vocal volume was definitely increased. However, the patient could not wear the valve for longer than approximately 20 minutes without complaining of shortness of breath. He did not demonstrate changes in the noninvasive monitoring measures. As it was theorized that the size of the current tracheostomy tube was affecting the exhaled airflow, the tracheostomy tube was downsized. JW tolerated a #6 Shiley tracheostomy tube without difficulty and wore the valve for extended hours during the day. He was also able to begin physical therapy off the ventilator, wearing his speaking valve, when given frequent rest periods. Oxygen saturation was monitored via pulse oximetry.

The patient was then evaluated for speaking valve use while he was on the ventilator. This was done to facilitate communication with the evening staff and the patient's nephew, who visited primarily at night. The transition to valve use was not difficult; assessment was done after the tracheostomy tube was downsized, and the patient tolerated the valve for 25 minutes during the initial trial. Oximetry measures remained steady at 98% and PCO_2 increased only slightly from 42 to 45, acceptable for this patient. There were no special ventilator modifications needed.

b. Weaning to room air/tracheostomy capping

JW continued in the weaning protocol. He was transitioned to continuous positive airway pressure (CPAP) ventilation at night, with pressure support of 10. This was gradually reduced until he was ready for T-piece trials at night. After 72 hours without ventilatory support, he was pronounced officially weaned. He wore his speaking valve without difficulty during this time. The next goal was to reduce the amount of oxygen the patient received. This was reduced very slowly as the patient was assessed with noninvasive monitoring tools. His weaning to room air coincided with the interventions for swallowing described below. After about 4 months, he was weaned to room air. Since he was taking an oral diet well, without signs and symptoms of aspiration, he was transferred to a step-down unit and entered the capping protocol. His first trial of tracheostomy tube capping, monitored by a respiratory care practitioner, was completed without difficulty for a full 12 hours. About the same time that the PEG was removed, he tolerated capping for a full 24 hours. The tracheostomy tube was successfully removed.

2. Stages of Swallowing Intervention

a.   As noted, JW was admitted with a PEG in place. There was no premorbid history of dysphagia. A clinical swallowing evaluation was largely unremarkable. Oromotor structure and function were within normal limits. There were no overt difficulties demonstrated with ice chip swallows colored with blue dye, also used as an initial screening tool to assess ability to tolerate cuff deflation. A small puree bolus was also used in the initial screening. The blue dye screening was also negative for this consistency. However, when the speech-language pathologist checked the blue dye tracking sheet the day after the assessment, a positive result had been noted hours after the clinical evaluation. Nursing had suctioned moderate amounts of blue-dyed secretions mixed with puree from the patient's tracheostomy tube. Continued tube feeding was recommended. A fiberoptic assessment of swallowing was scheduled after consultation with the patient's pulmonologist. Because the patient felt quite discouraged by his inability to begin oral intake, he was seen by the facility psychologist for counseling and support.

b. The fiberoptic swallowing evaluation was performed with the patient off the ventilator (receiving oxygen via T-piece ventilation), fully deflated and with the Passy-Muir speaking valve in place. It was observed that when the examination started, the patient's heart rate increased and oxygen saturation decreased. The scope was removed. JW's oxygen flow was increased to 7 liters for the duration of the assessment. The respiratory care practitioner was asked to join the otolaryngologist and speech-language pathologist for the test. The patient was reassured, and oxygen increased to 98% saturation while heart rate stabilized. The examination continued. There was redness observed near the arytenoids. There was no evidence for pooled secretions. The patient managed an ice chip bolus without penetration or aspiration. Vocal folds were mobile. JW demonstrated a timely pharyngeal swallow and mild-moderate residue (vallecular and pyriform sinus) with semisolids and thick liquids. There was no initial penetration or aspiration, but after several swallows of the semi-solid, material re-entered the pharynx from the area of the pharyngo-esophageal segment. This material was not swallowed again. Rather, it was seen to penetrate and subsequently was aspirated. There was visible patient response in the form of a cough, but subglottic residue was viewed in the trachea, below the vocal cords (a 7 on the penetration-aspiration scale). Oral feeding was not recommended at this time. Because the issue appeared related to a potential esophageal component, a modified barium swallow was recommended.

c. The modified barium swallow was ordered by the primary care physician and scheduled at the affiliated acute care facility, on an outpatient basis. That examination conducted by speech pathology and radiology revealed functional oral preparation, good bolus transit, a timely swallow, and mild vallecular pooling of a thin liquid bolus. The liquid was given in graduated amounts, beginning with a 1-cc bolus, as per the protocol suggested by Logemann (1998). There was no primary aspiration. As larger amounts of liquids were given, they were also followed through the esophagus. There was significant stasis of liquid contrast in the cervical esophagus. There were tertiary, nonpropulsive contractions throughout the body of the esophagus. The tortuous pattern of the esophageal body suggested spasm. Intraesophageal reflux was seen, followed by sudden, extreme retrograde flow of liquid into the pharynx. A small amount of aspiration occurred, followed by coughing. Due to concern with further aspiration risk, the patient's esophagus was not assessed in a supine or side-lying position as would have been typical for the radiologist to recommend. Rather, the radiologist and speech-language pathologist suggested referral to gastroenterology for possible endoscopy and further motility testing.

d. JW's case was discussed with his primary care physician who agreed to a consultation with gastroenterology. The patient was referred to the assistant director of the Gastroenterology Department, also director of the GI Motility Laboratory. He reviewed the videotape and films from the modified barium swallow and esophagram with the speech-language pathologist and radiologist. He recommended direct visualization of the esophagus via endoscopy and motility testing via manometry. To expedite the examinations and reduce patient fatigue from traveling, both examinations were conducted on the same day. Endoscopy was significant for laryngeal and pharyngeal edema, gastritis, and a tortuous esophagus. Manometry findings revealed a major esophageal motility disorder consistent with esophageal spasm. The gastroenterologist and primary care physician decided on a course of medication, specifically calcium channel blockers, given 20 to 30 minutes prior to meals. After approximately 2 weeks, limited oral intake of liquids was begun. The patient initially experienced a feeling of fullness after even a few swallows of liquid. Medications were adjusted. The patient gradually tolerated more liquids by mouth. Tube feedings were decreased. Semisolids were introduced conservatively during supervised feedings. Eventually, while continuing medication, the patient advanced to a full oral diet of soft solids. He was educated on symptoms of reflux and monitored his rate of intake carefully. Approximately 5 months after his initial assessment, his PEG was removed.

JW's physical status improved rapidly as he was transitioned to more normal oral intake and weaned from the ventilator and tracheostomy. This was at least partially related to his emotional status, greatly enhanced by his progress. He continued physical therapy and increased his endurance significantly. JW was discharged from the extended care facility to an assisted living environment about 8 months after his admission.

VIII. TRACHEOSTOMIZED AND VENTILATOR-DEPENDENT PATIENTS: ETHICAL CONCERNS

A. Informed Consent

The cases in this chapter clearly illustrate the typical management scenario for tracheostomized and ventilator-dependent patients. The speech-language pathologist may recommend repeated diagnostic procedures as the patient moves through the Continuum of Disability. As a medical professional, the speech-language pathologist may face the ethical challenge of obtaining informed consent from these medically fragile individuals. The term informed consent is often reduced to mutual decision making (Beauchamp & Childress, 1994). True informed consent should be an individual's autonomous authorization of a medical intervention. Beauchamp and Childress (1994) stated that informed consent occurs only if a patient understands and independently authorizes a professional to perform an intervention. They emphasized that "one gives an informed consent to an intervention if (and perhaps and only if) one is competent to act, receives a thorough disclosure, comprehends the disclosure, acts voluntarily, and consents to the intervention" (p. 145). This challenges the speech-language pathologist, who must typically intervene with patients who are communicatively impaired, to ensure that all the elements of true informed consent are met. This pertains to speech pathology procedures such as fiberoptic endoscopic evaluations of swallowing safety, modified barium swallows, and speaking valve placement. However, the speech-language pathologist's role in informed consent for issues such as initiation of enteral feedings cannot be overlooked. As was illustrated through the case example BT, the speech-language pathologist served an important role as a member of the Bioethical Committee, conveying the intentions of the nonvocal patient.

When the speech-language pathologist is involved in clinical research trials, obtaining informed consent receives an even stronger emphasis. This is described by Villa et al. (2001). Managing tracheostomized and ventilator-dependent patients is much more than recommending procedure after procedure. It also means considering the unique needs of the individual and facilitating communication so that the person may participate in autonomous decision making.

10

Building a Program: Competencies to Policies

The development of any new clinical program requires time, coordination, and commitment from a variety of transdisciplinary team members. The development of a coordinated concept of care for the individual who is tracheostomized and/or ventilator dependent will occur only through this effort. Through inservices, team rounds, and during the daily clinical care of the patient, the team begins the education process that will ensure a successful program, one that meets the many needs of this complex population. Regulatory agencies, such as the Department of Health and the Joint Commission on Accreditation of Healthcare Organizations, emphasize comprehensive care planning and an interdisciplinary (transdisciplinary) team approach. This chapter will provide strategies for program development. Policies and procedures that highlight the roles of the many members of the transdisciplinary team will be included.

I. BEGINNING STAGES

A. Transdisciplinary Team Concept

A transdisciplinary team format is one in which all team members use their own expertise to work toward a common goal. After the goal is established, "one or two professionals assume the responsibility of implementing the treatment plan established by the team" (Voicing!, 1994, p. 8.11). For example, if the team wants to encourage an anxious ventilator-dependent patient to engage in recreational activities and leave the hospital room, the recreation therapist takes the primary responsibility of scheduling an event appropriate for the individual. Assistance from nursing (to determine a convenient time during the patient's daily care schedule), respiratory therapy (to place the patient on a portable ventilator with a tank of oxygen), speech pathology (to ensure that the patient has a method of communication), and social service (to reassure a nervous individual and invite a family member) will be requested. The physician will write any appropriate orders. All team members will reinforce the patient's success in attending an out of bed activity.

1. Scope of Practice

In the coordinated concept of care, team members work toward shared goals; however, professionals do not encroach on each other's roles. For example, although the speech-language pathologist and respiratory care practitioner must work together to achieve communication and swallowing goals with the ventilator-dependent patient, they maintain their scope of practice. It is not the role of the speech-language pathologist to change the tracheostomy tube, manipulate the ventilator, or perform tracheostomy care. Similarly, the respiratory care practitioner does not make recommendations regarding communication options or swallowing status. However, an informed respiratory care practitioner would certainly refer an appropriate candidate to a speech-language pathologist for an oral communication assessment. In addition, the speech-language pathologist might suction a patient (according to established facility policy and procedure) during a swallowing evaluation. The goal of the transdisciplinary team is not for team members to replace one another but to work *together* to maximize the patient's potential.

B. Raising Awareness

The transdisciplinary team must work together in establishing a treatment plan for the individual who is tracheostomized and/or ventilator-dependent. Unless key members of the team have an awareness of communication and swallowing issues, these specific problem areas may go unidentified or unaddressed.

1. Targeting Medical Staff to Inservice

Identifying the key members of the team who will aid the process of restoring communication and swallowing function is an initial step in program development. Targeting specific physicians and therapists who are willing to share information and are open to team building is necessary. After team members are targeted, the identification of a team leader is the next step. The team leader must agree with the team philosophy. Often the pulmonologist is identified as an appropriate team leader, as he or she will be able to integrate the pulmonary needs of the patient with the intervention necessary to maximize communication and swallowing. The process of inservicing may begin with daily clinical visits to a model patient who requires intervention and coordinated management in a variety of areas. Discussions with team members at bedside will allow the clinician to explain the rationale for communication intervention. As other issues arise, more formal inservice training can be scheduled. For example, the process of cuff deflation for oral communication can take place with the pulmonologist, respiratory care practitioner, nurse, and speech-language pathologist. Issues pertaining to maintenance of mechanical ventilation in the presence of deflated cuffs can be discussed further during a scheduled lecture.

2. Promoting Benefits of Communicative Intervention with This Population

Enticing team members with one illustrative, model case example is often the most effective way to highlight communication and swallowing issues. As each team member is exposed to the benefits of restoring communication and swallowing function, referrals for other cases will arise. Identification of potential patients for intervention occurs when team members have an understanding of what services the speech-language pathologist can provide. A successful case will make everyone aware that individuals who are tracheostomized and/or ventilator dependent may be able to communicate orally. Communication not only enhances the patient's quality of life, but can facilitate interaction with all team members. For example, the social worker will be able to communicate with the patient and obtain detailed information regarding advanced directives, the nurse can be quickly alerted to the patient's immediate needs, and the recreational therapist can integrate the patient into group activities.

C. Integration of the Transdisciplinary Team

The function of the transdisciplinary team is to create the treatment care plan. The team must review and prioritize the information from each discipline's assessment. For example, while the speech-language pathologist's initial recommendation is to downsize the tracheostomy tube to increase airflow for phonation, the respiratory care practitioner may wish to begin the weaning process. At the same time, the psychologist is concerned about decreasing the patient's anxiety through group therapy. It may not be possible to achieve these individual goals simultaneously. The team must determine the next action step together, ensuring that the needs of the resident, not the needs of each discipline, take precedence. Coordination and prioritization are best achieved during transdisciplinary team rounds.

1. Vent Team

The Vent Team is the group of individuals who meet during weekly and monthly rounds to:

- identify patient specific needs.
- establish a mission statement for the facility regarding the care of these complex patients.
- problem solve difficult cases and prioritize intervention strategies.

- identify the need for specific policies and procedures.

- introduce new clinical concepts and equipment.

- update the plan of care and establish appropriate treatment goals.

As was discussed in Chapter 9, the team consists of medical, allied medical, and rehabilitation professionals. The Vent Team meets in two separate forums, clinical care rounds and administrative team meetings.

a. Clinical care rounds

Clinical care rounds are held weekly to discuss and, at times, implement specific intervention techniques. Each member signs in. The team assigns a secretary to take the minutes regarding each patient's case. The previous week's minutes are available for review to ensure that prior suggestions and recommendations were implemented. The team may discuss each case at the patient's bedside or round via chart reviews. For each patient, the team leader facilitates discussion regarding many issues, including current ventilator settings, tolerance of modifications made to the ventilator or tracheostomy tube, current weight, status of oral intake, recommendations made by consultants, laboratory and x-ray results, and an action plan for the coming week. The patient often participates in this discussion by bringing questions and concerns to the team's attention. Physician orders for consultation from specialists or for introduction of a new medication are written during rounds. The team begins to prioritize goals and works to develop a schedule to implement strategies and intervention techniques. For example, in an extended care setting, the recreation therapist may work with nursing and respiratory therapy to determine the most optimal time for an out-of-bed leisure activity. The three disciplines might coordinate the daily care schedule with the proposed activity, place the resident on a portable ventilator, use a speaking valve in-line, and ensure that a suction machine is available at all times during the scheduled event.

Clinical care rounds are generally conducted for 1 to 1½ hours for approximately 20–25 tracheostomized and/or ventilator-dependent patients. During the initial stages, the rounds may be lengthy as each team member becomes familiar with the coordinated concept of care. In acute care settings, a predetermined list of patients can be sent to each discipline for review prior to rounds to expedite discussion of individuals who may be scattered throughout the hospital. In this setting, an increased number of team members can have input and take part in the team round with a minimum expenditure of time. For example, a list of individuals is reviewed by the respiratory therapy department, and during a staff meeting, each respiratory care practitioner is asked for input. The department representative who participates in the clinical care rounds may thus share information regarding an individual's readiness for weaning or possible evaluation for speaking valve use. This format can expedite discussion of a large number of individuals who may not be physically together in the hospital. However, the coordinated concept can be honored and information shared among team members.

b. Administrative team meetings

In addition to the clinical care team members, an administrative representative can often assist in initial policy making and support during administrative team meetings. In this forum, an administrative representative joins the transdisciplinary team to discuss specific issues. In addition to facilitating policy making decisions, participation in team meetings can ensure that the facility administration understands the special needs of this patient population. Administrative team meetings, held monthly, are often co-led by the leader of the clinical care rounds and administrative representative. Initial administrative meetings may occur bimonthly as policies and procedures are being created and reviewed. Prior to the administrative team meetings, an agenda is prepared. Each team member submits items for discussion such as purchase of a new piece of equipment, staffing concerns, or review of a new policy and procedure. During administrative team rounds the team leader facilitates discussion pertaining to agenda items. Table 10-1 illustrates a sample agenda from an initial administrative team meeting during the program development of a specialized unit for tracheotomized and ventilator-dependent patients. This agenda can be contrasted to the agenda shown in Table 10-2. At this point the team, with basic policy and procedures established, dealt with issues beyond the day-to-day operation of the unit. Thus, resident quality of life as well as continuing education for staff were the focus of the agenda.

Normally, direct patient care issues would not be discussed. However, if specific problems with patient care cannot be managed during the clinical care forum, they may be aired during the more formal discussion group. For example, at Silvercrest Extended Care Facility, the problem of patients who refuse to leave their rooms was discussed at the administrative meetings because it was a recurring theme during the clinical care rounds. From these discussions it was decided that a psychologist would be an essential addition to the team, at least in a consultant role. On the administrative level, funds were designated to make these services available to residents. The psychologist is now not only consulted to treat patients, but participates in clinical care rounds to discuss behavioral issues and management strategies.

Table 10-1. Sample Agenda: Administrative Vent Team Meeting (Initial Meeting).

Silvercrest Extended Care Facility
Subject: Vent Team Meeting
Date: August 28, 1992
Time: 2:00 p.m.–4:00 p.m.
Location: Administrative Conference Room

AGENDA

I. Coordination of Care
   A. Clinical Care Rounds
      1. Schedule
      2. Participants
      3. Objectives
      4. Record
   B. Identifying Resident Needs
II. Philosophy of Unit
III. Clarification/Assignment of Duties
IV. Use of Room
V. Equipment
VII. Census

Table 10-2. Sample Agenda: Administrative Vent Team Meeting (Later Stages).

Silvercrest Extended Care Facility
Subject: Vent Team Meeting
Date: January 23, 2002
Time: 2:00 P.M.–3:00 P.M.
Location: Administrative Conference Room

AGENDA

I. Review of minutes from previous meeting. (Administrator)
II. Updated physician coverage schedule. (Medical Director)
III. New portable (weaning) ventilators. (Director Respiratory)
IV. Tracheostomy tube changes—new protocol. (Director Respiratory)
V. Weaning and decannulation protocol. (Director Speech Pathology)
VI. Therapeutic recreation afternoon out of bed schedule for residents. (Director Therapeutic Recreation)
VII. New tube feeding formulary (pressure ulcers). (Chief Dietitian)

During administrative team meetings, opportunities for formal inservices and lectures are scheduled. Topics are often generated during both clinical care rounds and administrative team meetings. Team members also can distribute pertinent articles and references for discussion. The scheduling of team visits to other facilities may also take place. Administrative team meetings are generally 1 to 1½ hours in length. Less time may be spent in meetings as major policies are set and successfully implemented. In the acute care setting, this type of meeting may be feasible only in the formative stages of team development. It may be more typical of the extended care facility model. In the acute care setting the team attempts to identify tracheostomized and ventilator-dependent patients throughout the facility and determine their appropriateness for the ventilator unit. This facilitates more appropriate specialized care as well as expedites transfer to a subacute rehabilitation setting for ongoing weaning.

II. SPEECH PATHOLOGY COMPETENCIES

Speech-language pathologists as well as allied medical professionals must develop and adhere to competencies in their fields. The tracheostomized and ventilator-dependent population demands specific competencies that ensure the safe and appropriate treatment of the patient. Suggested competencies would include but not be limited to the following topics.

A. Safety

Examples include suctioning (oral and tracheal); general ability to troubleshoot a ventilator (e.g., reset alarm, check battery and tubing) and read a gauge on an oxygen tank; manual resuscitation and care of patients with IV lines, ventilator tubing, and oxygen masks.

B. Monitoring

Examples include assessing a patient's response to treatment via pulse oxymetry, capnography, and auscultation; ability to assess and describe clinical signs and symptoms to appropriate staff (nursing, physician).

C. Knowledge

Examples include working knowledge and clinical skills in the area of medical speech pathology, including anatomy and physiology and disease processes; the impact of tracheotomy and ventilator dependence upon speech and swallowing; understanding the limitations of the clinical assessment and the applicability of an objective evaluation.

D. Documentation

Examples include obtaining pertinent background information including intubation history, size/type of tracheostomy tube, ventilator settings; writing evaluations and goal setting for this specialized population (taking into account the interrelationship between speech, swallowing, and respiration).

III. POLICY AND PROCEDURES

As a need for specific policies and procedures is identified during clinical care rounds and administrative team meetings, each discipline becomes responsible for generating policies and procedures that address the needs of patients who are tracheostomized and ventilator dependent. The following are outlines of policies and procedures used with this population at one specialized tracheostomy and ventilator facility. Clinicians are encouraged to develop more individualized and detailed policies and procedures with their team members to meet the needs of other health care settings.

Title: Fenestrated Inner Cannulas

Policy: Tracheostomy tubes with fenestrated inner cannulas will be available on physician order, as clinically indicated, after evaluation by the speech-language pathologist (SLP) and respiratory care practitioner (RCP).

Purpose: To allow additional airflow through the upper airway for communication and weaning purposes. This occurs when the patient is unable to tolerate downsizing or occlusion of the tracheostomy tube, even after a downsize, does not appear to have sufficient leak around the sides of the tracheostomy tube, and/or requires connection to mechanical ventilation.

Procedure:

1. Members of the Vent Team will identify residents who are having difficulty tolerating occlusion of the tracheostomy tube, who can not be downsized or decannulated, or have insufficient air leak around the sides of the tracheostomy tube.
2. A consult will be generated by the attending physician to otolaryngology if vocal fold status is questionable.
3. An order will be generated to respiratory therapy and speech pathology. The patient will be evaluated for the appropriate tracheostomy tube size by the physician (MD), RCP, and SLP.
4. The RCP will place the recommended tracheostomy tube.
5. The patient will have the nondisposable fenestrated inner cannula placed by respiratory therapy or nursing during the period when oral communication is indicated and during weaning attempts. This will occur only during waking hours. The MD will indicate this in the orders.
6. Nursing will replace the nondisposable fenestrated inner cannula (green hub) with a nondisposable nonfenestrated inner cannula (white hub) after the specified time period (i.e., at night).
7. Nursing will clean the nondisposable inner cannula according to the established nursing policy and procedure (see nursing policy #00000).
8. A speaking valve or decannulation plug will be placed by nursing, respiratory therapy, or speech pathology if indicated and ordered by the attending MD.

Title: Talking Tracheostomy Tubes

Policy: Talking tracheostomy tubes will be available on physician order, as clinically indicated, after evaluation by speech-language pathologist (SLP) and respiratory care practitioner (RCP).

Purpose: To allow oral communication for patients who are unable to tolerate cuff deflation.

Procedure:

1. Members of the Vent Team will identify residents who are unable to tolerate cuff deflation.
2. An order will be generated to speech pathology and respiratory therapy. They will determine the appropriate size and type of the talking tracheostomy tube.
3. The RCP will place the talking tracheostomy tube.
4. The RCP will connect either compressed air or oxygen that is humidified to the external speaking air source. A bottle of sterile water can be used for humidification. Air tubing is used to connect the external air source to the speaking air connector.
5. Speech pathology and respiratory therapy will jointly conduct initial sessions to attach and maintain the air connection and to establish the proper airflow levels. Air flow should not exceed 14 liters.
6. Inservice training of all unit staff will be conducted by speech pathology regarding regulation of airflow for communication. Simple instructions which detail airflow control and manual occlusion of the external port will also be placed above the patient's bed (with patient consent) by speech pathology.
7. The SLP will train the patient in coordinating voice with airflow as per speech pathology treatment regime.
8. The MD will generate an order indicating daily use.

Title: Fiberoptic Evaluation of Swallowing (FEES and FEEST)

Policy: A fiberoptic evaluation of swallowing will be ordered by the primary care physician (MD) and performed by the speech-language pathologist (SLP) and otolaryngologist (ENT) as part of a comprehensive swallowing evaluation.

Purpose: A fiberoptic evaluation of swallowing will be performed for any individual who requires assessment of the oropharyngeal mechanism secondary to suspected pharyngeal stage dysphagia. In addition, these individuals may have limited physical mobility or decreased ability to follow directions that may preclude other assessment procedures (i.e., videofluoroscopy).

(continued)

Procedure:

1. The SLP will identify patients who require a fiberoptic evaluation following a clinical bedside evaluation of swallowing.
2. The MD will order a fiberoptic swallowing evaluation.
3. The primary care physician (MD) will order a consultation from ENT for "swallowing evaluation in joint consultation with speech pathology." Any possible contraindications for the procedure should be discussed at this time.
4. The SLP will bring to the bedside the following equipment: fiberoptic scope, light source, VCR, sensory box, disinfecting solutions, various bolus consistencies, and blue/green food coloring.
5. The ENT typically will meet the SLP at the bedside, assist with verifying informed consent, and answer any additional questions from the patient and family.
6. Prior to introduction of the scope, a baseline oxygen saturation level will be obtained via pulse oximetry. Additionally, the patient will be monitored for changes from baseline throughout the evaluation.
7. The ENT or SLP will introduce the fiberoptic scope transnasally. ENT and SLP will observe velopharyngeal closure, appearance of hypopharynx at rest, swallowing of saliva, presence of pooled secretions, respiration (abduction), airway protection (adduction), and phonation (abduction/adduction).
8. The patient's ability to tolerate a longer examination incorporating sensory testing is determined. Sensory testing is conducted prior to bolus feeding. Thresholds are obtained bilaterally.
9. The examination begins with dyed ice chips presented to the patient to rule out gross aspiration of secretions. In this case, the study may be halted unless therapeutic maneuvers can be utilized. The patient would also be suctioned.
10. The SLP will administer various dyed bolus consistencies in graduated size boluses. Amounts will be increased unless aspiration occurs.
11. The SLP will instruct the patient in therapeutic maneuvers during appropriate points in the examination to determine the efficacy of these techniques.
12. ENT will document results of the laryngeal examination on the consultation form.
13. SLP will write dysphagia evaluation results in the integrated progress notes and on a consultation form and indicate a recommendation for oral or nonoral feeding status with further dysphagia follow-up.
14. SLP will alert MD, nursing, and dietary services of the results of the examination.

Source: Adapted from Langmore, S. F. (2001). *Endoscopic Evaluation and Treatment of Swallowing Disorders.* New York: Thieme; and from Aviv, J. E., Kim, T., Thomson, J. E., Sunshine, S., Kaplan, S., & Close, L. G. (1998). Fiberoptic Endoscopic Evaluation of Swallowing with Sensory Testing (FEESST) in Healthy Controls. *Dysphagia, 13,* 87–92.

Title: Speaking Valves

Policy: Speaking valves will be available on physician order, as clinically indicated, after evaluation by speech pathology and respiratory therapy.

Purpose: Speaking valves will be provided to tracheostomized and ventilator-dependent patients who are considered candidates for oral communication.

Procedure:

1. The primary care physician (MD) will generate an order for a speaking valve evaluation.
2. The speech-language pathologist (SLP) and respiratory care practitioner (RCP) will schedule a joint session to obtain baseline objective measurements of oxygen saturation, carbon dioxide levels, and heart rate. Any possible contraindications will be discussed at this time. Additionally, the patient will be monitored for changes from baseline throughout evaluation.
3. The SLP and RCP will follow cuff deflation protocol to allow for airflow through the upper airway as well as modifications to the ventilator if indicated.
4. The otolaryngologist (ENT) will be consulted by the primary care physician (MD) if voice production is considered inadequate.
5. The SLP or RCP will place the speaking valve on the 15 mm hub of the tracheostomy tube.
6. The SLP will begin instruction in voicing techniques to facilitate coordination of phonation with respiration.
7. The MD will generate an order based on recommendations from the SLP and RCP for daily wear schedule. Wear schedule will be indicated on care plan and nursing treatment sheets.
8. For tracheostomized patients, once routine wear schedule is established, the nursing care assistant (CNA) can place the valve for the specified amount of time.
9. For ventilator-dependent patients, the RCP will place the speaking valve and make necessary modifications to the ventilator.

Title: Speaking Valve Cleaning Procedure

Policy: All speaking valves will be cleaned daily by primary nursing care assistants (CNA).

Purpose: To ensure proper functioning and fulfill lifetime use (2 months), the speaking valve should be cleaned daily.

Procedure:

1. Daily cleaning can be accomplished with warm water and any fragrance-free soap.
2. After the valve is removed, it should be rinsed in warm water and placed in the storage container with the lid open to air dry.
3. Lifetime of the valve with proper cleaning should be at least 2 months. Residents who use the valve daily or for extended periods can be issued two valves so that if one is in the cleaning cycle, another is available for use.
4. Valves should not be cleaned with nonapproved solutions (e.g., peroxide, bleach, vinegar, or alcohol). They should not be brushed or autoclaved.
5. Valves that are kept in the Speech Pathology office are cleaned by the speech pathologist. Valves on the units are cleaned daily by nursing and respiratory staff. This is noted on the daily nursing and respiratory treatment sheets.

Title: Blue Dye Test

Policy: A blue dye test will be performed, by the speech-language pathologist (SLP), for tracheostomized individuals who are considered at risk for gross aspiration.

Purpose: To detect gross aspiration of secretions or food.

Procedure:

1. The physician (MD) will order a blue dye assessment.
2. The SLP will place two to three drops (total) of blue food coloring with one to two ice chips on the patient's tongue or (for oral feeders) mixed in food to allow observation of this material in suctioned contents.
3. The nurse (RN) will be notified that the test has been performed. A blue dye test 24-hour tracking sheet will be placed at the patient's bedside.
4. Observation of any blue material obtained via the tracheostomy tube will be noted. Immediately following intake of food or swallowed saliva, the patient will be suctioned by the SLP or RN. Negative or positive findings will be documented on the blue dye test tracking sheet which will be located at the patient's bedside.
5. The patient will then be suctioned in 15–30 minute intervals for up to 2 hours by the SLP, RN, or respiratory care practitioner (RCP). Negative or positive findings during these periods or at any time will be documented on the tracking sheet. Time of suctioning will also be recorded. The primary care physician (MD) will be notified of results immediately.
6. The SLP will then make appropriate recommendations regarding the patient's gross airway protection status, potential for full/ongoing tracheostomy tube deflation, and candidacy for objective swallowing assessment.
7. Patients who are tolerating oral diets will have additional blue dye screenings with each consistency of food in their current diet prior to any diet upgrade. The amount of blue dye is kept to 1–2 drops per bolus.

IV. CONCERNS AND CLINICAL ISSUES

Initial attempts to coordinate the transdisciplinary team through clinical care rounds and administrative team meetings often trigger questions and concerns by administrators regarding time expenditure of participants. Weekly and monthly rounds do require time commitment from each member of the transdisciplinary team; however, the cost benefit easily outweighs the time allotment.

A. Performance Improvement

Ongoing performance improvement is part of good clinical practice. Moreover, it is mandated by regulatory agencies that review performance improvement plans during survey. Speech pathology performance improvement projects with the tracheostomized and ventilator-dependent population require the team approach stressed repeatedly throughout this text. Dikeman and Kazandjian's (2001) most recent performance improvement effort focused on cleaning of speaking valves. It became apparent that there was no standard system to ensure routine cleaning of the valves. The speaking valves were being cleaned in many different ways throughout the facility. An interdisciplinary project work group was formed to address this issue. A system that was neither complicated nor time consuming, but met the manufacturer's requirements was put into place to clean valves. This addressed infection control concerns and ensured longevity of the project. This performance improvement project includes regular follow-up to ensure training of new staff and reevaluation of the effectiveness of the current system.

B. Cost Benefits

1. Justification of Speech Pathology Services

The speech-language pathologist on the ventilator unit must capture time spent through statistics, even if the majority of patients will fall under all-inclusive payment systems, such as the prospective payment system (PPS). In these cases individual services cannot be billed. However, speech pathologists who keep careful statistics can support their time spent working with tracheostomized and ventilator-dependent patients with appropriate documentation. This might include number of patients transitioned from tube feeding to oral intake or any decrease in transfers from subacute settings to acute care for aspiration-related pneumonias. Evidence-based practice and outcome surveys are an essential part of this process. Kazandjian and Dikeman (2000) developed a practical dysphagia outcome survey measure on a subacute ventilator unit to both validate speech pathology services and meet performance improvement requirements. The dysphagia outcome survey was designed to compare the patients' perceived quality of life pre- and post-dysphagia treatment. Additionally, any change in their nonoral feeding status was correlated with these perceptions. Results of the survey for this group revealed that a patient's swallowing status appeared at least associated with the perception of overall health status. That perception improved after a successful treatment program. Surveys such as these justify speech pathology services as part of a customer service-oriented approach. Speech-language pathologists can develop their own outcome surveys or use validated measures such as the SWAL-QOL (McHorney et al., 2000; McHorney, Bricker, Kramer, Rosenbek, Robbins, Chignell, 2000).

2. Timely Resolution of Treatment Goals

Weekly clinical care rounds ensure that all members of the transdisciplinary team are aware of the complete treatment plan. The coordination of services allows each discipline to proceed to the next action step. For example, when the speech-language pathologist indicates that his or her goal for the week is cuff deflation, the respiratory care practitioner adjusts his or her schedule to coordinate a joint treatment session or works to maximize deflation time for a patient. Both team members will report the results of their intervention at the next clinical care rounds.

3. Less Duplication of Services

Because the transdisciplinary team members are aware of each other's treatment goals, service duplication and overall treatment time are reduced. For example, the patient who is tracheostomized may not require direct supervision with the nurse during weaning attempts because the respiratory care practitioner has already determined safety and a specific amount of wear time for a plug. The nurse needs only to monitor the patient.

C. Enhanced Service Delivery

1. Improved Quality of Life

When the transdisciplinary team coordinates efforts to allow patients to participate in activities important to them, quality of life improves. Birdsall and Gutekunst (1995) noted that in a well-integrated team concept:

> Staff at all levels have incorporated resident advocacy and family support in practice. When new challenges are identified, the staff respond appropriately meeting physiologic, psychologic, social, and spiritual needs of the ventilator residents who choose to come and live at the unit. (p. 43)

The following example illustrates the coordination of the team and a patient's response:

> I wanted to have my hair colored and set. I haven't had it done in the 6 months since I have been sick. My family keeps telling me that I don't

look like myself and to be honest with you, I don't feel like myself when
I look in the mirror.

This patient wanted to participate in the normal activity of keeping an appointment with a beautician. The members of the team including the respiratory care
practitioner, physical therapist, beautician, and nurse discussed how they could
coordinate efforts to allow this patient to have her hair done. Although the
beautician could have come to the patient's bedside for a cut and set, she required access to her salon equipment for coloring. An appointment was made
with the beautician in the facility. Extra time and space were allotted to accommodate the patient, ventilator, respiratory care practitioner, and suction equipment. The physical therapist provided a special chair with a back support that
could be removed for easy utilization of the beautician's sink. The respiratory
care practitioner adjusted his schedule so that he could help transport the patient and monitor her respiratory status. The nursing assistant accompanied the
patient throughout the visit. These team members worked together to ensure
that the patient could feel more positive about her appearance and improve her
quality of life while ventilator dependent in an extended care setting.

2. Overall Improved Service Delivery

Clinicians who do not work together as a team are not able to meet their individual goals. For example, the speech-language pathologist cannot place a
speaking valve in-line without the direct assistance and coordination of the
respiratory care practitioner. A transdisciplinary team effort allows the patient
to receive optimal care and to reach treatment goals in a timely manner.

R

References

Adams, L., & Connolly, M. A. (1993). Nonvocal treatments for short term and long term ventilator patients. In M. Mason (Ed.), *Speech pathology for the tracheostomized and ventilator dependent patient* (pp. 288–335). Newport Beach, CA: Voicing!

Adams, L., & Kazandjian, M. (2001). Managing communication and swallowing difficulties. In H. Mitsumoto & T. L. Munsat (Eds.), *Amyotrophic lateral sclerosis* (133–150). New York: Demos Medical Publishing.

Adler, J. A., & Zeides, J. (1986). Evaluation of the electrolarynx in the short-term hospital setting. *Chest, 89*(3), 407–409.

Adran, G. M., & Kemp, F. H. (1952). The protection of the laryngeal airway during swallowing. *British Journal of Radiology, 25,* 406–416.

Alba, A. (1986, Winter). Frog breathing can mean more time on your own. *Accent on Living,* pp. 74–76.

Alba, A., & Pilkington, L. A. (1984). Neuromuscular disease with respiratory insufficiency. In A. P. Ruskin (Ed.), *Current therapy in physiatry* (pp. 341–346). Philadelphia: W. B. Saunders.

Alba, A., Pilkington, L. A., Kaplan, E., Baum, J., Schultheiss, M., Ruggieri, A., & Lee, M. (1976, November/December). Long term pulmonary care in ALS. *Respiratory Therapy.*

American Speech-Language-Hearing Association, Ad Hoc Committee on Advances in Clinical Practice. (1992a). Instrumental diagnostic procedures for swallowing. *ASHA, 34*(7), 25–33.

American Speech-Language-Hearing Association, Ad Hoc Committee on Advances in Practice. (1992b). Sedation and topical anesthetics in audiology and speech-language pathology. *ASHA, 34*(7), 41–46.

American Speech-Language-Hearing Association, Ad Hoc Committee on Use of Specialized Medical Speech Devices. (1993). Position statement and guidelines for the use of voice prostheses in tracheostomized persons with or without ventilatory dependence. *ASHA, 36*(10), 17–20.

Andrews, M. L. (1999). *Manual of voice treatment: Pediatrics through geriatrics* (2nd ed.). Clifton Park, NY: Singular.

Aronson, A. E. (1985). *Clinical voice disorders: An interdisciplinary approach* (2nd ed.). New York: Thieme.

Arvedson, J. C., & Brodsky, L. (1993). *Pediatric swallowing and feeding: Assessment and management.* Clifton Park, NY: Singular Publishing Group.

Aviv, J. E., Kim, T., Thomson, J. E., Sunshine, S., Kaplan, S., & Close, L. G. (1998). Fiberoptic endoscopic evaluation of swallowing with sensory testing (FEESST) in healthy controls. *Dysphagia, 13,* 87–92.

Aviv, J. E., Martin, J. H., Keen, M. S., Debell, M., & Blitzer, A. (1993). Air pulse quantification of supraglottic and pharyngeal sensation: A new technique. *Annals of Otolaryngology, Rhinology, and Laryngology, 102*(10), 777–780.

Bach, J. R. (1993). Mechanical insufflation-exsufflation: Comparison of peak expiratory flows with manually assisted and unassisted coughing techniques. *Chest, 104*(5), 1553–1561.

Bach, J. R. (1996). Pathophysiology of paralytic-restrictive pulmonary syndromes. In J. R. Bach (Ed.), *Pulmonary rehabilitation: The obstructive and paralytic conditions* (pp. 275–284). Philadelphia: Hanley and Belfus.

Bach, J. R., & Alba, A. (1990a). Tracheostomy ventilation: A study of efficacy with deflated cuffs and cuffless tubes. *Chest, 97,* 679–683.

Bach, J. R., & Alba, A. (1990b). Noninvasive options for ventilatory support of the traumatic high level quadriplegic patient. *Chest, 98,* 613–619.

Bach, J. R., Alba, A., Bohatiuk, G., Saporito, L., & Lee, M. (1987). Mouth intermittent positive pressure ventilation in the management of postpolio respiratory insufficiency. *Chest, 91*(6), 859–864.

Bach, J. R., Alba, A., Mosher, R., & Delaubier, A. (1987). Intermittent positive pressure ventilation via nasal access in the management of respiratory insufficiency. *Chest, 92,* 168–170.

Bach, J. R., & Ishikana, Y. (2000). Respiratory insufficiency: Pathophysiology, indications, and other considerations for intervention. In D. Tippet (Ed.), *Tracheostomy and ventilator dependence* (pp. 29–45). New York: Thieme Medical Publishers.

Baken, R. J., & Orlikoff, R. F. (2000). *Clinical measurement of speech and voice.* Clifton Park, NY: Singular.

Balestrieri, F., & Watson, C. B. (1982). Intubation granuloma. *Otolaryngologic Clinics, 15,* 567–579.

Bastian, R. W. (1993). The videoendoscopic swallowing study: An alternate and partner to the videofluoroscopic swallowing study. *Dysphagia, 8,* 359–367.

Beauchamp, T. L., & Childress, J. F. (1994). *Principles of biomedical ethics* (4th ed.). New York: Oxford University Press.

Beckford, N. S., Mayo, R., Wilkinson, A., & Tierney, M. (1990). Effects of short-term endotracheal intubation on vocal function. *Laryngoscope, 100,* 331–336.

Bell, S. D. (1996, February). Use of the Passy-Muir tracheostomy speaking valve in mechanically ventilated neurological patients. *Critical Care Nurse, 16*(1), 63–68.

Beukelman, D. R., Yorkston, K. M., & Dowden, P. A. (1985). *Communication augmentation: A casebook of clinical management.* San Diego, CA: College-Hill Press.

Birdsall, C., & Gutekunst, M. (1995). Preparing staff for opening a new ventilator unit in long-term care. *Journal of Gerontological Nursing, 21*(5), 39–43.

Bishop, M. (1989). Mechanisms of laryngotracheal injury following prolonged tracheal intubation. *Chest, 96*(1), 185–186.

Bishop, M. J., Weymuller, E. A., & Fink, B. R. (1984). Laryngeal effects of prolonged intubation. *Anesthesiology Analogs, 63,* 335–342.

Bloodstein, O. (1979). *Speech pathology: An introduction.* Boston: Houghton Mifflin.

Bolton, P., & Kline, K. (1994, June). Understanding modes of mechanical ventilation. *American Journal of Nursing,* pp. 36–42.

Bonanno, P. C. (1971). Swallowing dysfunction after tracheotomy. *Annuals of Surgery, 174,* 29–33.

Bone, D. K., Davis, J. L., Zuidema, G. D., & Cameron, J. L. (1974). Aspiration pneumonia: Prevention of aspiration in patients with tracheostomies. *Annals of Thoracic Surgery, 18,* 30–37.

Borgstrom, P. S., Olsson, R., Sundkuist, S., & Ekberg, O. (1988). Pharyngeal and oesophageal function in patients with diabetes mellitus and swallowing complaints. *British Journal of Radiology, 61*(729), 817–821.

Bosma, J. F. (1992). Development and impairments of feeding in infancy and childhood. In M. Groher (Ed.), *Dysphagia diagnosis and management* (2nd ed., pp. 107–141). Stoneham, MA: Butterworth-Heinemann.

Brantigan, C. O., & Grow, J. B. (1976). Cricothyroidotomy: Elective use in respiratory problems requiring tracheostomy. *Journal of Thoracic and Cardiovascular Surgery, 71*(1), 72–80.

Brantigan, C. O., & Grow, J. B. (1980). Cricothyroidotomy revisited again. *Ear, Nose and Throat, 59*(6), 26–38.

Britton, D., Jones-Redmond, J., & Kasper, C. (2001). The use of speaking valves with ventilator dependent and tracheostomy patients. *Current Opinion in Otolaryngology & Head and Neck Surgery, 9,* 147–152.

Brook, A. D., Sherman, G., Malen, J., & Kollef, M. H. (2000). Early versus late tracheostomy in patients who require prolonged mechanical ventilation. *American Journal of Critical Care, 9*(5), 352–359.

Cameron, J. L., Reynolds, J., & Zuidema, G. D. (1973). Aspiration in patients with tracheostomies. *Surgical Gynecological Obstetrics, 136,* 68–70.

Casper, J. K., & Colton, R. H. (1993). *Clinical manual for laryngectomy and head and neck cancer rehabilitation.* Clifton Park, NY: Singular.

Chang, D. W. (2001). *Clinical application of mechanical ventilation* (2nd ed.). Clifton Park, NY: Delmar Learning.

Chi-Fishman, G., & Sonies, B. C. (2000, October). *Kinematic strategies in task accommodation: Discrete versus rapid sequential swallowing.* Paper presented at the Ninth Annual Dysphagia Research Society Meeting, Savannah, GA.

Cole, R., & Aguilar, E. (1988). Cricothyroidotomy versus tracheostomy: An otolaryngologist's perspective. *Laryngoscope, 98,* 131–135.

Colice, G. L. (1992). Resolution of laryngeal injury following translaryngeal intubation. *American Review of Respiratory Disease, 145,* 361–364.

Colice, G. L., Stukel, T. A., & Dain, B. (1989). Laryngeal complications of prolonged intubation. *Chest, 96,* 877–884.

Colodny, N. (2001). Effects of age, gender, disease, and multisystem involvement on oxygen saturation levels in dysphagic persons. *Dysphagia, 16,* 48–57.

Conetta, R., Barman, A. A., Iakovou, C., & Masakayan, R. J. (1993). Ventilatory failure from massive subcutaneous emphysema. *Chest, 104,* 978–980.

Conlan, A. A., & Kopec, S. E. (2000). Tracheostomy in the intensive care unit. *Journal of Intensive Care Medicine, 15,* 1–13.

Cook, I. J., Dodds, W. J., Dantas, R. O., Kern, M. K., Massey, B. T., Shaker, R., & Hogan, W. J. (1989). Timing of videofluoroscopic manometric events and bolus transit during the oral and pharyngeal phases of swallowing. *Dysphagia, 4,* 8–15.

Dikeman, K., Kazandjian, M., & Chua, R. (2000). Evaluation of the patient with impaired pulmonary function and dysphagia. In R. H. Mills (Ed.), *Evaluation of dysphagia in adults* (pp. 239–282). Austin, TX: Pro-Ed.

Donen, N., Tweed, W. A., Dashfsky, S., & Guttormson, B. (1983). The esophageal obturator airway: An appraisal. *Canadian Anaesthesiology Society Journal, 30,* 194–200.

Downs, A. M. (1996). Physiological basis for airway clearance techniques. In D. Frownfelter & E. Dean (Eds.), *Principles and practice of cardiopulmonary physical therapy* (3rd ed., pp. 321–338). St. Louis, MO: Mosby.

Drinker, P. A., & Krupoff, S. (1981). *Eyelink for non-vocal communication.* Paper presented at the Fourth Annual Conference on Rehabilitation Engineering, Washington, DC.

Edgar, J. D. (1994). *Meal related patterns of respiration and deglutition in patients with COPD.* Unpublished doctoral dissertation, University of Minnesota, Minneapolis.

Eibling, D. E., & Diez-Gross, R. D. (1996). Subglottic air pressure: A key component of swallowing efficiency. *Annals of Otology, Rhinology, and Laryngology, 105*(4), 253–258.

Ellis, E. R., Bye, P. T. P., Bruderer, J. W., & Sullivan, C. E. (1987). Treatment of respiratory failure during sleep in patients with neuromuscular disease. *American Review of Respiratory Disease, 135,* 148–152.

Escourrou, P. J. L., Delaperche, M. F., & Visseaux, A. (1990). Reliability of pulse oximetry during exercise in pulmonary patients. *Chest, 97,* 635–638.

Eubanks, D., & Bone, R. C. (1990). *Comprehensive respiratory care: A learning system* (2nd ed.). St. Louis, MO: C. V. Mosby.

Fagon, J., Chastre, J., Domart, Y., Trouillet, J., Pierre, J., Darne, C., & Gibert, C. (1989). Nosocomial pneumonia in patients receiving continuous mechanical ventilation. *American Review of Respiratory Disease, 139,* 877–884.

Feldman, S. A., Deal, C. W., & Urquhart, W. (1966). Disturbance of swallowing after tracheotomy. *Lancet, 1,* 954–955.

Fernandez, R., Blanch, L., Mancebo, J., Bonsoms, N., & Artigas, A. (1990). Endotracheal tube cuff pressure assessment: Pitfalls of finger estimation and need for objective measurement. *Critical Care Medicine, 18*(12), 1423–1426.

Feussner, H., Kauer, W., & Siewert, J. R. (1993). The place of esophageal manometry in the diagnosis of dysphagia. *Dysphagia, 8*(2), 98–104.

Fienberg, M. J. (1993). Radiographic techniques and interpretation of abnormal swallowing in adult and elderly. *Dysphagia, 8,* 356–358.

Finucane, B. T., & Santora, A. H. (1988). *Principles of airway management.* Philadelphia: F. A. Davis.

Fishman, A. P. (1980). *Pulmonary diseases and disorders.* New York: McGraw-Hill.

Fishman, I. (1987). *Electronic communication aids and techniques.* Boston, MA: College-Hill Press.

Fleming, R., & Sobel, E. (1997, September). Weaning outcomes and survival on a ventilator unit in a long-term care facility. *Chest, 112*(3), 1295.

Fleming, R., Sobel, E., & Chua, R. (1997, April). Long term care weaning outcome utilizing a respiratory therapist driven protocol. *American Journal of Respira-*

tory and Critical Care Medicine, 155(4), A411.

Fornataro-Clerici, L., & Zajac, D. (1993). Aerodynamic characteristics of tracheostomy speaking valves. *Journal of Speech and Hearing Research, 36,* 529–532.

Fried-Oken, M., Howard, J. M., & Stewart, S. R. (1991). Feedback on AAC intervention from adults who are temporarily unable to speak. *AAC, 7,* 43–50.

Froeschels, E., Kastein, S., & Weiss, D. A. (1955). A method of therapy for paralytic conditions of the mechanisms of phonation, respiration and glutination. *Journal of Speech and Hearing Disorders, 20,* 365–370.

Frownfelter, D., & Dean, E. (1996). *Principles and practice of cardiopulmonary physical therapy* (3rd ed.). St. Louis, MO: Mosby-Year Book.

Gilardeau, C., Kazandjian, M. S., Bach, J. R., Dikeman, K. J., Willig, T. N., & Tucker, L. M. (1995). The evaluation and management of dysphagia. *Seminars in Neurology, 15*(1), 46–51.

Groher, M. E. (Ed). (1992). *Dysphagia: Diagnosis and management* (2nd ed.). Stoneham, MA: Butterworth-Heinemann.

Groher, M. E. (1994). Determination of the risks and benefits of oral feeding. *Dysphagia, 9,* 233–235.

Groher, M. E. (2000). The case history. In R. H. Mills (Ed.), *Evaluation of dysphagia in adults* (pp. 1–26). Austin, TX: Pro-Ed.

Gross, R. G., Dettlebach, M. A., Zajac, D. J., & Eibling, D. E. (1994, September). *Measure of subglottic air pressure during swallowing in a patient with tracheostomy.* Paper presented at Annual Convention of the American Academy of Otolaryngology—Head and Neck Surgery, San Diego, CA.

Hamlet, S., Muz, J., Farris, R., Kumpuris, T., & Jones, L. (1992). Scintigraphic quantification of pharyngeal retention following deglutition. *Dysphagia, 7*(1), 12–16.

Hamlet, S., Penney, D. G., & Formolo, J. (1994). Stethoscope acoustics and cervical auscultation of swallowing. *Dysphagia, 9,* 63–68.

Hammon, W. E., & Martin, R. J. (1989). Chest physical therapy for acute atelectasis. *Physical Therapy, 59,* 1247–1248.

Heffner, J. E. (1989). Medical indications for tracheostomy. *Chest, 96*(1), 186–190.

Heffner, J. E. (1993). Timing of tracheotomy in mechanically ventilated patients. *American Review of Respiratory Disease, 147,* 768–771.

Heffner, J. E., Miller, S., & Sahn, S. A. (1986a). Tracheostomy in the intensive care unit. Part 1: Indications, technique, management. *Chest, 90*(2), 269–274.

Heffner, J. E., Miller, S., & Sahn, S. A. (1986b). Tracheostomy in the intensive care unit. Part 2: Complications. *Chest, 90*(3), 430–436.

Hendrix, T. (1993). Art and science of history taking in the patient with difficulty swallowing. *Dysphagia, 8,* 69–73.

Hess, D., Schlottag, A., Levin, B., Mathai, J., & Rexrode, W. O. (1991). An evaluation of the usefulness of end-tidal PCO_2 to aid weaning from mechanical ventilation following cardiac surgery. *Respiratory Care, 36,* 837–843.

Hough, A. (1991). *Physiotherapy in respiratory care: A problem solving approach.* London: Chapman & Hall.

Huckabee, M., & Pelletier, C. (1999). *Management of adult neurogenic dysphagia.* Clifton Park, NY: Singular.

Hudson, J. C., & Mills, R. H. (2000). Dental aspects of swallowing. In R. H. Mills (Ed.), *Evaluation of dysphagia in adults* (pp. 207–238). Austin, TX: Pro-Ed.

Huxley, E. J., Viroslav, J., Gray, W. R., & Pierce, A. K. (1978). Pharyngeal aspiration in normal adults and patients with depressed consciousness. *American Journal of Medicine, 64,* 564–568.

Ideno, K., Koghnali, H., Leachman, R., Rigs, S., Zeluff, S., Kolmansberger, B., Clark, M., & Adams, S. (1991). *Green discoloration phenomenon in a tube-fed patient.* ASPEN 15th Clinical Congress Conference Proceedings, 373. Silver Spring, MD.

Jubran, A., & Tobin, M. J. (1994). Monitoring gas exchange during mechanical ventilation. In M. J. Tobin (Ed.), *Principles and practice of mechanical ventilation* (pp. 919–944). New York: McGraw-Hill.

Kazandjian, M., & Dikeman, K. (1990, April). *Communication intervention with the ventilator dependent patient.* The ventilator: Psychosocial and medical aspects. Paper presented at the Foundation of Thanatology, Columbia Presbyterian Medical Center, New York, NY.

Kazandjian, M. S., & Dikeman, K. J. (1993). Transdisciplinary team concept. In M. Mason (Ed.), *Speech pathology for the tracheostomized and ventilator dependent patient* (pp. 256–287). Newport Beach, CA: Voicing!

Kazandjian, M. S., & Dikeman, K. J. (1998). Communication options for tracheostomy and ventilator-dependent patients. In E.N. Meyers, J. Johnson, & T. Murry (Eds.). *Tracheostomy: Airway management, communication and swallowing* (pp. 97–118). Clifton Park, NY: Singular.

Kazandjian, M., & Dikeman, K. (2000, November). *Developing a dysphagia outcome survey measure in a subacute/extended care setting.* Paper presented at the American Speech-Language Hearing Association Annual Convention, Washington, DC.

Kazandjian, M. S., Dikeman, K. J., & Adams, E. (1991, November). *Communication management of the ventilator-dependent and tracheostomized patient.* Paper presented at Annual Convention of the American Speech-Language-Hearing Association, Atlanta, GA.

Kazandjian, M. S., Dikeman, K. J., & Bach, J. R. (1995). Assessment and management of communication impairment in neurological disease. *Seminars in Neurology, 15*(1), 52–59.

Kent, R. (1997). *The speech sciences.* Clifton Park, NY: Singular.

King, S. A. (1994). The tracheostomized patient: Tracheal toilet and speech. *Clinical Pulmonary Medicine, 1*(6), 365–368.

Kirsch, C. M., & Sanders, A. (1988). Aspiration pneumonia: Medical management. *Otolaryngologic Clinics of North America, 21*(4), 677–689.

Kost, K. M. (1998). Tracheostomy in the intensive care setting. In. E. N. Myers, J. Johnson, &

T. Murry (Eds.), *Tracheostomy: Airway management, communication and swallowing* (pp. 75–96). Clifton Park, NY: Singular.

Laitman, J. T., & Reidenberg, J. S. (1993). Comparative and developmental anatomy. *Dysphagia, 8,* 318–325.

Langer, M., Mosconi, P., Cigada, M., Mandelli, M., & The Intensive Care Unit Group of Infection Control. (1989). Long-term respiratory support and risk of pneumonia in critically ill patients. *American Review of Respiratory Disease, 140,* 302–305.

Langmore, S. (1993, April). *Integrating fiberoptic endoscopy (FEES) into the assessment, treatment and management of dysphagia.* Paper presented at Annual Convention of the New York Speech-Language-Hearing Association, Lake Kiamesha, NY.

Langmore, S. (1996). Dysphagia in neurologic patients in the intensive care unit. *Seminars in Neurology, 16*(4), 329–340.

Langmore, S. (2000). Fiberoptic endoscopic evaluation of swallowing. In R. H. Mills (Ed.), *Evaluation of dysphagia in adults.* Austin, TX: Pro-Ed.

Langmore, S. (2001). *Endoscopic evaluation and treatment of swallowing disorders.* New York: Thieme.

Langmore, S., Schatz, K., & Olsen, N. (1988). Fiberoptic endoscopic examination of swallowing safety: A new procedure. *Dysphagia, 2,* 216–219.

Law, J. H., Barnhart, K., Rowlett, W., de la Rocha, O., & Lowenberg, S. (1993). Increased frequency of obstructive airway abnormalities with long-term tracheostomy. *Chest, 104*(1), 136–138.

Law, R. C., Carney, A. S., & Manara, A. R. (1997). Long-term outcome after percutaneous dilational tracheostomy. *Anaesthesia, 52,* 51–56.

Lazarus, C. L., Logemann, J. A., Rademaker, A. W., Kahrilas, P. J., Pajek, T., Lazar, R., & Halper, A. (1993). Effects of bolus volume, viscosity, and repeated swallows in nonstroke subjects and stroke patients. *Archives of Physical Medicine and Rehabilitation, 74,* 1066–1070.

Lazzara, G., Lazarus, C., & Logemann, J. A. (1986). Impact of thermal stimulation on the triggering of the swallowing reflex. *Dysphagia, 3,* 189–191.

Le, H. M., Aten, J. L., Chiang, J. T., & Light, R. W. (1993). Comparison between conventional cap and one-way valve in the decannulation of patients with long-term tracheostomies. *Respiratory Care, 38*(11), 1161–1167.

Leder, S. B. (1990). Verbal communication for the ventilator dependent patient: Voice intensity with the Portex "talk" tracheostomy tube. *Laryngoscope, 100,* 1116–1121.

Leder, S. B. (1991). Prognostic indicators for successful use of "talking" tracheostomy tubes. *Perceptual and Motor Skills, 73,* 441–442.

Leder, S. B. (1994). Perceptual rankings of speech quality produced with one-way tracheostomy speaking valves. *Journal of Speech and Hearing Research, 37,* 1308–1312.

Leder, S. (1996a, March–April). Gag reflex and dysphagia. *Head and Neck, 18*(2), 138–141.

Leder, S. B. (1996b). Comment on Thompson-Henry and Braddock: The modified Evan's blue dye procedure fails to detect aspiration in the tracheostomized patient: Five case reports. *Dysphagia, 11,* 80–81.

Leder, S. B. (1997). Videofluoroscopic evaluation of aspiration with visual examination of the gag reflex and velar movement. *Dysphagia, 12,* 21–23.

Leder, S. B., Joe, J. K., Hill, S. B., & Traube, M. (2001). Effect of tracheostomy tube occlusion on upper esophageal sphincter and pharyngeal pressures in aspirating and nonaspirating patients. *Dysphagia, 16,* 79–82.

Leder, S. B., & Ross, D. A. (2000). Investigation of the causal relationship between tracheotomy and aspiration in the acute care setting. *Laryngoscope, 110,* 641–644.

Leder, S. B., Tarro, J. M., & Burrell, M. I. (1996). Effect of occlusion of a tracheostomy tube on aspiration. *Dysphagia, 11,* 254–258.

Leder, S. B., & Traquina, D. T. (1989). Voice intensity of patients using a COMMUNItrach I® cuffed speaking tracheostomy tube. *Laryngoscope, 99,* 744–747.

Leverment, J. N., Pearson, F. G., & Rae, S. (1976). A manometric study of the upper esophagus in the dog following cuffed tube tracheostomy. *British Journal of Anaesthesiology, 48,* 83–89.

Levine, S. P., Koester, D. J., & Kett, R. L. (1987). Independently activated talking tracheostomy systems for quadriplegic patients. *Archives of Physical Medicine and Rehabilitation, 68,* 571–573.

Levine, S. A., & Niederman, M. S. (1991). The impact of tracheal intubation on host defenses and risks for nosocomial pneumonia. *Clinics in Chest Medicine, 12*(3), 523–543.

Levitzky, M. G. (1982). *Pulmonary physiology.* New York: McGraw-Hill.

Levitzky, M. G., Cairo, J. M., & Hall, S. M. (1990). *Introduction to respiratory care.* Philadelphia: W. B. Saunders.

Logemann, J. A. (1993, April). *Management of tracheostomy tubes, intubation, ventilators during swallowing assessment and treatment.* Paper presented at Special Consultations in Dysphagia, Northern Speech Services, Chicago, IL.

Logemann, J. A. (1998). *Evaluation and treatment of swallowing disorders* (2nd ed.). Austin, TX: Pro-Ed.

Long, J., & West, G. (1981). The Olympic Trach-Button as an interim airway following tracheostomy tube removal. *Respiratory Care, 26*(12), 1269–1272.

Maloney, J.; Halbower, A.; Fouty, B.; Fagan, K.; Balasubramaniam, V.; Pike, A.; Moss, M. (2000). Systematic absorption of food dye in patients with sepsis. *New England Journal of Medicine. 343* (14), 1047–1048.

Manzano, J. L., Lubillo, S., Henriquez, D., Martin, J. C., Perez, M. C., & Wilson, D. J. (1993). Verbal communication of ventilator dependent patients. *Critical Care Medicine, 21*(4), 512–517.

Marsh, H., Gillespie, D., & Baumgartner, A. (1989). Timing of tracheostomy in the critically ill patient. *Chest, 96*(1), 190–192.

Martin, B. J. W. (1991, October). *Advances in the understanding of swallowing and respiratory function.* Paper presented at Swallowing and Swallowing Disorders: From Clinic to Laboratory Conference, Northwestern University, Evanston, IL.

Martin, B. J. W. (1994, October). *Biomechanical and temporal characteristics of laryngeal closure in patients with pulmonary disease.* Paper presented at the Third Annual Dysphagia Research Society Meeting, McLean, VA.

Martin, B. J. W., Logemann, J. A., Shaker, R., & Dodds, W. J. (1993). Normal laryngeal valving patterns during three breath-hold maneuvers: A pilot investigation. *Dysphagia, 8,* 11–20.

Martin, B. J. W., Logemann, J. A., Shaker, R., & Dodds, W. J. (1994). Coordination between respiration and swallowing: Respiratory phase relationships and temporal integration. *Journal of Applied Physiology, 76,* 714–723.

Martin, B. J. W., & Robbins, J. (1995). Physiology of swallowing: Protection of the airway. *Seminars in Respiratory and Critical Care Medicine, 16*(6), 448–458.

Martin, R. E., Letsos, P., Taves, D. H., Inculet, R. L., Johnston, H., & Preiksaitis, H. G. (2001). Oropharyngeal dysphagia in esophageal cancer before and after transhiatal esophagectomy. *Dysphagia, 16,* 23–31.

Mason, M. (Ed). (1993). *Speech pathology for tracheostomized and ventilator dependent patients.* Newport Beach, CA: Voicing!

Mason, M., Watkins, C., & Romey, P. (1992a, March). *Communication for the tracheostomized and ventilator dependent patient utilizing the Passy-Muir speaking valve.* Paper presented at the Annual Conference of the Respiratory Nursing Society, Anaheim, CA.

Mason, M., Watkins, C., & Romey, P. (1992b). Protocol for use of the Passy-Muir tracheostomy speaking valve. *The European Respiratory Journal, 5*(15), 148–153.

Mayberry, J. C., Goldman, R. K., & Rehm, C. G. (1999, October). Percutaneous tracheostomy in the severely injured patient: Transition from the operating room to the intensive care unit. *Asian Journal of Surgery, 22*(4), 392–397.

Maynard, F. M., & Muth, A. S. (1987). The choice to end life as a ventilator dependent quadriplegic. *Archives of Physical Medicine and Rehabilitation, 68,* 862–864.

McConnel, F. M. S., Cerenko, D., & Mendelsohn, M. S. (1988). Manofluorgraphic analysis of swallowing. *Otolaryngologic Clinics of North America, 21*(4), 625–635.

McHorney, C. A., Bricker, D. E., Kramer, A. E., Rosenbek, J. C., Robbins, J., & Chignell, K. A. (2000). The SWAL-QOL outcomes tool for oropharyngeal dysphagia in adults II: Item reduction and preliminary scaling. *Dysphagia, 15*(3), 122–135.

McHorney, C. A., Bricker, D. E., Kramer, A. E., Rosenbek, J. C., Robbins, J., Chignell, K. A., Logemann, J. A., & Clarke, C. (2000). The SWAL-QOL outcomes tool for oropharyngeal dysphagia in adults I: Conceptual foundation and item development. *Dysphagia, 15*(3), 115–121.

Menon, A. S., Carlin, B. W., & Kaplan, P. D. (1993). Tracheal perforation: A complication associated with transtracheal oxygen therapy. *Chest, 104*(2), 636–637.

Metheny, N. A., & Clouse, R. E. (1997). Bedside methods for detecting aspiration in tube-fed patients. *Chest, 111*(3), 724–731.

Meyer, T. J., & Hill, N. S. (1994). Noninvasive positive pressure ventilation to treat respiratory failure. *Annals of Internal Medicine, 120,* 760–770.

Murray, J., Langmore, S., Ginsberg, S., & Dostie, A. (1996). The significance of accumulated oropharyngeal secretions and swallowing frequency in predicting aspiration. *Dysphagia, 11*(2), 99–103.

Muz, J., Mathog, R. H., Miller, P. R., Rosen, R., & Borrero, G. (1987). Detection and quantification of laryngotracheopulmonary aspiration with scintigraphy. *Laryngoscopy, 97,* 1180–1185.

Muz, J., Mathog, R. H., Nelson, R., & Jones, L. A. (1989). Aspiration in patients with head and neck cancer and tracheostomy. *American Journal of Otolaryngology, 10,* 282–286.

Nash, M. (1988). Swallowing problems in the tracheostomized patient. *Otolaryngologic Clinics of North America, 21*(4), 701–709.

Netsell, R. (1986). *A neurobiologic view of speech production and the dysarthrias.* San Diego, CA: College-Hill Press.

Netsell, R., & Hixon, T. J. (1978). A noninvasive method of clinically estimating subglottal air pressure. *Journal of Speech and Hearing Disorders, 43,* 326–330.

Neumann, S., Bartolome, G., Buchholtz, D., & Prosiegel, M. (1995). Swallowing therapy of neurologic patients: Correlation of outcomes with pretreatment variables and therapeutic methods. *Dysphagia, 10,* 1–5.

Niederman, M., Ferranti, R. D., Ziegler, A., Merrill, W. W., & Reynolds, H. Y. (1984). Respiratory infection complicating long term tracheostomy: The implication of persistent gram-negative tracheobronchial colonization. *Chest, 85*(1), 39–44.

Niederman, M., Merrill, W. M., Ferranti, R. D., Pagano, K. M., Palmer, L. B., & Reynolds, H. Y. (1984). Nutritional status and bacterial binding in the lower respiratory tract in patients with chronic tracheostomy. *Annals of Internal Medicine, 100,* 795–800.

Nilsson, H. Ekberg, O., Bulow, M., & Hindfelt, B. (1996, October). *Assessment of respiration in dysphagic patients.* Paper presented at the Fifth Annual Dysphagia Research Society Meeting, Aspen, CO.

Nishino, T., Yonezawa, T., & Honda, Y. (1985). Effects of swallowing on the pattern of continuous respiration in human adults. *American Review of Respiratory Disease, 132,* 1219–1222.

O'Connor, A. (1994, October). *Influence of eating and drinking on cardiopulmonary function in adults.* Paper presented at the Third Annual Dysphagia Research Society Meeting, McLean, VA.

Oppenheimer, E. A. (1993). Decision-making in the respiratory care of amyotrophic lateral sclerosis: Should home mechanical ventilation be used? *Palliative Medicine, 7*(2), 49–64.

Orenstein, D., Curtis, S. E., Nixon, P. A., & Hartigan, E. R. (1993). Accuracy of three pulse oximeters during exercise and hypoxemia in patients with cystic fibrosis. *Chest, 104*(4), 1187–1190.

Owens, G. R. (1992). Advances in the treatment of chronic obstructive pulmonary disease. *Hospital Formulas, 27,* 1012–1027.

Perkins, W. H., & Kent, R. D. (1986). *Functional anatomy of speech, language and hearing: A primer.* Boston, MA: College-Hill Press.

Perlman, A. L. (1993). Electromyography and the study of oropharyngeal dysphagia. *Dysphagia, 8,* 351–355.

Peruzzi, W. T. (1993, April). *Mechanical ventilatory support.* Paper presented at Special Consultations in Dysphagia, Northern Speech Services, Chicago, IL.

Pickersgill, T., Dawson, K., & Wiles, C. M. (1998, October). *Organization of breathing and swallowing: Abnormal patterns in central and peripheral neurological lesions.* Paper presented at the Seventh Annual Meeting of the Dysphagia Research Society, New Orleans, LA.

Pierce, L. (1995). *Guide to mechanical ventilation and intensive respiratory care.* Philadelphia, PA: W. B. Saunders Co.

Pineda, H. (1984). Pulmonary disorders. In A. P. Ruskin (Ed.), *Current theory in physiatry* (pp. 331–341). Philadelphia: W. B. Saunders.

Pothman, W., Tonner, P. H., & Schulte am Este, J. (1997). Percutaneous dilatational tracheostomy: Risks and benefits. *Intensive Care Medicine, 23,* 610–612

Potts, R. G., Zaroukian, M. D., Guerrero, P. A., & Baker, C. D. (1993). Comparison of blue dye visualization and glucose oxidase test strip methods for detecting pulmonary aspiration of enteral feedings in intubated adults. *Chest, 103*(1), 117–121.

Quartararo, C., & Bishop, M. J. (1990). Complications of tracheal intubation: Prevention and treatment. *Seminars in Anesthesiology, 9*(2), 119–127.

Robbins, J. (2000, October). *Evolution of swallowing over the adult age span.* Paper presented at the Ninth Annual Meeting of the Dysphagia Research Society, Savannah, GA.

Robbins, J., Ramig, L., Shaker, R. (1996, October). *Senescence and swallowing.* Symposia presented at the Fifth Annual Dysphagia Research Society Meeting, Aspen: CO.

Robbins, J., Coyle, J., Rosenbek, J., Roecker, E., & Wood, J. (1999). Differentiation of normal and abnormal airway protection during swallowing using a penetration-aspiration scale. *Dysphagia, 14* (4), 228–232.

Robbins, J., Ramig, L., & Shaker, R. (1996, October). *Senescence and swallowing.* Symposia presented at the Fifth Annual Dysphagia Research Society Meeting, Aspen, CO.

Robbins, M., & Fagerholm, M. (1992, November). *A collaborative role between the speech-language pathologist and the radiologist.* Paper presented at Annual Convention of the American Speech-Language-Hearing Association, San Antonio, TX.

Romney, D. (1987). (Morse code graphics). Unpublished pictorial representation system.

Rosenbek, J. C., Robbins, J., Fishback, B., & Levine, R. L. (1991). Effects of thermal stimulation on dysphagia after stroke. *Journal of Speech and Hearing Research, 34,* 1257–1268.

Rynders, A. (1992). Coordination of deglutition and phases of respiration: Effect of aging, tachypnea, bolus volume and chronic obstructive pulmonary disease. *American Journal of Physiology, 263,* 750–755.

Salciccia, C., Adams, L., & Kapassikis, G. (1986, December). *Communication management of respiratorily-involved quadriplegic adults.* Paper presented at Goldwater Memorial Hospital, New York.

Sasaki, C., Suzuki, M., Horiuchi, M., & Kirshner, J. (1977). The effects of tracheostomy on the laryngeal closure reflex. *Laryngoscope, 87,* 1428–1433.

Scanlan, C. L., Spearman, C. B., & Seldon, R. L. (Eds.), *Egan's fundamentals of respiratory care* (5th ed., pp. 683–699). St. Louis, MO: C. V. Mosby.

Scanlan, C. L. (1990b). Selection and application of ventilatory support devices. In C. L. Scanlan, C. B. Spearman, & R. L. Seldon (Eds.), *Egan's fundamentals of respiratory care* (5th ed., pp. 740–779). St Louis, MO: C. V. Mosby.

Scanlan, C. L., & Gupta, T. L. (1990). Synopsis of cardiopulmonary diseases. In C. L. Scanlan, C. B. Spearman, & R. L. Seldon (Eds.), *Egan's fundamentals of respiratory care* (5th ed., pp. 412–452). St. Louis, MO: C. V. Mosby.

Sellars, C., Dunnet, C., & Carter, R. (1998). A preliminary comparison of videofluoroscopy of the swallow and pulse oxymetry in the identification of aspiration in dysphagic patients. *Dysphagia, 13,* 82–86.

Selley, W. G., Ellis, R. E., Flack, F. C., Bayliss, C. R., Chir, B., & Pearce, V. R. (1994). The synchronization of respiration and swallow sounds with videofluoroscopy during swallowing. *Dysphagia, 9,* 162–167.

Selley, W. G., Flack, F. C., Ellis, R. E., & Brooks, W. A. (1989a). Respiratory patterns associated with swallowing: Part I: The normal adult pattern and changes with age. *Age and Ageing, 18,* 168–172.

Selley, W. G., Flack, F. C., Ellis, R. E., & Brooks, W. A. (1989b). Respiratory patterns associated with swallowing: Part II: Neurologically impaired dysphagic patients. *Age and Ageing, 18,* 173–176.

Shaker, R. (1995). Airway protective mechanisms: Current concepts. *Dysphagia, 10,* 216–227.

Shaker, R. (2000, October). *Functional relationships of the aerodigestive tract.* Paper presented at the Ninth Annual Meeting of the Dysphagia Research Society, Savannah, GA.

Shaker, R., Dodds, W. J., Dantas, R. O., Hogan, W. J., & Arndorfer, R. C. (1990). Coordination of deglutitive glottic closure with oropharyngeal swallowing. *Gastroenterology, 98,* 1478–1484.

Shaker, R., Li, Q., Ren, J., Townsend, W. F., Dodds, W. J., Martin, B. J., Kern, M. K., & Rynders, A. (1992). Coordination of deglutition and phases of respiration: Effect of aging, tachypnea, bolus volume and chronic obstructive pulmonary disease. *American Journal of Physiology, 263,* 750–755.

Siebens, A. A., Tippett, D. C., Kirby, N., & French, J. (1993). Dysphagia and expiratory airflow. *Dysphagia, 8,* 266–269.

Silver, K., & Nostrand, D. (1992). Scintigraphic detection of salivary aspiration: Description of a new diagnostic technique and case reports. *Dysphagia, 7*(1), 45–49.

Simmons, K. F. (1990). Airway care. In C. L. Scanlan, C. B. Spearman, & R. L. Seldon (Eds.), *Egan's fundamentals of respiratory care* (5th ed., pp. 483–512). St. Louis, MO: C. V. Mosby.

Smith, J., Wolkove, N., Colacone, A., & Kreisman, H. (1989). Coordination of eating, drinking and breathing in adults. *Chest, 96,* 578–582.

Snyderman, C. H., Johnson, J. T., & Eibling, D. E. (1994). Laryngotracheal diversion and separation in the treatment of massive aspiration. *Current Opinion in Otolaryngology—Head and Neck Surgery, 2,* 63–67.

Sobel, E., Fleming, R., Chua, R., & Leddy, P. (1998, May). *Age as a predictor of weaning outcome and survival on a ventilator unit in a long term care facility.* Poster presented at the American Geriatric Society Annual Meeting, Seattle, WA.

Sonies, B., & Baum, B. (1988). Evaluation of swallowing pathophysiology. *The Otolaryngologic Clinics of North America, 21*(4), 637–748.

Sottile, F. D., Marrie, T. J., Prough, D. S., Hobgood, C. D., Gower, D. J., Webb, L. X., Coserton, J. W., & Gristina, A. G. (1986). Nosocomial pulmonary infection: Possible etiologic significance of bacteria adhesion to endotracheal tubes. *Critical Care Medicine, 14*(4), 265–270.

Stachler, R. J., Hamlet, S. L., Choi, J., & Fleming, S. M. (1994, September). *Scintigraphic quantification of aspiration with the Passy-Muir valve.* Paper presented at the Annual Convention of the American Academy of Otolaryngology—Head and Neck Surgery, San Diego, CA.

Stachler, R. J., Hamlet, S. L., Choi, J., & Fleming, S. (1996). Scintigraphic quantification of aspiration reduction with the Passy-Muir valve. *Laryngoscope, 106,* 231–234.

Stauffer, J. L., Olson, D. E., & Petty, T. L. (1981). Complications and consequences of endotracheal intubation and tracheostomy. *The American Journal of Medicine, 70,* 65–75.

Takahashi, K., Groher, M. E., & Michi, K. (1994). Symmetry and reproducibility of swallowing sounds. *Dysphagia, 9,* 168–173.

Tamura, F., Shishikura, J., Mukai, Y., & Kaneko, Y. (1999). Arterial oxygen saturation in severely disabled people: Effect of oral feeding in the sitting position. *Dysphagia, 14*(4), 204–211.

Tesoriero, J. V., & Dail, D. H. (1990). Functional anatomy of the respiratory system. In C. L. Scanlan, C. B. Spearman, & R. L. Seldon (Eds.), *Egan's fundamentals of respiratory care* (5th ed., pp. 111–152). St. Louis, MO: C. V. Mosby.

Thompson-Henry, S., & Braddock, B. (1995). The modified Evan's blue dye procedure fails to detect aspiration in the tracheostomized patient: Five case reports. *Dysphagia, 10,* 172–174.

Tippett, D., & Siebens, A. (1991). Speaking and swallowing on a ventilator. *Dysphagia, 6,* 94–99.

Tippett, D. C., & Siebens, A. (1996). Reconsidering the value of the modified Evan's blue dye test: A comment on Thompson-Henry and Braddock. *Dysphagia, 11,* 78–81.

Tippett, D. C., & Vogelman, L. (2000). Communication, tracheostomy and ventilator dependency. In D. Tippett (Ed.), *Tracheostomy and ventilator dependency: Management of breathing, speaking and swallowing* (pp. 93–142). New York: Thieme Medical Publishers.

Tolep, K., Getch, C. G., & Criner, G. J. (1996). Swallowing dysfunction in patients receiving prolonged mechanical ventilation. *Chest, 109,* 167–172.

Valles, J., Artigas, A., Rello, J., Bonsoms, N., Fontanals, D., Blanch, L., Fernandez, R., Baigorri, F., & Mestre, J. (1995). Continuous aspiration of subglottic secretions in preventing ventilator-associated pneumonia. *Annals of Internal Medicine, 122*(3), 179–186.

Villa, M., Newman, S., Kazandjian, M., Belozerco-Tracey, L., Dikeman, K., & Logemann, J. (2001, October). Ethical issues in clinical trials. *ASHA Special Interest Division 13 Newsletter, 10*(4), 20–22.

Voicing! (1994). *Communication approaches for tracheostomized and ventilator dependent patients.* Newport Beach, CA: Voicing!.

Weller, J., Siebens, A., Marshall, T., et al. (1995). The effect of position on the cross sectional area of the pharynx. *Proceedings of the 5th International Conference on Pulmonary Rehabilitation and Home Ventilation, 106.*

Weymuller, E. A. (1992). Prevention and management of intubation injury of the larynx and trachea. *American Journal of Otolaryngology, 13*(3), 139–144.

Williams-Colon, S., & Thalken, F. (1990). Management and monitoring of the patient in respiratory failure. In C. L. Scanlan, C. B. Spearman, & R. L. Seldon (Eds.), *Egan's fundamentals of respiratory care* (5th ed., pp. 780–835). St. Louis, MO: C. V. Mosby.

Wilson-Pauwels, L., Akesson, B. A., & Stewart, P. A. (1988). *Cranial nerves: Anatomy and clinical comments.* Toronto: B. C. Decker.

Wright, P. E., Marini, J. J., & Bernard, G. R. (1989). In vitro versus in vivo comparison of endotracheal airflow resistance. *American Review of Respiratory Disease, 140,* 10–16.

Yung, M. W., & Snowdon, S. L. (1984). Respiratory resistance of tracheostomy tubes. *Archives of Otolaryngology, 110,* 591–595.

Zaidi, N. H., Smith, H. A., King, S. C., Park, C., O'Neill, P. A., & Connolly, M. J. (1995). Oxygen desaturation on swallowing as a potential marker of aspiration in acute stroke. *Age and Ageing, 24,* 267–270.

Zemlin, W. R. (1981). *Speech and hearing science: Anatomy and physiology* (2nd ed.). Englewood Cliffs, NJ: Prentice-Hall.

Zenner, P. M. (1992, April). *Using a tracheostomy cuff deflation technique to improve swallowing with ventilator dependent adults.* Paper presented at Fourth Multidisciplinary Symposium on Dysphagia, Baltimore, MD.

Zenner, P. M. (2000). The clinical examination for dysphagia. In R. H. Mills (Ed.), *Evaluation of dysphagia in adults* (pp. 27–63). Austin, TX: Pro-Ed.

Zenner, P. M., Losinski, D. S., & Mills, R. H. (1995). Using cervical auscultation in the clinical dysphagia examination in long-term care. *Dysphagia, 10,* 27–31.

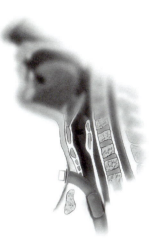

G

Glossary

access method (scanning, direct select, encoding): refers to the way that an individual will use (access) an alternative or augmentative communication device.

acidosis: a condition, of either respiratory or metabolic origin, in which there are excessive quantities of acids in the blood. Conversely, alkaline levels will be abnormally low.

adult respiratory distress syndrome: a syndrome occurring in people with no prior history of lung disease who have a catastrophic occurrence of high oxygen demands and then hypoxia of body tissues. Some common etiologies or predisposing conditions are sepsis, shock, burns, lung trauma (such as inhaled toxins), or a near drowning. The patient will require respiratory support of varying duration to ensure oxygenation of the tissues.

aerobic: an organism, such as a bacteria, that requires molecular oxygen to live. It is the aerobic bacteria, such as those of the Pseudomonas species, which appear to bind to cells of the trachea.

albumen: a protein found in mammals, often measured in a blood analysis to determine an individual's nutritional needs. Low levels of albumen can impede the weaning process by decreasing

inspiratory muscle strength and affecting the ability to tolerate increases in the work of breathing.

alkalosis: a condition, of either respiratory or metabolic origin, in which there is an excessive alkaline content of the blood. Conversely, there is a reduction of the acid content of the blood.

alternative communication: a method of communication other than oral; one that replaces oral-verbal communication.

alveoli: the end of the respiratory tract. Alveoli are the terminal air sacs where gas exchange with the blood takes place.

anaerobic: an organism, such as a bacteria, that cannot live in the presence of molecular oxygen. Anaerobic bacteria are usually cultured from saliva.

aphonia: loss of voice or phonation due to various causes such as tracheostomy tube placement with diversion of airflow from the vocal folds. Also caused by complete paralysis of vocal fold function (see **dysphonia**).

apnea: a transitory cessation of respiration. Apnea during the respiratory cycle usually results from lack of stimulation to the respiratory center, secondary to inadequate CO_2 levels in the blood. The apneic interval during swallowing refers to the pause time that occurs, usually between inspiration and expiration, to allow the bolus to pass over the closed airway.

arterial blood gases (ABG): a term identifying the gases dissolved in the arterial blood, usually measuring concentration (in percent) and partial pressure of O_2 and CO_2; also includes pH.

artificial airway: a means of securing an airway to insure patency (e.g., an endotracheal tube). Often used to connect with mechanical ventilation.

aspiration: the entry of foreign material into the airway, past the level of the vocal folds.

assist control (A/C): a mode of mechanical ventilatory support. The ventilator will respond to the patient's spontaneous breathing efforts by delivering volume, and provide a preset number of breaths if the patient fails to inspire within a set time period.

atelectasis: an area of collapsed lung (alveoli) which occurs when all of the oxygen in the tissue is absorbed by the blood, and access to further oxygenation through the bronchioles is blocked. This may occur, for example, when there are excessive secretions in portions of the lungs preventing gas exchange.

augmentative communication: to supplement or augment speech/voice or oral communication.

auscultation: a method of listening to body sound, especially sounds in the lungs, for purposes of diagnosis. Cervical auscultation involves the placement of a stethoscope on the larynx to listen to the sounds of the swallow paired with inspiration and exhalation.

autoclaving: a method of heat sterilization that utilizes moist heat under high pressure.

auto-PEEP: a physiological term which refers to the amount of air left in the lungs after a maxi-

mum expiration; positive end expiratory pressure ensures that the lungs do not collapse after a maximum expiration. The placement of a one-way valve (Passy-Muir) in the ventilatory circuit may create additional auto-PEEP over what is supplied from the ventilator.

bilevel ventilation (BiPAP™): a method of non-invasive mechanical ventilation which provides an inspiratory pressure as well as a lower expiratory pressure. It is a variation of CPAP (see **continuous positive airway pressure**).

bronchospasm: reflex constriction of the airways often related to irritation from inhaled particles; the airway narrows and constricts. In chronic disease this mechanism is exaggerated. The effort to breathe out against narrowed airways creates a prolonged expiration and the sense of struggling just to breathe.

button: decannulation plug for a tracheostomy tube alternately referred to as a cork, plug, or cap, depending upon the type of tracheostomy tube. Used during the weaning and decannulation process to assist the patient in learning to breathe solely though the upper airway, caps seal off the outer or inner cannula of the tracheostomy tube.

capnography: a device used to monitor CO_2 levels. Capnography may be noninvasive, measuring exhaled $PetCO_2$ at the nose, mouth, or tracheal stoma; transcutaneous; or invasive. The $PetCO_2$ values obtained with capnography generally trend with changes in $PACO_2$, which may reflect changing $PaCO_2$ levels.

cardiopulmonary disorders: diseases characterized by impairment in cardiovascular function related to pulmonary disease (see **cor pulmonale**). The close proximity of the heart and lungs often leads to problems with vascular pressures and fluid retention in the lungs. For example, during left ventricular failure of the heart, backup of (blood) pressure into the lungs may occur, with resultant pulmonary hypertension and hypoxia.

chemoreceptors: specialized cells (i.e, neural receptors) in the central nervous system which respond to gas levels in the blood, especially levels of CO_2, in order to activate the muscles of inspiration.

chronic bronchitis: see **chronic obstructive pulmonary disease.**

chronic obstructive pulmonary disease (COPD) (emphysema, bronchitis, asthma): a diagnosis that includes generalized airway obstruction; a combination of emphysema and bronchitis, sometimes with components of asthma. Emphysema is chronic alveolar distension caused by destruction of the lung tissue. Bronchitis is usually defined as the presence of a productive cough three months out of the year for a period of two years (consecutively) and excessive mucus production. Asthma is a narrowing of the bronchi. These conditions may be partly reversible with treatment, but severe COPD is usually considered irreversible.

cilia: hair-like projections from certain epithelial cells; usually serve a filtering and protective function.

compliance: the technical definition of compliance refers to forces that oppose expansion of a substance. Specifically, lung compliance refers to the ability of the lung to inflate during inspiration. The lungs should inflate easily; however, this normal lung expansion or compliance is affected by many types of pulmonary disease.

congestive heart failure (CHF): a chronic failure of the heart to pump adequate amounts of blood throughout the body; congestion and fluid accumulation in various organs in the body (such as the lungs) result.

connective tissue disorders: diseases characterized by impairment of the immune system leading to chronic connective tissue inflammation and damage. A variety of severe conditions with cardiopulmonary complications fall under this general description, such as systemic lupus, scleroderma, and ankylosing spondylitis.

continuous positive airway pressure (CPAP): a mode of mechanical ventilatory support that is noncycled; the ventilator provides a continuous flow of air to maintain a fairly constant pressure in the airway and at the alveolar level.

controlled mode ventilation (CMV): a mode of ventilation that cycles to provide inspiratory breaths independent of the breathing efforts of the patient.

cor pulmonale: heart disease that occurs following lung disease and strains the right ventricle.

cricothyroidotomy: procedure performed as an emergency airway management technique; the creation of an incision between the cricoid and thyroid cartilages.

cuff: the balloon-like part of an artificial airway (i.e., endotracheal tube, tracheostomy tube) that is inflated in the trachea to provide a seal in the airway; usually used during mechanical ventilatory support or in the presence of copious aspiration.

cyanosis: a blue discoloration of the skin, nail beds, and lips, caused by unsaturated hemoglobin in the blood. The condition is common in patients with heart or lung disease or anyone deprived of oxygen for a prolonged period.

dead space: refers to the nongas exchange portion of the airway. Anatomic dead space refers to the conducting airways (i.e., trachea, bronchi). Mechanical dead space refers to the space created by the presence of the ventilator circuitry, causing rebreathing of expired air.

decannulation: the removal of a tracheostomy tube.

dedicated communication system: a device that is used solely for the purposes of communication.

demulcent: a slippery fluid that prevents irritation and decreases irritation of mucous membranes (e.g., saliva).

dysphonia: impairment in voice or phonation due to various causes, such as partial diversion of airflow from tracheostomy, or partial vocal fold paralysis. May reduce vocal volume and affect voice quality.

dyspnea: labored breathing.

emollient: a softening agent for a mucous membrane (e.g., saliva).

emphysema: see **chronic obstructive pulmonary disease.**

endotracheal intubations: see **intubation.**

enteral: refers to the delivery of nutrition and hydration via an alternate means, such as a nasogastric or gastrostomy tube, for patients who cannot take adequate nutrition or hydration via mouth. Utilizes the preferred route of the GI tract to supply nutrients.

environmental control unit (ECU): a unit that is used to control a separate device or devices in the physical environment (e.g., a light or a television set).

exhaled tidal volume: the amount of volume that a patient receiving mechanical ventilation exhales or returns to the ventilator. The exhaled tidal volume display on the ventilator is monitored to assess if the patient is receiving adequate amounts of air. If a leak develops in this system, the exhaled tidal volume return alarm will sound. A leak deliberately created in the system (e.g., by cuff deflation) can be compensated for with increased volume from the ventilator.

expiration: the act of breathing out.

faucial arches: the anterior and posterior pillars at the posterior portion of the oral cavity, referred to as the fauces (i.e., the opening into the pharynx). The anterior faucial arches are usually the site for application of thermal stimulation during dysphagia treatment.

fenestration: an opening or window. Fenestrations are placed in tracheostomy tubes to aid in passage of air through the cannula.

fistula: an abnormal opening or hole created between two structures (e.g., a tracheoesophageal fistula).

flange: the portion of a tracheostomy tube that assists in fastening the tube around the neck; may be rigid or flexible.

gas sterilization: a chemical method of sterilization most typically used for devices that are sensitive to heat and moisture sensitive devices.

glossopharyngeal breathing: a substitute method of breathing. Also called frog breathing, it utilizes air injected into the lungs through the gulping action of the oral and pharyngeal muscles. It may decrease an individual's dependence on mechanical ventilatory support.

glottic closure response: the adduction of the vocal folds in response to the entry of foreign material into the larynx; a protective mechanism that may become less effective during periods of chronic airflow redirection, as in the presence of tracheostomy.

glottic control: a learned technique in which the vocal folds are kept adducted to assist in controlling airflow through the glottis and upper airway. May be utilized by individuals who are ventilator dependent during periods of cuff deflation.

goblet cells: mucus-secreting cells in the airway.

granuloma: the growth of connective tissue and capillaries, in a small grain-like structure, from an open wound, usually forming after repeated irritation. May occur, for example, at a tracheotomy stoma site or on the vocal folds after intubation (i.e., intubation granuloma).

Heat moisture exchange filter (HME): a type of humidification device which is placed in-line with ventilatory tubing. It collects warmth and humidity from the patient's breaths which are then used to moisten the next breath on inspiration.

hemodynamics: having an effect on blood flow.

hemoglobin (Hb): the respiratory pigment in red blood cells that combines with oxygen to transport it through the circulatory system. May be reflected in the results of an arterial blood gas.

hypercapnia: the presence of excessively high levels of CO_2 in the blood.

hypertension: abnormally high blood pressure levels; may relate to pulmonary pathology. The latter occurs when resistance to blood flow by constriction of blood vessels in the lungs increases pressures in the right cardiac ventricle.

hyperventilation: ventilation that exceeds the needs of the body. Reflected in abnormally low levels of CO_2 in the arterial blood.

hypotension: abnormally low blood pressure levels. Blood circulation may therefore be inadequate to circulate oxygen throughout the body.

hypoventilation: ventilation that is inadequate to meet the needs of the body. Reflected by increased levels of CO_2 in the arterial blood.

hypoxia: a decreased amount of oxygen at the level of body tissues. May have differing causes (e.g., anemic hypoxia results from a hemoglobin deficiency).

hypoxemia: a decreased amount of oxygen in the arterial blood.

incentive spirometry: see **spirometry.**

inner cannula: the internal portion of a tracheostomy tube that fits within the main or external structure of the tube. May be disposable or nondisposable.

inspiratory/expiratory ratio (I:E ratio): the relationship, in the breath cycle, of the length of the inspiratory phase to the length of the expiratory phase during mechanical ventilatory support. It is expressed as a numeric ratio (e.g., 1:4).

intermittent mandatory ventilation (IMV): a mode of cycled ventilation where the patient may breathe spontaneously between timed mandatory breaths.

intubation: the insertion of a tube into the body, as during endotracheal intubation (i.e., the insertion of an endotracheal tube into the trachea).

laryngeal vestibule: the area above the true vocal folds in the larynx, bounded by the underside of the epiglottis superiorly. Often referenced during a videofluoroscopic evaluation.

laryngectomy tube: an artificial airway utilized only after laryngectomy, the removal of the larynx, to assist in maintaining stoma opening. Because they do not have to extend into the airway, laryngectomy tubes are shorter in design than regular tracheostomy tubes.

laryngoscope: a device used for directly viewing the larynx and glottis for proper placement of an endotracheal tube in the airway.

laryngospasm: involuntary muscular contraction of the larynx. This usually includes tight closure of the glottis, and may occur during a procedure such as a fiberoptic examination of the larynx if the scope touches the false vocal folds, arytenoid cartilages, or true vocal folds.

lower respiratory tract: the portion of the respiratory tract that consists of the trachea and lungs; also referred to as the tracheobronchial tree.

manometer: an instrument used for measuring the pressure exerted by a liquid or a gas.

manual bagging: the process of supplying breaths by a manual resuscitation bag, often used to oxygenate the patient before attempting intubation or when the patient is temporarily disconnected from mechanical ventilation.

mean airway pressure: average airway pressure during both inspiration and expiration (the respiratory cycle). Although adequate mean airway pressure is important in providing delivery of oxygen to the patient, it may also create high positive pressure in the chest, leading to multiple cardiac and respiratory complications. Mean airway pressure must be carefully monitored for patients receiving positive pressure mechanical ventilation.

mechanical exsufflation: a technique which utilizes a device to apply a positive pressure, followed by a negative pressure, to simulate a cough and clear secretions from the distal airways.

mechanical ventilation (ventilator-dependent): mechanical assistance in the breathing process; it may be used to augment the efforts of a patient who has spontaneous, but weak, breaths or for individuals who do not breathe on their own.

minimal leak technique: the process of maintaining cuff inflation while maintaining a small air leak, confirmed during tracheal auscultation, to ensure that the cuff does not place excessive pressure on the tracheal walls.

minimal occluding volume: the minimal amount of volume needed to inflate a tracheostomy tube cuff. Obtained during auscultation by placing a stethoscope on the side of the neck and inflating the cuff to the point that air is no longer heard.

minute ventilation: the volume of air breathed in one minute; for a patient on mechanical ventilatory support, minute volume is a function of respiratory rate and tidal volume.

minute volume: see **minute ventilation.**

mucolytic: a pharmalogical agent used to loosen mucus for easier removal from the airway.

nasogastric tube (NGT): a temporary, artificial means of providing nutrition and hydration via a tube inserted through the nose and into the aerodigestive tract. Complications include aspiration, especially if a patient is reclined too soon after receiving a feeding, and localized irritation of the nares.

nasopharyngolaryngoscopy: a direct visualization of the nares, nasopharynx, pharynx, and larynx utilizing a flexible fiberoptic scope with a light source. The positioning of the scope within the nares allows the patient to perform speech and nonspeech activities. A modification of this procedure is utilized during the fiberoptic evaluation of swallowing.

negative pressure ventilation: negative pressure ventilation is a noninvasive mode of ventilatory support which utilizes negative pressure around the thorax to decrease intrathoracic pressure in relation to atmospheric pressure, causing inspiration. Expiration is passive. As a noninvasive mode, negative pressure ventilation does not require an endotracheal tube or tracheostomy, but can be physically restricting to the patient and carries with it other complications.

neuromuscular diseases/conditions: disease processes that affect the central or peripheral nervous system and spinal cord, which may create respiratory dysfunction. May be progressive (e.g., amyotrophic lateral sclerosis) or static (e.g., cerebral vascular accident).

nosocomial: an infection acquired in a hospital, appearing 72 hours after admission.

obturator: a device that closes an aperture (e.g., the obturator of a tracheostomy tube, which is placed in the outer cannula of the tracheostomy tube to extend past the blunted end, rounding it and easing insertion of the tube into the stoma site).

odynophagia: the sensation of pain upon swallowing.

one-way speaking valve: a one-way valve which is placed upon the hub of a tracheostomy tube to allow air to enter on inspiration. On expiration, the valve is closed and air cannot escape out through the tracheostomy tube. Rather, it is redirected through the vocal folds and into the upper airway, available for speaking and swallowing.

outer cannula: the portion of the tracheostomy tube that forms the actual body of the tube (i.e., the external structure of the tube into which the inner cannula fits).

PaCO$_2$: the partial pressure of carbon dioxide in the arterial blood, represents the amount of carbon dioxide dissolved in blood plasma. PaCO$_2$ is one of the values reflected in an arterial blood gas.

PaO$_2$: the partial pressure of oxygen in the arterial blood, represents the amount of oxygen dissolved in blood plasma. PaO$_2$ is one of the values reflected in an arterial blood gas.

partial pressure: refers to the pressure or tension needed to move a gas (i.e., O$_2$ or CO$_2$) from air to blood and then to body tissues.

peak inspiratory pressure: the highest measured airway pressure during the inspiratory phase of mechanical ventilatory support; pressures significantly exceeding this level will cause the high pressure alarm on the ventilator to sound.

pentaplegia: paralysis of all extremities and bulbar motor functions.

percussion: sometimes referred to as chest clapping. The use of mechanical stimulation on the chest wall, either manually or via various devices, to loosen secretions from the bronchi and possibly increase the ease of their removal during suctioning or coughing. Vibration is sometimes used synonymously with percussion as part of chest physical therapy. Vibration applies gentle compression, coupled with rapid friction of the practitioner's upper extremities, to the chest wall. These techniques are often applied while the patient is in a postural drainage position.

percutaneous gastrostomy tube (PEG): an artificial means of taking nutrition and hydration via a tube placed percutaneously, via endoscopy, in the stomach. This type of tube is generally more comfortable for a patient than an NGT. It appears to carry the same risk of aspiration, especially if aspiration precautions (i.e., elevation of the head during feeding) are not followed.

percutaneous tracheotomy: a method of providing adult intubated patients with a tracheostomy; involves progressive dilation of an initial tracheotomy puncture with various size catheters. Can be performed at the patient's bedside with relatively low complication rate by a skilled practitioner,

pH: a value representing the acidity or alkalinity of a substance (e.g., blood). pH levels express the hydrogen ion concentration of a solution.

pleura: the membrane that lines the inside of the thorax and outside surfaces of the lungs.

pneumonia: inflammation of the lung, usually of infectious (i.e., viral or bacterial) origin. Pneumonia can also be related to aspiration of either gastric contents, with high acid levels, or oropharyngeal contents, containing bacteria.

pneumothorax: the presence of trapped air in the pleural space of the thorax. This may occur when a lung has ruptured after barotrauma, allowing air to escape into the pleural space.

polyp: a pedunculated growth arising from a mucosal surface (e.g., the vocal folds).

positive end expiratory pressure (PEEP): the maintenance of airway pressures above atmospheric throughout the expiratory phase of a ventilator; designed to improve oxygenation. PEEP can be set at differing levels according to patient need.

positive pressure ventilation: a means of mechanical ventilation that can be administered via invasive or noninvasive means by creating higher pressure than atmospheric and pushing air into the lungs.

pressure support ventilation (PSV): the addition of preset positive pressure breaths to the inspiratory phase of ventilation; helps reduce the work of breathing. Can be used with cycled ventilatory modes or with CPAP.

pulmonary edema: swelling of alveoli in the lung that occurs when they fill with fluid leaking from the capillaries. Can lead to significant respiratory distress.

pulmonary function tests (PFTs): a variety of assessment techniques that can provide both diagnostic and therapeutic information. These involve tests of lung volumes and capacities and expired airflow.

pulse oximetry: pulse oximetry is a noninvasive method of determining arterial oxygen saturation via a probe placed upon a highly oxygenated area of the body. Infrared light is released and analyzed by recording its changing absorption in the arterial blood.

respiratory control center: the part of the central nervous system that coordinates the control of respiration; the reticular formation in the brainstem mediates the automatic control of breathing, responding to the specialized chemoreceptors.

respiratory rate: the number of breaths per minute that a patient breathes, either spontaneously or assisted (by mechanical ventilation).

SaO_2: the percentage of saturation of hemoglobin with oxygen in the blood. This reflects the ability of the blood to transport oxygen.

spirometry: an instrumental procedure for measuring the capacity of the lungs. Incentive spirometry is a technique to encourage maximal deep breathing.

stretch receptors: specialized neural cells in the walls of the lung and the thorax. During inspiration, these cells respond to the movement of these structures by sending impulses to the respiratory center to cease movement of the inspiratory muscles.

stroboscopy: a technique that provides a visualization of the vibratory mode of the vocal folds via a sampling of vocal fold position at different intervals in the vibratory cycle. This technique is helpful in the diagnosis and treatment of voice disorders.

stylet: a rigid probe used to assist in the insertion of a flexible tube, such as an endotracheal tube, into the body.

surfactant: an agent that lowers surface tension. Surfactant is secreted by the epithelial cells of the alveoli and allows ease of movement as well as maintaining surface tension and decreasing the risk of alveolar collapse.

synchronized intermittent mandatory ventilation (SIMV): a mode of cycled ventilation where the patient may breathe spontaneously between timed breaths. Unlike IMV, this mode of ventilation will synchronize with the spontaneous breathing efforts of the patient and wait, within a preset time, to allow the patient to inspire, without necessarily imposing a preset breath.

tachycardia: abnormally high heart rate (over 100–120 beats per minute), usually associated with an increased work of breathing.

tachypnea: abnormally rapid respiration.

talking tracheostomy tube: a tracheostomy tube that has been adapted to permit phonation in the presence of an inflated cuff. Talking or speaking tracheostomy tubes contain an external air port which connects to a separate air source and allows air to enter the airway above the level of the tracheostomy tube cuff.

tidal volume: the amount of air that moves in and out of the lungs during respiration. For mechanically ventilated patients, this value is set on the ventilator to ensure that a patient is adequately ventilated.

tracheal button: a closure plug used to close the stoma of a tracheostomized patient; often utilized during the decannulation process.

tracheomalacia: the softening of cartilaginous rings of the trachea, usually related to repeated trauma, possibly related to the presence of artificial airways.

tracheostomy: an artificial airway; the tube used to secure the stoma after a tracheotomy. Tracheostomy tubes vary in size, composition (material), cuff design, and angle of placement in the airway.

tracheotomy: the surgical creation of an opening in the trachea, performed to create a patent airway and provide a means of pulmonary toilet.

Valsalva maneuver: the closure of the true and false vocal folds to assist in fixing the thorax for effortful activities (i.e., coughing and lifting).

vasoconstrictor: an agent that produces constriction of blood vessels; often used to treat hypotension.

ventilation: the movement of gas in and out of the lungs.

ventilator dependence: see **mechanical ventilation.**

vibration: see percussion.

weaning: the process of removing a patient from mechanical ventilatory support. May be a gradual reduction of support, as with levels of IMV/SIMV, or a more abrupt process. This may depend on both the physician's training and philosophy and patient tolerance. Also describes the process of gradually decannulating a patient from a tracheostomy.

work of breathing: the work done by the respiratory muscles during breathing; is present in normal quiet breathing to overcome the forces (e.g., gravity, etc.) that resist inspiration. The work of breathing may be increased in patients with diseases of the respiratory musculature.

xerostomia: a condition of excessively dry mouth caused by abnormal saliva production.

A

Appendix A: Resources

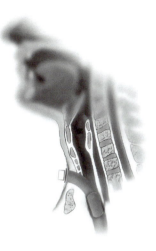

ORAL COMMUNICATION OPTIONS
AND TRACHEOSTOMY TUBE MANAGEMENT

Ballard Medical Products
12050 Lone Peak Parkway
Draper, UT 84020
(800) 345-8865
http://www.bmed.com

Boston Medical Products, Inc.
117 Flanders Rd.
Westborough, MA 01581
(800) 433-2674
http://www.bosmed.com

Hood Laboratories
575 Washington St.
Pembroke, MA 02359
(800) 942-5227
http://www.hoodlabs.com

Kay Elemetrics Corp.
2 Bridgewater Lane
Lincoln Park, NJ 07035
(800) 289-5297
(973) 628-6200
http://www.kayelemetrics.com

Nellcor Puritan Bennett Inc.
(Nellcor, Puritan Bennett, Shiley, and
   Mallinckrodt products)
4280 Hacienda Drive
Pleasanton, CA 94588
(800) 635-5267
http://www.nellcor.com

Olympic Medical Corp.
5900 First Avenue South
Seattle, WA 98108
(800) 426-0353
(206) 767-3500
http://www.olymed.com

Passy-Muir Inc.
PMB 273
4521 Campus Drive
Irvine, CA 92612
(800) 634-5397
(949) 833-8255
http://www.passy-muir.com

Pentax Precision Instrument Corp.
30 Ramland Rd.
Orangeburg, NY 10962
(800) 431-5880
http://www.pentaxmedical.com

Pilling Surgical
200 Precision Rd.
Suite 200
Horsham, PA 19044
(800) 523-6507
http://www.pillingsurgical.com

Portex, Inc.
(Smiths Medical Group)
(Portex and Bivona products)
10 Bowman Drive
Keene, NH 03431
(800) 258-5361
http://www.portexusa.com

Siemens Hearing Instruments Inc.
10 Constitution Ave.
Piscataway, NJ 08854
(800) 766-4500
http://www.siemens-hearing.com

Voicing!
c/o Passy-Muir Inc.
PMB 273
4521 Campus Drive
Irvine, CA 92612
(800) 634-5397
(949) 833-8255
http://www.passy-muir.com

MECHANICAL VENTILATION

J. H. Emerson Company
22 Cottage Park Ave.
Cambridge, MA 02140-1691
(800) 252-1414
http://www.jhemerson.com

Nellcor Puritan Bennett Inc.
(Nellcor, Puritan Bennett, Shiley, and
Mallinckrodt products)
4280 Hacienda Drive
Pleasanton, CA 94588
(800) 635-5267
http://www.nellcor.com

Posey Company
5635 Peck Rd.
Arcadia, CA 91006
(800) 447-6739
http://www.posey.com

Pulmonetic Systems, Inc.
(portable ventilators)
930 South Mount Vernon St.
Suite 100
Colton, CA 92324
(800) 754-1914
http://www.pulmonetic.com

Respironics, Inc.
1501 Ardmore Blvd.
Pittsburgh, PA 15221
(800) 638-8208
(412) 731-2100
http://www.respironics.com

NONORAL COMMUNICATION

Crestwood Communication Aids, Inc.
6625 N. Sidney Place
Milwaukee, WI 53209-3259
(414) 352-5678
http://www.communicationaids.com

Dynavox Systems LLC
2100 Wharton St., Suite 400
Pittsburgh, PA 15203
(800) 344-1778
http://www.dynavoxsys.com

Mayer-Johnson Company
P.O. Box 1579
Solana Beach, CA 92075-1579
(800) 588-4548
http://www.mayer-johnson.comPrentke Romich

Company
1022 Heyl Rd.
Wooster, OH 44691
(800) 262-1984
http://www.prentrom.com

Zygo Industries, Inc.
P.O. Box 1008
Portland, OR 97207-1008
(800) 234-6006
http://www.zygo-usa.com

ASSISTIVE TECHNOLOGY

AAC (Augmentative and Alternative
   Communication) Institute
338 Meadville Street
Edinboro, PA 16412
(814) 392-6625
http://www.aacinstitute.org

Communication Aid Manufacturers Association
P.O. Box 1039
Evanston, IL 60204
(800) 441-2262
http://www.aacproducts.org

COMMUNICATION RESOURCES
FOR NEUROLOGICALLY IMPAIRED ADULTS

American Speech-Language-Hearing
   Association
10801 Rockville Pike
Rockville, MD 20852-3279
(800) 498-2071
http://www.asha.org

Communication Independence for the
   Neurologically Impaired
116 John St., Suite 1304
New York, NY 10038
(212) 385-8045
http://www.cini.org

DYSPHAGIA

Dysphagia Research Society
c/o International Meeting Managers, Inc.
4550 Post Oak Place, Suite 342
Houston, TX 77027
http://www.als.uiuc.edu/drs

Steris Corporation
(Hausted chair)
5960 Heisley Rd.
Mentor, OH 44060
(800) 428-7833
http://www.steris.com

Appendix B: Communication Needs Assessment

Needs Assessment

AUGMENTATIVE COMMUNICATION CENTER
DEPARTMENT OF REHABILITATION MEDICINE
UNIVERSITY OF WASHINGTON HOSPITAL

Name:

Date:

Interviewer:

Responders:

Please indicate whether the needs listed are:
    M – Mandatory
    D – Desirable
    U – Unimportant
    F – May be mandatory in the future

Positioning

In bed:
    While supine
    While lying prone
    While lying on side
    While in a Clinitron bed
    While in a Roto bed
    While sitting in bed
    While in arm restraints
    In a variety of positions

Related to mobility:
    Carry the system while walking
    Independently position the system
    In a manually controlled wheelchair
    In an electric wheelchair
    With a lapboard
    While the chair is reclined
    Arm troughs

Other equipment:
    With hand mitts
    With arterial lines
    Orally intubated
    While trached
    With oxygen mask

Source: From *Communication Augmentation: A Casebook of Clinical Management* by D. R. Beukelman, K. M. Yorkston, & P. A. Dowden, pp. 209–211. San Diego: College-Hill Press. Copyright 1985 by Pro-Ed. Reprinted with permission.

With electric wheelchair controls
Environmental control units

Other needs related to positioning:

_____

_____

_____

Communication Partners

Someone who cannot read (e.g., child or nonreader)
Someone with no familiarity with the system
Someone who has poor vision
Someone who has limited time or patience
Someone who is across the room or in another room
Someone who is not independently mobile
Several people at a time
Someone who is hearing impaired

Other needs related to partners:

_____

_____

_____

Locations

Only in a single room
In multiple rooms within the same building
In dimly lit rooms
In bright rooms
In noisy rooms
Outdoors
While traveling in a car, van, and so forth
While moving from place to place within a building
At a desk or computer terminal
In more than two locations in a day

Other needs related to locations:

_____

_____

_____

Message Needs

> Call attention
> Signal emergencies
> Answer yes-no questions
> Provide unique information
> Make requests
> Carry on a conversation
> Express emotion
> Give opinions
> Convey basic medical needs
> Greet people
> Prepare messages in advance
> Edit texts written by others
> Edit texts prepared by the user
> Make changes in diagrams
> Compile lists (e.g., phone numbers)
> Perform calculations
> Take notes

Other needs related to messages:

_____

_____

_____

Modality of Communication

> Prepare printed messages
> Prepare auditory messages
> Talk on the phone
> Communicate with other equipment (e.g., environment control units)
> Communicate privately with some partners
> Switch from one modality to another during communication
> Via several modalities at a time (e.g., taking notes while talking on the phone)
> Communicate via an intercom
> Via formal letters or reports
> On pre-prepared worksheets

Other needs related to modality of communication:

_____

_____

_____

C

Appendix C: Sample Communication and Swallowing Evaluation Form for Tracheostomized and Ventilator-Dependent Patients

Communication/Swallowing Evaluation for Tracheostomized and Ventilator-Dependent Patients

Name _____ Room _____ Date _____

BACKGROUND INFORMATION

Medical DX _____

Physical-motor status _____

Tracheostomy tube type _____ Size _____ Cuff status _____

Ventilator settings: Mode _____ FIO_2 _____ TV _____

"Freetime" _____ PEEP _____

Status of current p.o. intake: Diet _____ IV _____ NGT _____ GT _____

Frequency of suctioning _____

Quality of secretions _____

Chest X-ray results _____ Date _____

SPEECH AND LANGUAGE

Receptive Language Function:

   Auditory Comprehension _____

   _____

   Auditory Retention _____

   _____

Expressive Language Function:

   Spontaneous Language _____

   _____

   Repetition _____

   Word Finding _____

   Automatic Speech _____

Visual Language Function _____

_____

BEHAVIORAL CHARACTERISTICS

Attention Span _____

Anxiety _____

    Expressed verbally _____ Expressed behaviorally _____

COGNITION

Orientation: Person _____ Place _____ Time _____

Memory: Immediate _____ Recent _____ Remote _____

Response Reliability: _____

ORAL PERIPHERAL MECHANISM

Labial: Symmetrical _____ Asymmetrical _____

           Protrusion _____ Retraction _____

           Saliva Management _____

Lingual: Protrusion _____ Deviation _____ Lateralization _____

           Elevation _____ Retraction _____

           Strength _____ Bite block used? _____

Mandibular: Depression _____ Elevation _____

Velum: Evaluation _____ Deviation _____

Gag: Present _____ Absent _____ Reduced _____

Dentition _____ Dentures _____ Edentulous _____ Gingiva _____

Voice quality: Liquids _____ Cervical auscultation _____

Semisolids _____ Cervical auscultation _____

Solids _____ Cervical auscultation _____

Cough reflex _____ Timing _____

Expulsion of bolus: trach tube _____

Stoma site _____ Timing _____

Compensatory strategies and results _____

_____

_____

Comments _____

_____

_____

Impressions _____

_____

_____

RECOMMENDATIONS

Speech: Fiberoptic Evaluation _____

               Speaking Valve Assessment _____

Language: Augmentative Communication Evaluation _____

Swallowing: Blue Dye Screening _____

               Fiberoptic Study_____

SPEECH/VOICE

Tracheostomized Patient:

    Cuff inflated: with tracheal occlusion

        Full inflation _____ Partial inflation _____

        Aphonic _____ Leak speech _____

    Cuff deflated: with tracheal occlusion

        Aphonic _____ Dysphonic _____

        Vocal quality (harsh, wet, etc.) _____

        Maximum sustained phonation _____

Ventilator Patient:

    Cuff inflated: Aphonic _____ Dysphonic _____

    Cuff deflated: Aphonic _____ Dysphonic _____

        Vocal quality (harsh, wet, etc.) _____

        _____

        Vocal volume _____

        Coordination of respiration/phonation _____

        Tolerance of cuff deflation _____

        Intelligibility _____

        Ventilator modifications: TV _____ PSV _____

                                    Rate _____ FIO_2

SWALLOWING

Previous dysphagia evaluation and history _____

_____

_____

Date and type of last evaluation _____

History of aspiration _____

History of pneumonia_____

Dysphagic complaint _____

_____

Food and liquid noted in tracheostomy _____

Around stoma _____

Cough: Volitional _____   Reflexive_____

Throat clear: Volitional _____   Reflexive_____

Oral Stage: WFL   _____   Mastication _____ Retention _____

Oral Transit _____   Bolus control _____

Pharyngeal Stage:

Pharyngeal Swallow (secs) _____

Absent Swallow _____

Trial Swallows: Liquids_____   Suctioning _____

                 Semisolids _____   Suctioning _____

                 Solids _____   Suctioning _____

Laryngeal Evaluation _____

Cuff: Inflated _____ Deflated _____

Tracheal occlusion_____

Speaking valve _____

Videofluoroscopy _____

P.O. status: P.O. _____   N.P.O. _____

Liquids: Thin _____   Thick _____

_____
Signature/Title

D

Appendix D:
Blue Dye
Tracking Sheet

Name _____   Date of Test _____

Room Number _____

Time/Date Initiating Dye Test	Test Consistency	Time/Date Suctioning	Blue Dye Presence at Suction				
			Location	Minimal	Moderate	Significant	None

Index